Menschen mit neurodegenerativen Erkrankungen

Menschen mit neurodegenerativen Erkrankungen
Katharine Preissner

Programmbereich Gesundheitsberufe

Wissenschaftlicher Beirat Programmbereich Gesundheitsberufe
Sophie Karoline Brandt, Bern; Heidi Höppner, Berlin, Christiane Mentrup, Zürich;
Sascha Sommer, Bochum; Birgit Stubner, Coburg; Markus Wirz, Zürich; Ursula Walkenhorst, Osnabrück

Katharine Preissner

Menschen mit neurodegenerativen Erkrankungen

Leitlinien der Ergotherapie Band 8

Deutschsprachige Ausgabe herausgegeben von Mieke le Granse

Aus dem Amerikanischen von Sabine Brinkmann und Anja Kirchner

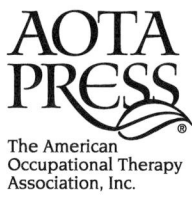

Mit freundlicher Unterstützung von ergotherapie austria

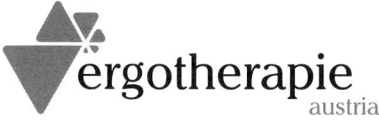

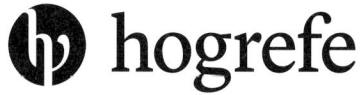

Katharine Preissner, EdD, OTR/L, Clinical Associate Professor and Academic Fieldwork Coordinator, Department of Occupational Therapy, College of Applied Health Sciences, University of Illinois at Chicago, Chicago

The American Occupational Therapy Association, Inc.
4720 Montgomery Lane
Bethesda, MD 20814
301-652-AOTA (2682)
TDD: 800-377-8555
Fax: 301-652-7711
http://www.aota.org

Wichtiger Hinweis: DDer Verlag hat gemeinsam mit den Autoren bzw. den Herausgebern große Mühe darauf verwandt, dass alle in diesem Buch enthaltenen Informationen (Programme, Verfahren, Mengen, Dosierungen, Applikationen, Internetlinks etc.) entsprechend dem Wissensstand bei Fertigstellung des Werkes abgedruckt oder in digitaler Form wiedergegeben wurden. Trotz sorgfältiger Manuskriptherstellung und Korrektur des Satzes und der digitalen Produkte können Fehler nicht ganz ausgeschlossen werden. Autoren bzw. Herausgeber und Verlag übernehmen infolgedessen keine Verantwortung und keine daraus folgende oder sonstige Haftung, die auf irgendeine Art aus der Benutzung der in dem Werk enthaltenen Informationen oder Teilen davon entsteht. Geschützte Warennamen (Warenzeichen) werden nicht besonders kenntlich gemacht. Aus dem Fehlen eines solchen Hinweises kann also nicht geschlossen werden, dass es sich um einen freien Warennamen handelt.

> **Bibliografische Information der Deutschen Nationalbibliothek**
> Die Deutsche Nationalbibliothek verzeichnet diese Publikation in der Deutschen Nationalbibliografie; detaillierte bibliografische Daten sind im Internet über http://www.dnb.de abrufbar.

Dieses Werk einschließlich aller seiner Teile ist urheberrechtlich geschützt. Jede Verwertung außerhalb der engen Grenzen des Urheberrechtes ist ohne Zustimmung des Verlages unzulässig und strafbar. Das gilt insbesondere für Kopien und Vervielfältigungen zu Lehr- und Unterrichtszwecken, Übersetzungen, Mikroverfilmungen sowie die Einspeicherung und Verarbeitung in elektronischen Systemen.

Anregungen und Zuschriften bitte an:
Hogrefe AG
Lektorat Gesundheitsberufe
z.Hd.: Barbara Müller
Länggass-Strasse 76
3000 Bern 9
Schweiz
Tel: +41 31 300 45 00
E-Mail: verlag@hogrefe.ch
Internet: http://www.hogrefe.ch

Lektorat: Barbara Müller, Diana Goldschmid
Bearbeitung: Mieke le Granse, Barbara Müller
Herstellung: Daniel Berger
Umschlagabbildung: © Goodluz, istockphoto.com
Umschlag: Claude Borer, Riehen
Satz: Claudia Wild, Konstanz
Druck und buchbinderische Verarbeitung: AZ Druck und Datentechnik GmbH, Kempten
Printed in Germany

Dieses Buch ist eine Übersetzung aus dem Amerikanischen. Der Originaltitel lautet: Preissner, K. (2014). *Occupational therapy practice guidelines for adults with Neurodegenerative Diseases* (AOTA Practice Guidelines Series). Bethesda, MD: AOTA Press.

© 2014 by the American Occupational Therapy Association, Inc.
ISBN-13: 978-1-56900-458-6 (E-Book)

1. Auflage 2018
© 2018 Hogrefe Verlag, Bern

(E-Book-ISBN_PDF 978-3-456-95779-1)
ISBN 978-3-456-85779-4
http://doi.org/10.1024/85779-000

Inhaltsverzeichnis

Danksagung		7
Geleitwort		9
1	**Einführung**	13
1.1	Zweck und Anwendung dieser Veröffentlichung	13
1.2	Gegenstandsbereich und Prozess der Ergotherapie	14
1.2.1	Gegenstandsbereich	14
1.2.2	Prozess	15
2	**Überblick zu neurodegenerativen Krankheiten (NDK)**	19
2.1	Multiple Sklerose (MS)	19
2.2	Idiopathisches Parkinsonsyndrom (IPS)	20
2.3	Amyotrophe Lateralsklerose (ALS)	20
2.4	Transverse Myelitis (TM)	21
3	**Der ergotherapeutische Prozess bei Klienten mit NDK**	23
3.1	Settings	23
3.2	Aktivitätsanforderungen	24
3.3	Screening	24
3.4	Überweisung	24
3.5	Evaluation	24
3.5.1	Betätigungsprofil	26
3.5.2	Analyse der Betätigungsperformanz	32
3.5.3	Betätigungsbereiche	32
3.5.4	Performanzfertigkeiten	33
3.5.5	Performanzmuster	33
3.5.6	Klientenfaktoren	33
3.5.7	Kontext und Umwelt	33
3.5.8	Überlegungen zu Assessments	35
3.6	Intervention	35
3.6.1	Interventionsplan	36
3.6.2	Implementierung der Intervention	36
3.6.3	Überprüfung der Intervention	36
3.7	Ergebnis und Ergebniskontrolle	37
3.8	Abschluss, Entlassungsplanung und Nachsorge	37
4	**Best Practice und Zusammenfassung der Evidenz**	39
4.1	Interventionen für Klienten mit MS	39
4.1.1	Interventionen mit Fokus auf Aktivität und Partizipation	40

4.1.2	Interventionen mit Fokus auf Performanzfertigkeiten	43
4.2	Interventionen für Klienten mit IPS	45
4.2.1	Übung und körperliche Aktivität	45
4.2.2	Umweltbedingte Reize, Stimuli und Objekte	47
4.2.3	Selbstmanagement und kognitive Verhaltensstrategien	47
4.3	Interventionen für Klienten mit ALS	48
4.3.1	Übung	48
4.3.2	Hilfsmittel und Rollstühle	48
4.3.3	Multidisziplinäre Programme	49
4.3.4	Palliativpflege	49
4.3.5	Vorbereitende Methoden	49
4.4	Zusammenfassung	49
5	**Schlussfolgerung für Praxis, Ausbildung und Forschung**	**53**
5.1	Schlussfolgerung für die Praxis	53
5.2	Schlussfolgerung für die Ausbildung	53
5.3	Schlussfolgerung für die Forschung	54
6	**Anhänge**	**57**
A	Vorbereitung und Qualifikationen von Ergotherapeuten und Ergotherapie-Assistenten	57
B	Selected CPT TM Codes ...	59
C	Evidenzbasierte Praxis	63
D	Übersicht zur Evidenz	67

Literatur	165
Sachwortverzeichnis	175
Glossar	179
Personenindex	187

Danksagung

The series editor for this Practice Guideline is

Deborah Lieberman, MHSA, OTR/L, FAOTA
Director, Evidence-Based Practice Staff Liaison to the Commission on Practice American Occupational Therapy Association Bethesda, MD

The issue editor for this Practice Guideline is

Marian Arbesman, PhD, OTR/L
President, ArbesIdeas, Inc. Consultant, AOTA Evidence-Based Practice Project Clinical Assistant Professor, Department of Rehabilitation Science, State University of New York at Buffalo

The authors acknowledge the following individuals for their contributions to the evidence-based literature review:

Marian Arbesman, PhD, OTR/L
Kendra L. Sheard, OTR/L
Virgil Mathiowetz, PhD, OTR/L, FAOTA
Chih-Huang Yu, MSc(OT), OT (Taiwan)
Linda Tickle-Degnen, PhD, OTR/L, FAOTA
Mayuri Bedekar, MA, OT

The authors acknowledge and thank the following individuals for their participation in the content review and development of this publication:

Susan Forwell, PhD, OT(C), FCAOT
Erin R. Foster, OTD, MSCI, OTR/L
Emily Frank, MS, OTR/L
Virgil Mathiowetz, PhD, OTR/L, FAOTA
Lauro A. Munoz, OTR, MOT, CHC
Kendra L. Sheard, OTR/L
Linda Tickle-Degnen, PhD, OTR/L, FAOTA
Jennifer Hitchon, JD, MHA
V. Judith Thomas, MGA
Madalene Palmer

The authors thank the following individuals for their contribution:

Cathleen Jensen, OTR/L
Nancy Z. Richman, OTR/L, FAOTA

Note. The authors of this Practice Guideline have signed a Conflict of Interest statement indicating that they have no conflicts that would bear on this work.

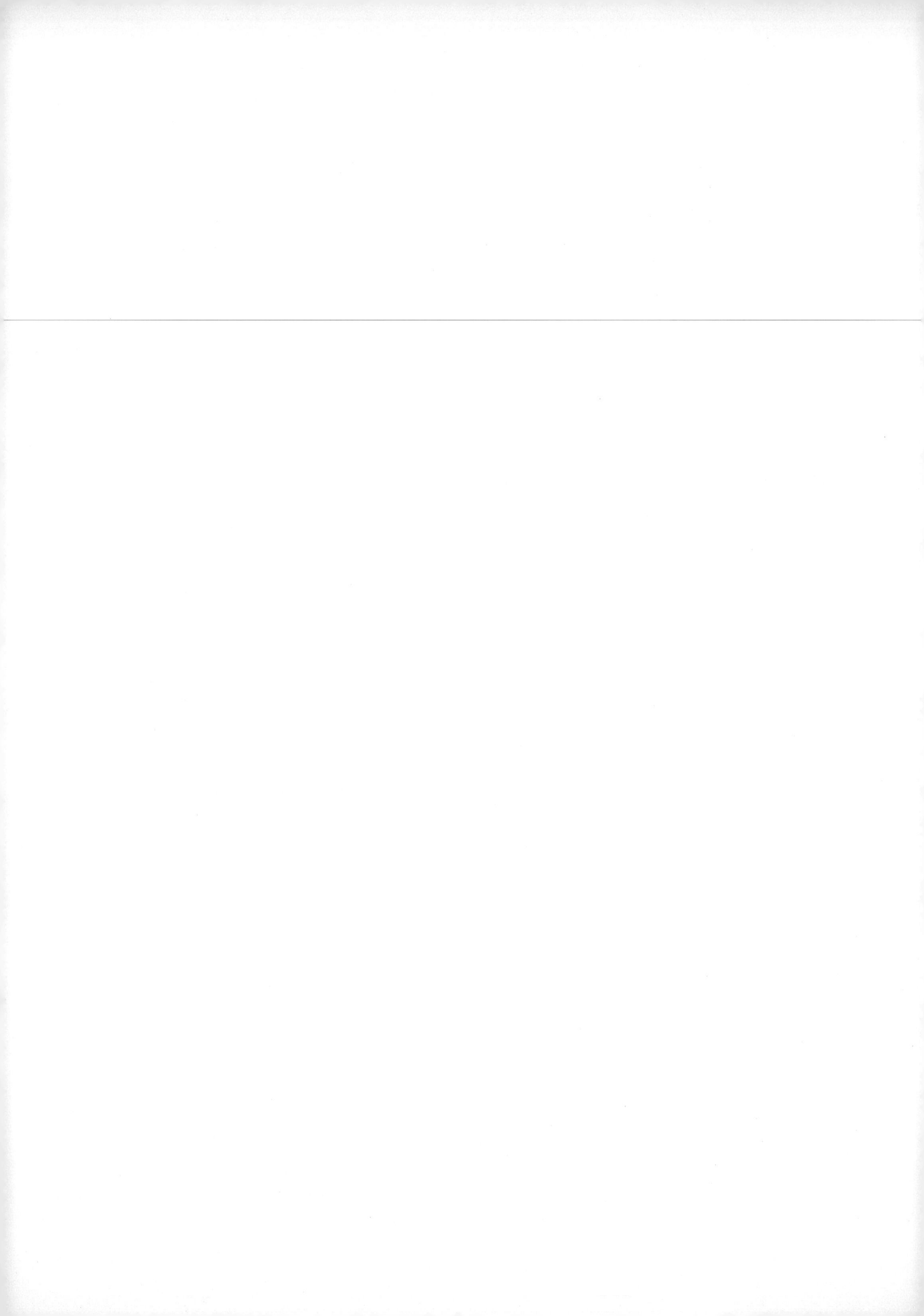

Geleitwort

Mieke le Granse

Vor Ihnen liegt eine der Praxisleitlinien aus der Reihe *The AOTA Practice Guidelines Series* des amerikanischen Berufsverbandes der Ergotherapie, der AOTA. Diese Reihe von Praxisleitlinien wurde entwickelt als eine Antwort auf die Veränderungen der Gesellschaft, des Gesundheitswesens und damit natürlich auch der Ergotherapie.

Durch diese Entwicklung von Praxisleitlinien erhofft man sich, die Qualität der ergotherapeutischen evidenzbasierten Angebote zu verbessern, die Zufriedenheit der Klienten zu erweitern, den Gewinn und Nutzen der Inhalte der Praxisleitlinien zu unterstützen und durch effektive und effiziente ergotherapeutische Angebote die Kosten im Gesundheitswesen zu reduzieren.

Viele amerikanische Experten aus der ergotherapeutischen Praxis, Lehre und Forschung haben diese AOTA-Praxisleitlinien entwickelt, um so eine hohe Qualität zu gewährleisten und fortlaufend die Praxisleitlinien zu aktualisieren oder neue zu entwickeln und herauszugeben. Sie bieten einen Überblick über den ergotherapeutischen Prozess und die dazugehörenden möglichen Interventionen bei einer Anzahl von Krankheitsbildern und beruhen alle auf der Perspektive von Evidence based Practice.

Ziel der AOTA ist, durch das Entwickeln von Praxisleitlinien, die Ergotherapeutinnen zu unterstützen, ihre Angebote zu verbessern und Entscheidungen zu erleichtern, sodass die ergotherapeutischen Angebote sich optimal dem Bedarf der Klienten und der Angehörigen der Berufsgruppe anpassen und für sie zugänglich sind. Daneben entspricht es der Intention der AOTA, nicht nur den Ergotherapeutinnen, sondern auch den Klienten, Studenten, Dozenten, Forschern, anderen professionelle Berufsgruppen und Dienstleistern wie Krankenkassen optimal begreifbar und verstehbar zu machen, was Ergotherapie zu bieten hat.

Und Ergotherapie hat viel zu bieten, sie ist die Expertin für das tägliche Handeln! Und damit wird sie immer mehr ein wichtiger Team Player im Gesundheitswesen. Ergotherapeutinnen sind überall präsent, zeigen ihre Bedeutung und ihren Einfluss in interprofessionellen Teams als Generalisten und Spezialisten. Die Ergotherapeutinnen, die wissenschaftlich arbeiten, werden immer mehr herausgefordert, Nachweise zu liefern für eine betätigungsorientierte Ergotherapie. Mit Hilfe der vielen wissenschaftlichen Nachweise sind Ergotherapeutinnen in der Lage, den Wert der von ihnen angebotenen Dienstleistungen zu rechtfertigen und ihre Qualität zu zeigen.

Für die Praxis bedeutet die Entwicklung und die Verwendung der Praxisleitlinien, dass es immer mehr signifikante Evidenz gibt für die zahlreichen Interventionen innerhalb des ergotherapeutischen Prozesses, welche die Betätigungsperformanz des Klienten effektiv verbessern. Dies bedeutet auch, dass Ergotherapeutinnen sach- und fachkundig sein müssen auf dem Gebiet der evidenzbasierten Forschungsergebnisse: Sie müssen sie verstehen und ethisch und angemessen anwenden können, um die Ergotherapie mit den besten Praxisansätzen durchführen zu können.

Diese Entwicklungen haben Auswirkungen auf die ergotherapeutische Ausbildung: die Dozenten sollten ihre Auszubildenden und Studierenden die aktuellsten evidenzbasierten Praktiken lehren, damit sichergestellt wird, dass sie gut vorbereitet werden auf eine evidenzbasierte Praxis. Durch den Einsatz von wissenschaftlicher Literatur im Unterricht kann man nicht nur den Wert der ergotherapeutischen Angebote legitimieren und argumentieren, sondern die Auszubildenden und Studierenden lernen, wie sie die Ergebnisse aus der wissenschaftlichen Literatur in der Praxis anwenden können.

Da diese Praxisleitlinien so wichtig sind für die Weiterentwicklung der Ergotherapie hat sich der Hogrefe Verlag entschieden, diese Praxisleitlinien übersetzen zu lassen durch Ergotherapie-Experten aus der Praxis, Lehre und Forschung aus Deutschland, Österreich und der Schweiz, und sie zu publizieren, damit auch die deutschsprachigen Ergotherapeutinnen profitieren können von dem schon erforschten Wissen der amerikanischen Kolleginnen.

So publizierte der Hogrefe Verlag im Herbst 2017 für die deutschsprachigen Länder die ersten vier Praxisleitlinien: Menschen mit Schlaganfall, Wohnraumanpassung, Menschen mit einer Autismus-Spektrum-Störung und Menschen mit schweren psychischen Erkrankungen.

Im Februar 2018 erschien die erste deutsche Übersetzung des OTPF (Occupational Therapy Practice Framework: Domain and Process, 3rd Edition) inklusive vieler Praxisbeispiele aus den Settings und Bereichen der Ergotherapie.

Das *Framework der AOTA* (OTPF) dient als wichtige Basis für alle Praxisleitlinien. Es beschreibt das zentrale Konzept der Ergotherapie-Praxis (die Betätigungsperformanz) und die positive Beziehung zwischen Handeln, Gesundheit und Wohlbefinden. Das OTPF gibt einen Einblick über den Anteil der Ergotherapeutinnen, um gemeinsam mit ihren Klienten die Gesundheit zu verbessern, die Partizipation und soziale Teilhabe von Menschen zu erhöhen und Organisationen und Populationen durch Engagement im täglichen Handeln zu ermutigen. Diese dritte Ausgabe des OTPFs baut auf der ersten und zweiten Ausgabe auf und begründet sich auf den Uniform Terminology for Occupational Therapists (AOTA, 1994) und der International Classification of Functioning, Disability and Health (ICF; WHO, 2001).

Es folgen noch eine große Reihe von übersetzten Praxisrichtlinien:
- Klienten mit Sehstörungen
- Aktives Altern zuhause
- Klienten mit Alzheimer Krankheit
- Klienten mit Schädel Hirn Trauma
- Autofahren und Mobilität für den älteren Menschen
- Arbeitsbedingte Verletzungen und Krankheiten
- Die frühe Kindheit: von der Geburt bis 5 Jahre
- Kinder und Klienten mit Herausforderungen in Bezug zu sensorische Verarbeitung und sensorische Integration
- Psychische Gesundheitsförderung – Prävention und Intervention für Kinder und Jugendliche
- Rehabilitation bei Krebserkrankungen
- Muskuloskelettale Krankheiten
- Arthritis

Die Praxisleitlinien sind so aufgebaut, dass sie mit einer Einführung beginnen, in der Ziel und Zweck der Praxisleitlinien beschrieben wird und einer Kurzversion vom Gegenstandsbereich und Prozess der Ergotherapie. Danach folgt eine Darstellung des/der spezifischen Krankheitsbildes(er), gefolgt durch die Darstellung und Auseinandersetzung des ergotherapeutischen Prozesses (von Überweisung bis zu Evaluation, Intervention und Ergebnis). Ein weiterer Textteil umfasst die Best Practices und Zusammenfassungen der Evidenz und die Implikationen der Evidenz für die ergotherapeutische Praxis, Ausbildung und Forschung. Jede Praxisleitlinie hat verschiedene Anhänge, unter anderen eine sehr ausführliche Evidenztabelle, mit vielen Beispielen von überwiegend Forschungsartikeln (meist mit einem Evidenzlevel von I, II oder III), welche die auf Handeln und Partizipation basierte ergotherapeutische Interventionen in Bezug zu dem betreffenden Krankheitsbild darstellen.

Da die Praxisleitlinien übersetzt werden aus den Situationen der amerikanischen Ergotherapie, bedeutet dies, dass der Leser auch Inhalten begegnen wird, die vielleicht anders sind als man im eigenen Umgang gewohnt ist. Einerseits bereichert dies natürlich das eigene Vorgehen um neue Perspektiven, aber erfordert auch vom Leser den Transfer von den Praxisleitlinien zur eigenen Tätigkeit. Wo es notwendig erscheint, unterstützen Fußnoten der Übersetzerinnen, der Herausgeberin und des Lektorats diesen Transferprozess, um den Unterschied aufzuzeigen zwischen der amerikanischen Praxis und der ergotherapeutischen Praxis in den deutschsprachigen Ländern. Beispielsweise wird in den USA unterschieden zwischen den ausführenden Aktivitäten von Ergotherapeutinnen und Ergotherapie-Assistentinnen. Auch gibt es viele Unterschiede in den gesetzlichen Vorgaben und den Institutionen. Auch die verwendete Terminologie ist in der Übersetzung verschieden. So ist jeder Praxisleitlinie ein Glossar angehängt mit den wichtigsten Begriffen aus der Terminologie des OTPF.

Die Praxisleitlinien sind in der weiblichen Form geschrieben, wenn sie die Person im Singular ansprechen, da die Mehrheit der Ergotherapeutinnen Frauen sind, bei der Beschreibung der Klienten wechselt die Anrede. Selbstverständlich ist in jedem Fall das jeweilig andere Geschlecht miteinbezogen und gleichermaßen benannt.

Ein ganz großes Dankeschön geht an die Kolleginnen der Ergotherapie, die die unterschiedlichen Praxisleitlinien übersetzt haben und ihre Zeit, Engagement und Expertise eingebracht und geschenkt haben, um den Beruf weiterzuentwickeln und ihren Kollegen das umfassende Material und Wissen der Praxisleitlinien in ihrer eigenen Sprache zur Verfügung zu stellen. Ein weiteres großes Dankeschön gilt den Kolleginnen vom Hogrefe Verlag, Barbara Müller und Diana Goldschmid, die mit großem Einsatz unermüdlich dafür gesorgt haben, dass diese wichtige und höchst interessante Reihe an Praxisleitlinien publiziert werden.

Wir wünschen allen Lesern viel Inspiration beim Lesen der Praxisleitlinien und sind offen für Feedback, Verbesserungsvorschläge und Tipps.

„Wissen schafft Nutzen – wenn es erschlossen, in eine anwendbare Form gebracht und verbreitet wird. Erst dann ermöglicht es einen konstruktiven Austausch, der wiederum neues Wissen hervorbringt.", Vision Hogrefe Verlag.

Ihre Herausgeberin
Mieke le Granse

1 Einführung

1.1 Zweck und Anwendung dieser Veröffentlichung

Praxisleitlinien sind vielfach als Antwort auf die Gesundheitsreformbewegung in den Vereinigen Staaten entwickelt worden. Solche Leitlinien können ein nützliches Instrument sein, um die Qualität der Gesundheitsversorgung zu verbessern, die Zufriedenheit der Verbraucher zu steigern, den angemessenen Einsatz der Dienstleistungen zu fördern und die Kosten zu reduzieren. Der Amerikanische Ergotherapieverband (American Occupational Therapy Association, AOTA) der nahezu 150 000 Ergotherapeuten, Ergotherapie-Assistenten (siehe **Anhang A**) und Ergotherapie-Studenten vertritt, möchte Informationen bereitstellen, um Entscheidungen zu unterstützen, die ein hochqualifiziertes System der Gesundheitsversorgung fördern, das für alle erschwinglich und zugänglich ist.

Aus evidenzbasierter Perspektive unter Einbeziehung der Schlüsselkonzepte aus der dritten Auflage des *Occupational Therapy Practice Framework: Domain und Process* (OTPF: AOTA, 2014) bietet eine solche Leitlinie einen Überblick über den ergotherapeutischen Prozess für Menschen mit neurodegenerativen Erkrankungen. Sie definiert den ergotherapeutischen Gegenstandsbereich und Prozess und die Interventionen, die innerhalb der Grenzen akzeptabler Praxis vorgenommen werden. Diese Leitlinie behandelt nicht alle Methoden der Versorgung, die möglich sind; sie empfiehlt zwar einige spezifische Methoden der Versorgung, aber welche der möglichen Interventionen angemessen ist für die Gegebenheiten einer bestimmten Person oder Gruppe, für ihre Bedürfnisse und die verfügbare Evidenz, beurteilt letztendlich die Ergotherapeutin[1].

Mit dieser Publikation möchte die AOTA Ergotherapeuten und Ergotherapie-Assistenten und auch denjenigen, die die Kosten tragen oder die ergotherapeutischen Dienstleistungen regeln, helfen, den Beitrag der Ergotherapie zur Arbeit mit alten Menschen in unterschiedlichen Settings zu erkennen. Diese Leitlinie kann ebenfalls als Empfehlung für Leistungserbringer und Heimleiter aus dem Gesundheitsbereich, Gesetzgeber für Gesundheit und Ausbildung, Kostenträger und Pflegeorganisationen dienen[2].

Diese Publikation kann angewandt werden, um:
- Ergotherapeuten und Ergotherapie-Assistenten zu helfen, sich mit externen Institutionen über ihre Intervention auszutauschen;
- Praktikern in anderen Gesundheitsberufen, Fallmanagern, Klienten, Familien und Angehörigen und Heimleitern aus dem Gesundheitsbereich bei der Entscheidung zu helfen, ob eine Überweisung zur Ergotherapie angemessen ist;
- Kostenträger bei der Entscheidung zu unterstützen, ob medizinische Notwendigkeit für Ergotherapie gegeben ist;
- Gesetzgebern, Kostenträgern, Bundes-, Landes- und lokalen Agenturen zu helfen, die Ausbildung und die Fertigkeiten von Ergotherapeuten und Ergotherapie-Assistenten zu verstehen;
- Planungsteams in Sozial- und Gesundheitsdiensten zu helfen, die Notwendigkeit von Ergotherapie festzustellen;
- Entwicklern von Gesundheitsprogrammen, Verwaltungen, Gesetzgebern, Landes- und kom-

---

1 Die Berufsangehörigen der Ergotherapie im Singular werden in diesem Dokument in der weiblichen Form bezeichnet; Klientenbezeichnungen der Ergotherapie im Singular stehen in diesem Dokument in männlicher oder in weiblicher Form, im Plural beide in der allgemeinen männlichen Form. Sie gelten selbstverständlich auch für das jeweilige andere Geschlecht.

2 In der Originalausgabe werden Informationen zu ausgewählten Diagnosen und Abrechnungsmodalitäten für Evaluation und Intervention im Anhang B aufgelistet. Sie haben für den deutschsprachigen Markt keine Relevanz. (Anmerkung des Lektorats)

munalen Agenturen und Kostenträgern zu helfen, das Spektrum ergotherapeutischer Dienstleistungen zu verstehen;
- Forschern, Ergotherapeuten, Ergotherapie-Assistenten, Programmauswertern und -analysten in diesem Praxisbereich zu helfen, Ergebnismessinstrumente festzulegen, die die Effektivität von ergotherapeutischer Intervention analysieren;
- Bewerten von Planung, Ausbildung und Gesundheitsfinanzierung zu helfen, die Angemessenheit von ergotherapeutischer Intervention für Menschen mit neurodegenerativen Erkrankungen zu verstehen;
- Politikern, Gesetzgebern und Organisationen zu helfen, den Beitrag zu verstehen, den Ergotherapie zu Gesundheitsförderung, Programmentwicklung und Gesundheitsreform für Menschen mit neurodegenerativen Erkrankungen leisten kann und
- ergotherapeutischem Lehrpersonal zu helfen, angemessene Curricula zu entwerfen, die die Rolle der Ergotherapie für Menschen mit neurodegenerativen Erkrankungen einbeziehen.
- den Klienten der Ergotherapie zu helfen, die Tiefe und Breite des Wissens und der Dienstleistungen zu verstehen, die im Rahmen der Ergotherapie von Menschen mit neurodegenerativen Erkrankungen zu erhalten sind.

Die Einführung dieser Leitlinien erläutert im Folgenden kurz den Gegenstandsbereich und den Prozess der Ergotherapie. Dann folgt eine detaillierte Beschreibung des ergotherapeutischen Prozesses für Menschen mit neurodegenerativen Erkrankungen. Darin finden sich auch Zusammenfassungen von Ergebnissen systematischer Evidenzreviews aus wissenschaftlicher Literatur zu Interventionen nach der besten ergotherapeutischen Praxis. Die Anhänge schließlich enthalten Tabellen zu Methoden (**Anhang C**) und Evidenz (**Anhang D**) für die Reviews.

1.2 Gegenstandsbereich und Prozess der Ergotherapie

Die Fachkompetenz von Ergotherapeuten[3] liegt in ihrem Wissen über Betätigung und wie das Betätigen genutzt werden kann, um zu Gesundheit und Teilhabe zuhause, in der Schule, am Arbeitsplatz und in der Gemeinde beizutragen.

Die Delegiertenversammlung des AOTA nahm 2013 das *Occupational Therapy Practice Framework: Domain und Process* (3rd ed.; AOTA, 2014) an. Auf der Grundlage der ersten und zweiten Ausgabe des *Occupational Therapy Practice Framework: Domain und Process* (AOTA, 2002, 2008), der früheren *Uniform Terminology for Occupational Therapy* (AOTA, 1989, 1994) und der *International Classification of Functioning, Disability and Health* (ICF; WHO, 2001) der WHO legt das Framework den Gegenstandsbereich des Berufes und den darin enthaltenen Therapieprozess dar.

1.2.1 Gegenstandsbereich

Der *Gegenstandsbereich* eines Berufes gliedert dessen Wissensbereich, seinen gesellschaftlichen Beitrag und seine intellektuellen oder wissenschaftlichen Aktivitäten. Der Gegenstandsbereich der Ergotherapie richtet sich darauf, anderen zur Teilhabe an alltäglichen Aktivitäten zu verhelfen. Der übergeordnete Begriff, den der Beruf zur Beschreibung von alltäglichen Aktivitäten nutzt, ist *Betätigung*. Wie im *Framework* dargelegt, arbeiten Ergotherapeuten und Ergotherapie-Assistenten zusammen mit Klienten, Organisationen und Populationen (Klienten), damit diese sich an Aktivitäten oder Betätigungen, die sie tun möchten oder tun müssen, so beteiligen können, dass Gesundheit und Partizipation unterstützt werden (siehe **Abb. 1-1**). Ergotherapeuten benutzen Betätigung sowohl als erwünschtes Ergebnis der Intervention als auch als Methode für die Intervention selbst; Ergotherapeuten[4] sind erfahren darin, die subjektiven und die objektiven Aspekte von Performanz zu erfassen, und sie verstehen Betätigung aus dieser

---

3 *Ergotherapeuten* sind für alle Aspekte der ergotherapeutischen Intervention verantwortlich und zuständig für die Sicherheit und Effektivität des ergotherapeutischen Interventionsprozesses. *Ergotherapie-Assistenten* behandeln ergotherapeutisch unter der Supervision von und in Partnerschaft mit einem Ergotherapeuten (AOTA, 2009)

4 Wenn hier der Begriff *Ergotherapeuten* gebraucht wird, sind sowohl *Ergotherapeuten* als auch *Ergotherapie-Assistenten* gemeint.

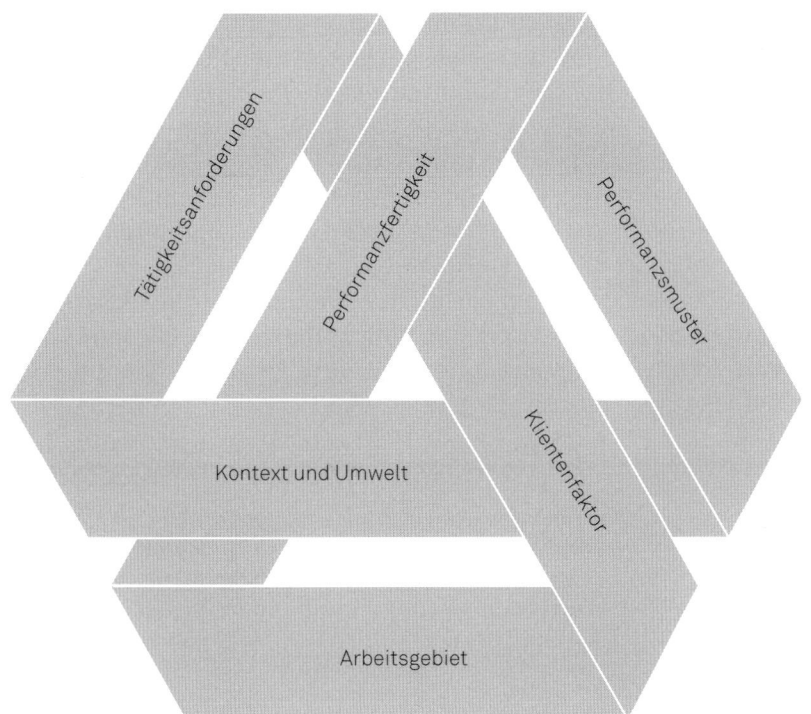

Abbildung 1-1: Ergotherapeutischer Gegenstandsbereich
Zur Beachtung. ADLs = Aktivitäten des täglichen Lebens. IADLs = Instrumentelle Aktivitäten des täglichen Lebens. Quelle: Occupational Therapy Practice Framework: Domain und Process (3rd ed. S. 55) des Amerikanischen Ergotherapieverbandes, 2014, American Journal of Occupational Therapy, 68 (Suppl. 1) S1-S48. Abdruck mit freundlicher Genehmigung.

zweifachen, aber dennoch ganzheitlichen Sicht. Die übergeordnete Aufgabe, Gesundheit, Wohlbefinden und Teilhabe am Leben durch Beteiligung an Betätigung zu unterstützen, umreißt den Gegenstandsbereich des Berufes, und sie betont, wie wichtig der Einfluss von Umwelt- und Lebensbedingungen darauf ist, wie Menschen ihre Betätigungen ausführen. Schlüsselaspekte des ergotherapeutischen Gegenstandsbereiches werden in **Tabelle 1-1** definiert.

1.2.2 Prozess

Viele Berufe nutzen den Prozess der Evaluation, Intervention und Outcome, der im *Framework* dargestellt wird. Die Anwendung dieses Prozesses durch die Ergotherapie ist jedoch durch seine Fokussierung auf Betätigung einzigartig (siehe **Abb. 1-2**). Der Prozess klientenzentrierter ergotherapeutischer Intervention beginnt üblicherweise mit dem Betätigungsprofil, ei-

Tabelle 1-1: Aspekte des ergotherapeutischen Gegenstandsbereichs

Betätigung	Klientenfaktoren	Performanzfertigkeiten	Performanzmuster	Kontext und Umwelt
Aktivitäten des täglichen Lebens (ADLs)*	Werte, Überzeugungen und Spiritualität	Motorische Fertigkeiten	Gewohnheiten	Kulturell
Instrumentelle Aktivitäten des täglichen Lebens (IADLs)	Körperfunktionen	Prozessbezogene Fertigkeiten	Routinen	Personbezogen
Ruhe und Schlaf	Körperstrukturen	Soziale Interaktionsfertigkeiten	Rituale	Physisch
Bildung			Rollen	Sozial
Arbeit				Zeitlich
Spiel				Virtuell
Freizeit				
Soziale Teilhabe				

*auch als Basisaktivitäten des täglichen Lebens (BADLs) oder personbezogene Aktivitäten des täglichen Lebens (PADLs) bezeichnet.
Quelle. Occupational Therapy Practice Framework: Domain and Process (3rd ed. S. S4) des Amerikanischen Ergotherapieverbandes, 2014, American Journal of Occupational Therapy, 68 (Suppl. 1) S1-S48. Abdruck mit freundlicher Genehmigung.

ner Erhebung der Betätigungsbedürfnisse, -probleme und -anliegen des Klienten und der Analyse der Betätigungsperformanz. Zu letzterer gehören Fertigkeiten, Muster, Kontext und Umwelt, Aktivitätsanforderungen und Klientenfaktoren, die zur Zufriedenheit des Klienten mit seiner Fähigkeit, an wertgeschätzten Alltagsaktivitäten teilzunehmen, beitragen oder sie behindern. Die Analyse von Betätigungsperformanz erfordert nicht nur, die komplexe und dynamische Interaktion zwischen Klientenfaktoren, Performanzfertigkeiten, Performanzmustern und Kontext und Umwelt zu durchschauen, sondern auch die Aktivitätsanforderungen der ausgeführten Betätigung. Therapeuten planen die Intervention und setzen sie mit vielerlei Ansätzen und Methoden um, bei denen Betätigung sowohl das Mittel als auch der Zweck ist (Trombly, 1995).

Ergotherapeuten überprüfen ständig die Effektivität der Intervention und die Fortschritte auf die vom Klienten erwünschten Ergebnisse. Von der Gesamtsicht auf die Intervention hängt die Entscheidung ab, ob letztere fortgeführt oder beendet und eine Überweisung an andere Gesundheitsdienstleister oder -berufe empfohlen wird.

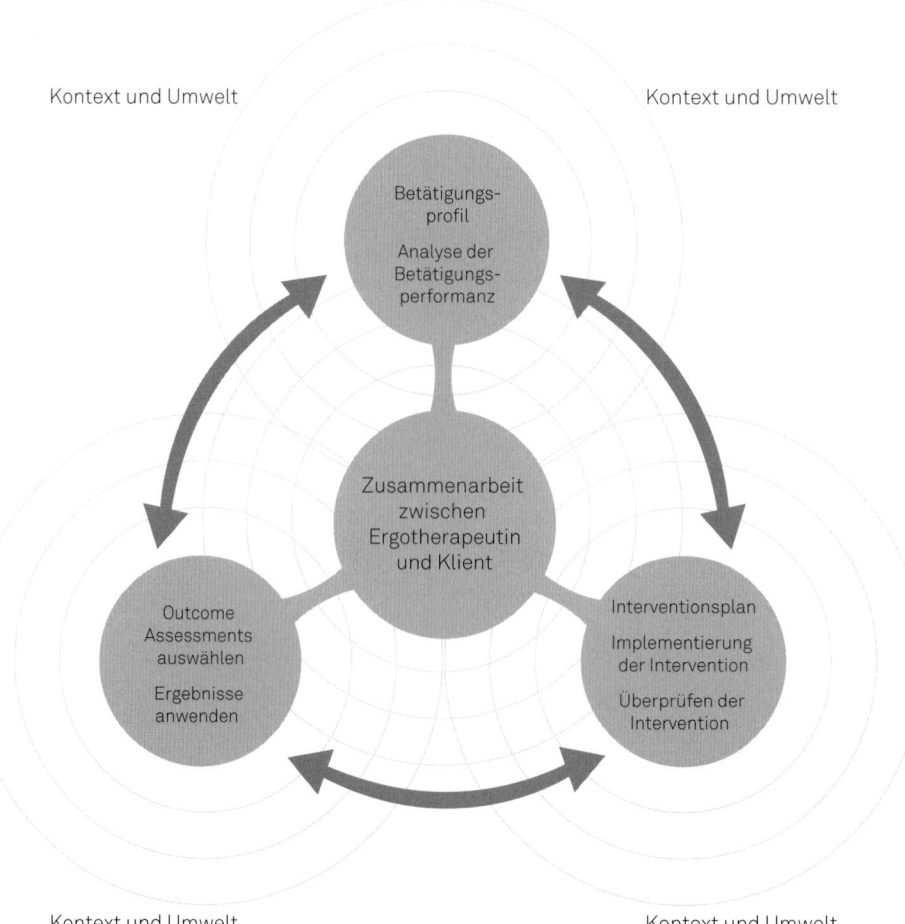

Abbildung 1-2:
Ergotherapeutischer Prozess
Quelle. *Occupational Therapy Practice Framework: Domain und Process* (3rd ed. S. 55) des Amerikanischen Ergotherapieverbandes, 2014, American Journal of Occupational Therapy, 68 (Suppl. 1) S1-S48. Abdruck mit freundlicher Genehmigung.

Tabelle 1-2: Prozess der ergotherapeutischen Dienstleistung

Evaluation
Betätigungsprofil – Der erste Schritt im Evaluationsprozess, durch den die Betätigungsvorgeschichte und Erfahrungen des Klienten, seine Alltagsmuster, Interessen, Werte und Bedürfnisse klar werden. Ebenso werden die Gründe deutlich, warum der Klient zur Ergotherapie kommt, seine Stärken und Sorgen in Bezug auf die Ausführung von Betätigungen und alltäglichen Aktivitäten, Bereiche möglicher Störungen, Unterstützungen und Barrieren sowie seine Prioritäten. *Analyse der Betätigungsperformanz* – Der Schritt im Evaluationsprozess, mit dem die Stärken und Probleme oder potentielle Probleme des Klienten genauer herausgefunden werden. Die derzeitige Performanz wird oft direkt im Kontext beobachtet, um Unterstützung bzw. Barrieren bei der Performanz des Klienten festzustellen. Performanzfertigkeiten, Performanzmuster, Kontext oder Umwelt, Klientenfaktoren und Aktivitätsanforderungen werden alle bedacht, aber nur bestimmte Aspekte werden möglicherweise genauer untersucht. Angestrebte Ergebnisse werden festgelegt.

Intervention
Interventionsplan – Der Plan leitet die Maßnahmen, die zusammen mit dem Klienten entwickelt und dann vorgenommen werden. Er beruht auf ausgewählten Theorien, Bezugsrahmen und Evidenz. Anzustrebende Ergebnisse werden bestätigt. *Umsetzung der Intervention* – Aktionen, die die Performanz des Klienten beeinflussen und unterstützen, um seine Performanz und Partizipation zu verbessern. Interventionen beziehen sich auf die erwünschten Ergebnisse. Die Reaktion des Klienten wird überwacht und dokumentiert. Überprüfung der Intervention – Überprüfung des Interventionsplans und der Fortschritte im Hinblick auf die angestrebten Ergebnisse.

Anstreben von Ergebnissen
Ergebnisse – Erfolgsdeterminanten beim Erreichen des erwünschten Endresultats des ergotherapeutischen Prozesses. Die Informationen aus dem Outcome Assessment leiten die Planungen zukünftiger Maßnahmen mit dem Klienten und evaluieren das Interventionsprogramm (Programmevaluation).

Quelle: *Occupational Therapy Practice Framework: Domain and Process* (3rd ed., p. S10), by American Occupational Therapy Association, 2014, *American Journal of Occupational Therapy, 68*(Suppl. 1), S1–S48. http://dx.doi.org/10.5014/ajot.2014.682006. Copyright © 2014 by the American Occupational Therapy Association.

2 Überblick zu neurodegenerativen Krankheiten (NDK)

Dieses Kapitel der Leitlinien beginnt mit einem breiten Überblick über neurodegenerative Krankheiten (im Folgenden auch: NDK). Darauf folgen spezifische Hintergrundinformationen zu vier NDK: Multiple Sklerose (im Folgenden auch: MS), idiopathisches Parkinsonsyndrom (im Folgenden auch: IPS), amyotrophe Lateralsklerose (im Folgenden auch: ALS) und transverse Myelitis (im Folgenden auch: TM). NDK können fortschreitende Schäden an Funktionen, Strukturen oder beiden Neuronen nach sich ziehen (Ahmad, 2012). Die Neuronen (Nervenzellen) des zentralen Nervensystems (ZNS), des peripheren Nervensystems (PNS) oder beide können betroffen sein. NDK neigen dazu, chronisch, fortschreitend und im Allgemeinen unheilbar und manchmal tödlich zu sein (Forwell, Copperman & Hugos, 2008). Zudem unterscheiden sich Formen und Schweregrad der Beeinträchtigungen sowie der Einfluss davon auf den Alltag von Klient zu Klient in hohem Maße. Des Weiteren sehen sich Menschen mit NDK oft mit wechselnden Niveaus an Beeinträchtigungen konfrontiert und müssen lernen, mit ihnen zurechtzukommen und sie zu bewältigen.

Die folgenden Kapitel beinhalten eine kurze Beschreibung der vier NDK einschließlich ihrer Ätiologie, Epidemiologie und Inzidenz, um den Lesern Hintergrundinformationen zu bieten, wie jede der Krankheiten zu Beeinträchtigungen und zum Bedarf an Ergotherapie führen kann.

2.1 Multiple Sklerose (MS)

MS ist eine chronische, meist fortschreitende entzündliche NDK, die Schäden am ZNS verursacht (Atkins, Amor, Fletcher & Mills, 2012; Oger & Al-Araji, 2006); im Besonderen im Gehirn, Rückenmark und den kranialen Nerven (National Multiple Sclerosis Society, 2013c). MS beschädigt Axone (Nervenfasern) und Neuronen (Cohen & Rudick, 2011), was zur Bildung von Narbengewebe oder Plaques führt, was die Leitfähigkeit der Axonen beeinträchtigt (Kenealy, Pericak-Vance & Haines, 2003). Trotz vieler Forschungen ist die Ursache von MS unbekannt (Atkins et al., 2012; Cohen & Rudick, 2011). Es gibt wissenschaftliche Hinweise, dass die Autoimmunität beteiligt ist und dass genetische Faktoren eine Rolle spielen könnten.

MS betrifft ungefähr 0,1 % der Menschen in den USA (Hanson & Cafruny, 2002) und mehr als 2,3 Millionen Menschen weltweit (National Multiple Sclerosis Society, 2013d). Es betrifft häufiger Frauen (Hanson & Cafruny, 2002), Menschen aus Bevölkerungsgruppen mit weißer Hautfarbe in gemäßigten Klimazonen (Atkins et al., 2012) und Menschen schottischer oder schwedischer Volkszugehörigkeit (Cohen & Rudick, 2011). MS tritt gewöhnlich im Alter zwischen 20 und 40 Jahren zum ersten Mal auf und ist die führende Ursache für Beeinträchtigungen bei Menschen unter 40 Jahren in den Industrieländern (Atkins et al., 2012). Die Lebenserwartung von Menschen mit MS ist ähnlich derjenigen der normalen Bevölkerung.

Es gibt vier Verläufe bei MS:
(1) schubförmig remittierend
(2) primär progredient
(3) sekundär progredient und
(4) progredient schubförmig (National Multiple Sclerosis Society, 2013c).

Menschen mit schubförmig remittierender MS erleben akute Schübe der Krankheit, gefolgt von entweder gänzlicher Erholung oder mit einigen Restdefiziten. Der primär progrediente Typ der Krankheit nimmt einen fortschreitend beeinträchtigenden Verlauf ohne

Schübe und intermittierender Erholung. Menschen mit sekundär progredienter MS erleben anfänglich einen schubförmig remittierenden Verlauf, wechseln dann aber zu einem fortschreitend beeinträchtigenden Verlauf, der mit oder ohne Schübe und Erholung verlaufen kann. Bei Menschen mit einem progredient schubförmigen Verlauf erfolgen die Schübe mit oder ohne anschließender vollständiger Erholung. Der schubförmig remittierende Krankheitsverlauf ist der häufigste (Atkins et al., 2012; Cohen & Rudick, 2011). Die meisten Menschen mit MS werden anfänglich mit schubförmig remittierender MS diagnostiziert, aber etwa die Hälfte dieser Klienten entwickelt innerhalb von 10 Jahren den sekundär progredienten Typ (National Multiple Sclerosis Society, 2013c). Ungefähr 10 % der Menschen mit MS werden mit dem sekundär progredienten Typ diagnostiziert und etwa 5 % der Menschen haben den progredient schubförmigen Typ.

MS kann zu einer Vielfalt von Anzeichen und Symptomen führen. Die häufigsten Symptome sind Fatigue, Taubheit, Probleme mit dem Gleichgewicht und Gehen, Darm- und Blasenfehlfunktionen, visuelle Probleme, Schwindel, Schmerz, Spastizität, sexuelle, kognitive und emotionale Veränderungen und Depression (National Multiple Sclerosis Society, 2013b; Oger & Al-Araji, 2006). Fatigue ist das häufigste dieser Symptome und mehr als die Hälfte der Menschen mit MS berichtet, dass Fatigue eines ihrer schlimmsten Symptome ist (National Multiple Sclerosis Society, 2012).

2.2 Idiopathisches Parkinsonsyndrom (IPS)

IPS ist eine chronisch fortschreitende NDK, in deren Verlauf die Neuronen im Gehirn angegriffen werden. Im Speziellen sterben Neuronen der Substantia nigra in den Basalganglien ab (Lang & Lozano, 1998; National Research Council, 2006), was eine verminderte Produktion des Neurotransmitters Dopamin zur Folge hat (Zhang, Dawson & Dawson, 2000). Obwohl es Interventionen für die Symptome von IPS gibt, ist die Ursache unbekannt.

IPS betrifft nicht weniger als eine Million Menschen in den USA (Okun, Fernandez, Grosset & Grosset, 2009). Es betrifft häufiger Menschen aus Bevölkerungsgruppen mit weißer Hautfarbe und Männer. Die Inzidenz steigt mit dem Alter (Okun et al., 2009). Die Krankheit selbst ist nicht tödlich, aber ihre Symptome können zu Komplikationen führen (zum Beispiel Thrombosen, Pneumonien, Stürze), die zu einer erhöhten Sterberate gegenüber derjenigen der Normalbevölkerung führen (Rajput, Rajput & Rajput, 2007).

Menschen mit IPS erleben Bradykinese (verlangsamte Bewegungen) und zumindest eines der folgenden Symptome: Tremor (Zittern), Rigor (Muskelstarre) oder posturale Instabilität (Haltungsinstabilität) (Chaudhuri, Clough & Sethi, 2011). Andere Merkmale von IPS sind die gebeugte Haltung, ein schleppender Gang, Hypomimie (*Maskengesicht*), Darm- und Blasenprobleme, Schmerzen sowie mentale und kognitive Veränderungen. Tremor ist das auffälligste und häufigste Symptom von IPS.

2.3 Amyotrophe Lateralsklerose (ALS)

ALS, auch bekannt als das *Lou-Gehrig-Syndrom*, ist eine schnell fortschreitende, normalerweise tödlich verlaufende NDK, welche die Neuronen angreift, die für die Kontrolle der Willkürmotorik verantwortlich sind (National Institute of Neurological Disorders and Stroke [NINDS], 2013a). Diese Krankheit der Motoneuronen verursacht die allmähliche Degeneration und letztendlich das Absterben sowohl der oberen als auch der unteren Motoneuronen. Die Muskeln, die keine Nervensignale mehr erhalten können, werden allmählich schwächer und atrophieren und letztendlich geht die Willkürkontrolle der motorischen Funktion verloren.

Nicht weniger als 20 000 bis 30 000 Menschen in den USA sind an ALS erkrankt (Cohen & Rudick, 2011; NINDS, 2013a), mit einer Prävalenz von etwa 1:7 pro 100 000 Menschen weltweit (Cwik, 2009). Die Inzidenz von ALS ist weltweit gleich, unabhängig von Kultur, Klima, Geografie, Rasse oder Ernährung. Meist tritt ALS zum ersten Mal zwischen 40 und 60 Jahren auf (NINDS, 2013a). Bei jüngeren Menschen tritt sie häufiger bei Männern auf, aber dieser Unterschied verschwindet bei älteren Menschen (Cwik, 2009).

Menschen mit ALS erleben Muskelschwäche, Krämpfe oder Zuckungen, Schwierigkeiten beim Sprechen und Kau- und Schluckprobleme (NINDS, 2013a). Zu Beginn ist es abhängig davon, welche Neuronen und Muskeln zuerst betroffen sind und welche Körperteile betroffen sind, aber letztendlich verbreitet es sich im ganzen Körper. Schäden an den oberen Motoneuronen verursachen Spastizität und Hyperreflexivität; Schäden an den unteren Motoneuronen führen zu Muskelkrämpfen und Zuckungen, Muskelschwäche und letztendlich Muskelatrophie (Muskelschwund). Mit dem Fortschreiten der Krankheit werden die Muskeln schwächer und atrophischer und die Sprech- und Schluckprobleme nehmen zu. In den späteren Stadien von ALS wird die Atemmuskulatur schwächer und Klienten verlieren ihre Fähigkeit, selbstständig zu atmen. Zusätzlich zu den körperlichen Symptomen weisen aktuelle Studien darauf hin, dass einige Menschen mit ALS Depressionen oder kognitive Veränderungen (zum Beispiel Beeinträchtigungen bei Entscheidungen und verminderte Gedächtnisleistungen; NINDS, 2013a) erleben können. Die häufigste Todesursache bei Menschen mit ALS ist Atemstillstand und die durchschnittliche Überlebensrate nach der Diagnose beträgt drei bis fünf Jahre (Rowland & Shneider, 2001).

2.4 Transverse Myelitis (TM)

TM ist eine neurologische Krankheit, bei der die Nervenfasern des Rückenmarks durch akute Entzündungen beeinträchtigt werden. Diese Entzündungen können einige Stunden bis Wochen dauern (Bhat, Naguwa, Cheema & Gershwin, 2010; NINDS, 2013b). Die Entzündung kann durch unterschiedliche Gegebenheiten wie Virusinfektionen, Autoimmunerkrankungen oder Rückenmarksinfarkte verursacht werden. In manchen Fällen kann die Ursache nicht identifiziert werden. Die Inzidenz von TM wird auf zwischen 1,34 und 4,6 Millionen Fälle pro Jahr geschätzt (Bhat et al., 2010). Es können keine genderbezogenen, genetischen oder ethnischen Muster sowie geografische Faktoren an die Inzidenz von TM gekoppelt werden.

Die Symptome von TM beinhalten beidseitige Schwäche, sensorische Defizite und Darm- und Blasenfehlfunktionen (Bhat et al., 2010). Das Maß der Erholung ist unterschiedlich. Einige Menschen mit TM erholen sich vollkommen, aber andere behalten bleibende Beeinträchtigungen (NINDS, 2013b).

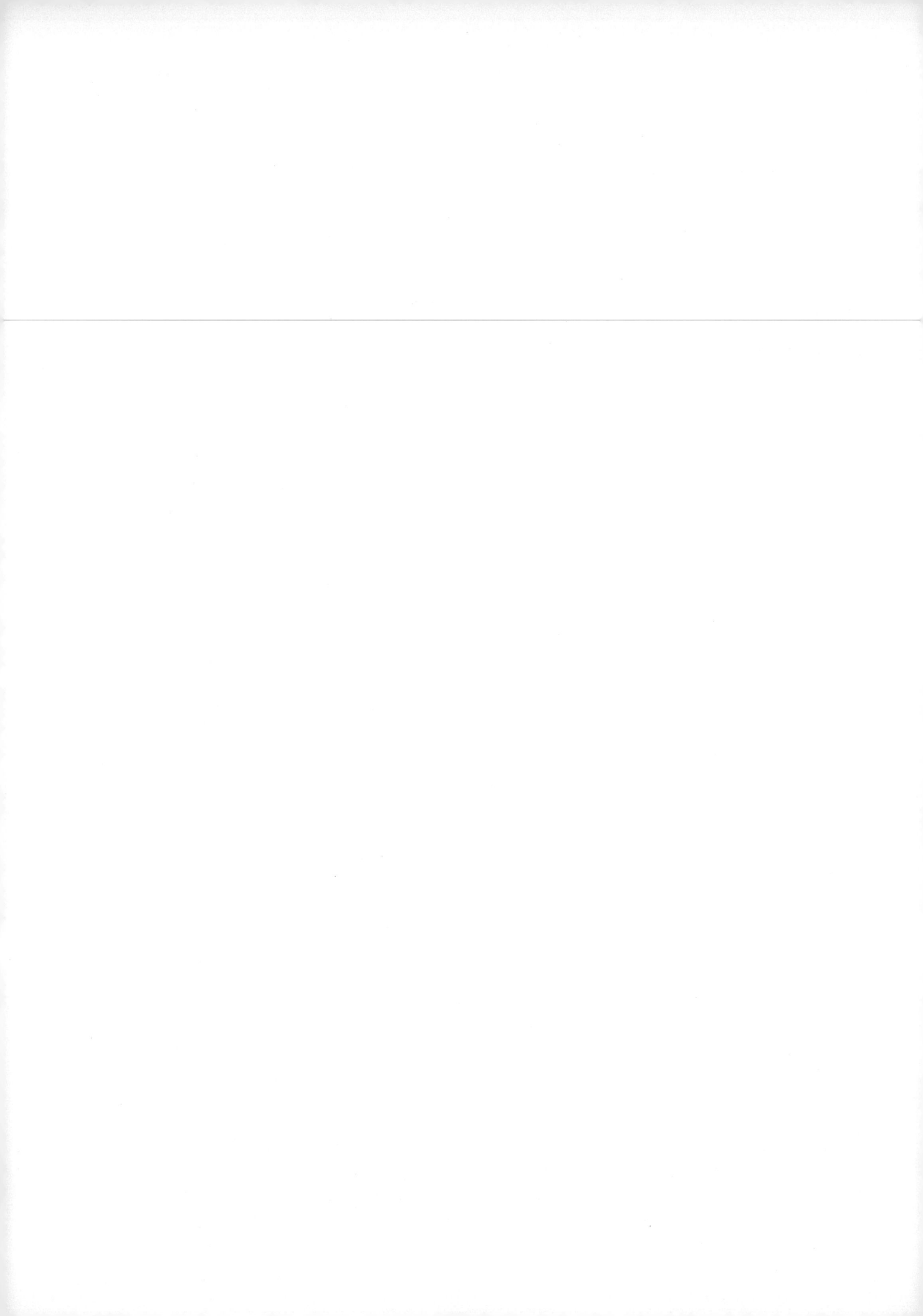

3 Der ergotherapeutische Prozess bei Klienten mit NDK

Dieses Kapitel beschreibt den Prozess der Dienstleistungen der Ergotherapie für Klienten mit NDK; speziell die Überweisung, Evaluation und Interventionen. Es beginnt mit einer kurzen Beschreibung der üblichen Settings, in denen Ergotherapeuten mit Klienten mit NDK arbeiten. Im Kapitel *Interventionen* sind Zusammenfassungen der Resultate systematischer Literaturübersichtsarbeiten wissenschaftlicher Artikel bezogen auf die Best Practice in der Ergotherapie bei Klienten mit NDK aufgenommen. Anschließend folgt eine Erläuterung zur Ergebnisüberwachung und zum Abschluss der Ergotherapie.

3.1 Settings

Ergotherapeuten arbeiten mit Klienten mit NDK und ihren Angehörigen in einer Vielzahl von *Settings*. Praxissettings sind die Kontexte des ergotherapeutischen Prozesses (Pendleton & Schultz-Krohn, 2013). Der Fokus der Ergotherapie ist in allen Settings der gleiche: Menschen ermöglichen, sich an Alltagsaktivitäten oder Betätigungen zu beteiligen, um Gesundheit, Wohlbefinden und Partizipation zu Hause, in der Schule, am Arbeitsplatz und im gesellschaftlichen Leben zu erreichen (AOTA, 2014). Ergotherapeuten arbeiten mit Klienten mit NDK in *medizinischen* und in *gemeindenahen* Settings.

Medizinische Settings beinhalten Krankenhäuser, stationäre Rehabilitation, Frührehabilitation, ambulante Rehabilitation und Pflegeeinrichtungen. Zum Beispiel könnte ein Klient mit ALS mit einer Lungenentzündung oder verschlechterter Mobilität in ein Krankenhaus eingewiesen werden. Dort könnte eine Ergotherapeutin beauftragt werden, die Klienten zu evaluieren und Interventionen anzubieten, mit dem Fokus auf Klienten- und Angehörigenedukation, zur angepassten Ausführung von Alltagsaktivitäten (ADL) wie baden, Toilettengang oder ankleiden. Ein hospitalisierter Klient beim Ausbruch einer TM könnte in eine stationäre Rehabilitation verlegt werden, um das vorherige Funktionsniveau erreichen zu können oder um die Funktionsfähigkeit mit den neuen Beeinträchtigungen zu maximieren.

Klienten mit NDK werden auch von Ergotherapeuten in gemeindenahen Settings aufgesucht. Dies betrifft beispielsweise Klienten mit NDK nach einem Klinikaufenthalt, welche zu Hause ergotherpeutisch therapiert werden, beispielsweise bei IPS zur Edukation kompensatorischer Techniken und Hilfsmittel, um die Effekte der Bradykinese während der Selbstversorgungs- und Haushaltsaktivitäten zu reduzieren, und für Empfehlungen in der häuslichen Umwelt, um die Sicherheit und Performanz zu erhöhen.

In anderen Situationen könnte eine Ergotherapeutin mit einem Klienten mit NDK an seinem Arbeitsplatz arbeiten wie bei Klienten mit Fatigue, Gleichgewichts- und Mobilitätsproblemen und kognitiven Veränderungen aufgrund einer MS-Erkrankung. Verschiedene Interventionen könnten angeboten werden, um es dem Klienten zu ermöglichen, weiterhin zu arbeiten. Diese Interventionen könnten Empfehlungen zu Anpassungen der physischen Umwelt beinhalten (zum Beispiel Organisation von Schränken und Regalen, um die körperliche Belastung zu reduzieren und um die am häufigsten benutzten Gegenstände einfach erreichen zu können), zum Einsatz von Hilfsmitteln (zum Beispiel eine Sackkarre, um Gegenstände zu transportieren) oder zum Einsatz von Technologien (zum Beispiel Telefonapplikationen oder Apps zur Erinnerung an Verabredungen und Aufgaben).

Schließlich erhalten manche Klienten mit NDK und ihre Angehörigen Ergotherapie durch gemeindenahe Dienstleister. Zum Beispiel könnte ein Klient mit MS eine Schulung über Fatigue-Management besuchen, die durch eine Ergotherapeutin angeboten wird, die bei einem Dienstleister angestellt ist. Und die Partnerin oder der Partner könnte an einer Schulung für betreuende Angehörige von kranken Menschen teilnehmen.

3.2 Aktivitätsanforderungen

Entscheidend dafür, ob ein Klient eine Aktivität ausführen kann, sind nicht nur die Performanzfertigkeiten, Performanzmuster und Klientenfaktoren eines Menschen, sondern auch die Anforderungen, die eine Aktivität an einen Klienten stellt. Die *Aktivitätsanforderungen* sind Aspekte einer Aktivität sowie die zur Ausführung dieser Aktivität benötigten Werkzeuge, der Raum und die sozialen Anforderungen, die die Aktivität erfordert, und die notwendigen Aktionen und Performanzfertigkeiten, um sich an dieser Aktivität zu beteiligen. Während des Evaluierungsprozesses identifiziert die Ergotherapeutin, ob die Partizipation eines Klienten aufgrund von Performanzfertigkeiten, Performanzmustern, Klientenfaktoren, Aktivitätsanforderungen oder von einer Kombination dieser Faktoren eingeschränkt ist. Falls die Aktivitätsanforderungen die volle Partizipation beeinträchtigen, werden Ergotherapeuten eine Aktivitätsanalyse zur Identifikation der Aktivitätsanforderungen an die Klienten durchführen, um festzulegen, was notwendig ist, um die Beteiligung an der gewünschten Aktivität zu ermöglichen (AOTA, 2014).

Manchmal werden die Aktivitätsanforderungen die individuelle Fähigkeit übersteigen, sich vollständig oder teilweise an der gewünschten Betätigung zu beteiligen. Außerdem wird sich die Fähigkeit eines Klienten mit NDK, die Anforderungen einer gewünschten Aktivität zu erfüllen, im Laufe der Zeit verändern, aufgrund des fortschreitenden Charakters der Krankheit. Mit einer Aktivitätsanalyse kann die Ergotherapeutin möglicherweise Aspekte der Aufgabe identifizieren, die angepasst werden können (z. B. Veränderungen an den Werkzeugen, am Raum und an den sozialen Anforderungen, die die Aktivität erfordert, oder an den notwendigen Aktionen und Performanzfertigkeiten, um sich an dieser Aktivität beteiligen zu können). Während des Prozesses der Intervention kann sie die Aktivität anpassen, damit die Fähigkeiten des Klienten mit den Aktivitätsanforderungen besser übereinstimmen.

3.3 Screening

Screening in der Ergotherapie verweist auf den Prozess, in dem relevante Informationen gefiltert werden, um festzulegen, ob ein potenzieller Klient eine ergotherapeutische Evaluierung benötigt oder, falls dies nicht der Fall ist, ihn an andere Berufsgruppen im Gesundheitswesen weiterzuverweisen (AOTA, 2013a). Screenings sind normalerweise knappe Durchsichten und können sich auf die Sichtung der Klientenakten beschränken: Ein Beispiel: Eine Ergotherapeutin im Akutbereich ist verantwortlich für die Analyse der medizinischen Akten aller Klienten auf der neurologischen Abteilung. Sie könnte beispielsweise die Akte eines Klienten mit IPS screenen, der wegen Stürzen und verminderten Funktionsfähigkeiten im häuslichen Bereich in die Klinik aufgenommen wurde, und eine ergotherapeutische Evaluierung empfehlen. In einem anderen Setting könnte das Screening einen direkten Klientenkontakt beinhalten: Eine MS-Ambulanz bei einem Neurologen könnte auch eine Ergotherapeutin im Team haben. Diese kann alle Klienten der Klinik screenen, beispielsweise durch ein Gespräch über ihre täglichen Betätigungen zu Hause und einige kurze Assessments (zum Beispiel zu Koordination, Kognition, Gleichgewicht).

3.4 Überweisung

Eine *Überweisung* eines Klienten mit NDK an die Ergotherapie ist dann notwendig, wenn ein Klient Beeinträchtigungen erfährt in der Beteiligung an Betätigungen wie Performanzeinschränkungen in den ADL oder instrumentellen ADL (IADL), bei Freizeitaktivitäten, Arbeit oder Bildungsaktivitäten, in der sozialen Partizipation oder bei Pausen und Schlaf. Eine Überweisung zur Ergotherapie kann durch einen Arzt oder andere Gesundheitsberufe, durch Angehörige oder den Klienten selbst initiiert werden. Ergotherapeuten müssen die staatlichen Gesetze und Verordnungen zum Zugang zu Ergotherapie kennen sowie die Praktiken der Kostenträger wie der Versicherungsgesellschaften (AOTA, 2010a).

3.5 Evaluation

Ergotherapeuten evaluieren in Zusammenarbeit mit dem Klienten und suchen spezifische Informationen zum gewünschten Ergebnis. Die zwei Elemente ergotherapeutischer *Evaluierung* sind (1) das Betätigungsprofil und (2) die Analyse der Betätigungsperformanz

(AOTA, 2014). Beispiele zu den erhobenen Informationen aus dem Betätigungsprofil und der Analyse der Betätigungsperformanz sind in den Fallstudien der **Tabellen 3-2 bis 3-6** enthalten.

Ergotherapeuten, die mit Klienten mit NDK arbeiten, können standardisierte und nichtstandardisierte Assessments verwenden. Es wird empfohlen, klinische Beobachtungen mit Daten standardisierter Assesments zu validieren. Der zuverlässige Gebrauch standardisierter Assessments im Verlauf der Betreuung während des Krankheitsprozesses erhöht die Kontinuität der Betreuung und erlaubt rückblickende Analysen der Ergebnisse, was zur Sammlung praxisunterstützender Evidenz beiträgt. **Tabelle 3-1** bietet

Tabelle 3-1: Ausgewählte Assessments, welche in der Ergotherapie bei Klienten mit neurodegenerativen Erkrankungen verwendet werden

Domäne der Ergotherapie	Beispiele innerhalb jeder Domäne für spezifische Funktionen, die häufig bei Klienten mit neurodegenerativen Erkrankungen betroffen sind	Beispiele von spezifischen Assessments, angewendet bei Klienten mit neurodegenerativen Erkrankungen
Betätigung	• Aktivitäten des alltäglichen Lebens (ADLs) • Instrumentelle Aktivitäten des alltäglichen Lebens (IADLs) • Bildung • Arbeit • Freizeit • Soziale Teilhalbe • Erholung und Schlafen	• Activity Card Sort (Baum & Edwards, 2008) • Arnadottir OT–ADL Neurobehavioral Evaluation (Gardarsdóttir & Kaplan, 2002) • Barthel Index (Mahoney & Barthel, 1965) • Canadian Occupational Performance Measure (COPM; Law et al., 2005) • Executive Function Performance Test (EFPT; Baum, Morrison, Hahn & Edwards, 2003) • FIM™ (Uniform Data System for Medical Rehabilitation, 1997) • Kohlman Evaluation of Living Skills (KELS; Thomson, 1993) • Multiple Errands Test–Revised (MET–R; Morrison et al., 2013) • Occupational Performance History Interview–II (OPHI–II; Kielhofner et al., 2004) • Occupational Self Assessment (OSA; Baron & Kielhofner, 2006) • Performance Assessment of Self-Care Skills (Rogers & Holm, 1994) • Worker Role Interview (WRI; Braveman et al., 2005)
Performanzfertigkeiten	• Motorische Fertigkeiten • Prozessbezogene Fertigkeiten • Soziale Interaktionsfertigkeiten	• Arnadottir OT–ADL Neurobehavioral Evaluation (Gardarsdóttir & Kaplan, 2002) • Assessment of Motor and Process Skills (AMPS; Fisher & Jones, 2012) • Assessment of Social and Interaction Skills (ASIS; Forsyth, Salamy, Simon & Kielhofner, 1998) • Disabilities of the Arm, Shoulder, and Hand Questionnaire (DASH; Solway et al., 1997) • Manual Ability Measure–36 (MAM–36; Chen & Bode, 2010)
Performanzmuster	• Gewohnheiten • Routinen • Rollen • Rituale	• COPM (Law et al., 2005) • The Model of Human Occupation Screening Tool (MOHOST; Parkinson, Forsyth & Kielhofner, 2006) • Role Checklist (Oakley, Kielhofner & Barris, 1985) • OPHI–II (Kielhofner et al., 2004)
Kontext und Umwelt	• Kulturell • Persönlich • Physisch • Sozial • Zeitlich • Virtuell	• Safety Assessment of Function and the Environment for Rehabilitation (SAFER; Oliver, Blathwayt, Brackley & Tamaki, 1993) • Westmead Home Safety Assessment (WeHSA; Clemson, 1997)

Domäne der Ergotherapie	Beispiele innerhalb jeder Domäne für spezifische Funktionen, die häufig bei Klienten mit neurodegenerativen Erkrankungen betroffen sind	Beispiele von spezifischen Assessments, angewendet bei Klienten mit neurodegenerativen Erkrankungen
Klientenfaktoren	• Werte, Überzeugungen und Spiritualität • Körperfunktionen • Körperstrukturen	• Berg Balance Scale (Berg, Wood-Dauphinee, Williams & Gayton, 1989) • The Fatigue Severity Scale (Krupp, LaRocca, Muir-Nash & Steinberg, 1989) • Manual muscle testing • Nine-Hole Peg Test (Mathiowetz, Weber, Kashman & Volland, 1985) • Paced Auditory Serial Addition Test (Gronwell, 1977) • Goniometry
Aktivitäten und Betätigungsanforderungen	• Verwendete Objekte und ihre Eigenschaften • Räumliche Anforderungen • Soziale Anforderungen • Sequenzierung und Timing • Erforderliche Aktionen • Erforderliche Körperfunktionen • Erforderliche Körperstrukturen	• Observational assessment during task performance • In-Home Occupational Performance Evaluation (I-HOPE; Stark, Somerville & Morris, 2010) • Interview

einen kurzen Überblick zu ausgewählten Assessments, die bei Klienten mit NDK genutzt werden können.

3.5.1 Betätigungsprofil

Das Ziel des Betätigungsprofils ist es, zu ermitteln, wer der Klient ist, was seine Bedürfnisse oder Sorgen sind und inwiefern diese mit der Beteiligung an Betätigungen zusammenhängen. Informationen für das Betätigungsprofil werden durch formelle und informelle Gespräche mit Klienten und Angehörigen erhoben. Formelle Assessments können das *Canadian Occupational Performance Measure* (COPM; Law et al., 2005), die *Activity Card Sort* (ACS; Baum & Edwards, 2008) oder das *Occupational Self Assessment* (OSA; Baron & Kielhofner, 2006) beinhalten. Gespräche mit Klienten helfen Ergotherapeuten zu verstehen, wie diese ihre Zeit verbringen, welche Aktivitäten sie ausführen möchten oder müssen und inwieweit die Umwelt die Beteiligung an Betätigungen unterstützt oder einschränkt. Folgende Schritte führen zur Entwicklung des Betätigungsprofils:

1. *Identifikation von Klienten*
2. *Identifikation des Anlasses für Ergotherapie:* Im Rahmen von Gesprächen oder anhand von Variablen der Checklisten wird ein Klient bei der Identifikation seiner aktuellen Probleme auf dem Gebiet der Betätigung und der Performanz unterstützt. Dies ist ein kritischer Teil der Evaluierung. Falls es sich um Klienten mit NDK mit kognitiven Beeinträchtigungen handelt, kann es nützlich sein, Angehörige oder andere Betreuende miteinzubeziehen, um den Grund für die Visite zu ermitteln. Assessments wie das *COPM* (Law et al., 2005) oder *OSA* (Baron & Kielhofner, 2006) können hilfreich sein, wenn klientenzentrierte Ziele zur Betätigungsperformanz aufgestellt werden.
3. *Identifikation von erfolgreichen und risikobehafteten Betätigungsbereichen:* Auf der Grundlage der aktuellen Probleme der Klienten erarbeiten Ergotherapeuten gemeinsam mit ihnen eine Analyse der Stärken und Schwächen in den Ausführungen der Aktivitäten und ermitteln die Barrieren, die die Aussicht auf Erfolg beeinflussen. Auch werden Informationen über Umweltaspekte erhoben, die die Beteiligung unterstützen oder hindern.
4. *Identifikation von signifikanten Aspekten der Betätigungsgeschichte:* Signifikante Aspekte können Lebenserfahrungen (zum Beispiel medizinische Interventionen, berufliche Laufbahn, arbeitsbezogene Vorlieben), Betätigungsrollen, Werte, Interessen und frühere Betätigungsmuster beinhalten, die dem Leben des Klienten Bedeutung verleihen. Das *Occupational Performance History Interview-II* (OPHI-II; Kielhofner et al., 2004) ist ein Beispiel eines Assessments, das bei der Ermittlung signifikanter Aspekte der Betätigungsgeschichte und der Darstellung der Betätigungsperformanz im zeitlichen Verlauf nützlich sein kann.
5. *Identifikation von Prioritäten und Zielen der Klienten:* Während des Interventionsprozesses werden Ergotherapeutin und Klient die Ziele besprechen

Tabelle 3-2: Fallstudie: Klientin mit Multipler Sklerose: gruppenbasiertes Fatigue-Management in der Gemeinde (Community)

Hintergrund	Ergotherapeutische Evaluation	Ergotherapeutische Intervention
Karen ist eine 33-jährige Frau mit primär progredienter MS, welche vor sechs Jahren diagnostiziert wurde. Karen besucht eine MS-Selbsthilfegruppe in ihrer Gemeinde. Hier hat sie Informationen über ein gruppenbasiertes Fatigue-Management-Programm erhalten und sich angemeldet. Das Programm wird von der regionalen Ortsgruppe einer nationalen MS-Organisation angeboten.	Ein kurzes Interview mit Karen vor Beginn der Gruppe ergab folgende Informationen: • Karen lebt gemeinsam mit ihrem Ehemann in einem Haus in einem Vorort der Gemeinde. • Sie hat einen Bachelor-Abschluss und arbeitete früher als Leiterin in einem Einzelhandelsgeschäft, vor Kurzem hat sie jedoch ihren Job aufgegeben und erhält seitdem Erwerbsunfähigkeitsleistungen. • Sie berichtet, dass ihre MS-Symptome, einschließlich der Fatigue, viele ihrer täglichen Aktivitäten beeinträchtigten. Karen benutzt einen Gehstock für die Mobilität draußen. Sie erhält Hilfe bei ADLs, einschließlich baden (auf einem Duschstuhl sitzend) und ankleiden. Sie kocht aufgrund der Fatigue nur vorbereitete Mahlzeiten und findet Einkaufen extrem anstrengend. Sie berichtet zudem von der Vermeidung sozialer Situationen aufgrund der Fatigue. • Karen bemerkte, dass sie ihre MS-Fatigue nicht gut beherrscht und war neugierig, mehr über das Fatigue-Management zu erfahren. • Karen füllte die 9-Item *Fatigue Severity Scale* (Krupp, LaRocca, Muir-Nash, & Steinberg, 1989) aus und erhielt ein Ergebnis von 6,8. Dieses Ergebnis deutet darauf hin, dass Karen die Fatigue als sehr erheblich erlebt. Aufgrund ihrer Punktzahl war sie berechtigt, am Gruppen-Fatigue-Management-Programm teilzunehmen. • Karen füllte das 14-Item *Self-Efficacy for Energy Conservation Questionnaire* (Liepold & Mathiowetz, 2005) aus. Darin werden die Teilnehmer gebeten, ihr Vertrauen in ihre Fähigkeit zu bewerten, die im Kurs vorgestellten Fatigue-Management-Strategien anzuwenden.	• Maria ist Ergotherapeutin. Sie leitet zusätzlich zu ihrer Vollzeittätigkeit in einer großen Rehabilitationsklinik gelegentlich Bildungsprogramme für die regionale Ortsgruppe einer nationalen MS-Organisation. Maria leitete den sechswöchigen Kurs *Managing Fatigue* (Packer, Brink & Sauriol, 1995), bei dem Karen eine der acht Teilnehmer war. Maria folgte dem Instructor-Manual und passte das Programm an die Bedürfnisse von Menschen mit MS an (Mathiowetz, Finlayson, Matuska, Chen & Luo, 2005; Sauter, Siebenholzer, Hisakawa, Zeitlhofer & Vass, 2008). Das Programm umfasste die folgenden sechs Sitzungen: 1. Die Bedeutung von Pausen 2. Kommunikation und Körpermechanik 3. Aktivitätsstationen 4. Prioritäten und Standards 5. Balancieren Sie Ihren Zeitplan 6. Kurszusammenfassung und Zukunftspläne • Karen war eine sehr aktive Teilnehmerin in der Gruppe. Sie hat immer die Hausaufgaben gemacht und oft ihre Erfolge und Herausforderungen mit der Gruppe geteilt. • Am Ende des Programms berichtet Karen über mehr Selbstvertrauen in ihre Fähigkeiten, die Fatigue zu bewältigen. Maria füllte das *Self-Efficacy for Energy Conservation Questionnaire* erneut aus. Die Ergebnisse zeigten, dass sich Karens Vertrauen in die Nutzung von Fatigue-Management-Strategien deutlich verbessert hat. • Karen berichtete, dass sie aufgrund ihrer Teilnahme folgende spezifischen Änderungen vorgenommen hätte: – Umgestaltung ihrer häuslichen Umgebung (zum Beispiel Platzieren häufig benutzter Gegenstände in leichter erreichbare Schubladen) – Änderung ihrer Standards und Prioritäten (zum Beispiel Häufigkeit der Hausarbeit) – Abbau von ermüdenden Aufgaben in kleinere, weniger ermüdende (zum Beispiel Wäsche waschen) – Planung wöchentlicher Aktivitäten zur Bewältigung der Fatigue – Ausgleich zwischen Aktivitäten und Pausen.

Hinweis. ADLs = Aktivitäten des alltäglichen Lebens; MS = Multiple Sklerose

Tabelle 3-3: Fallstudie: Klientin mit Multipler Sklerose: subakute Rehabilitationseinrichtung

Hintergrund	Ergotherapeutische Evaluation	Ergotherapeutische Intervention
Barbara ist eine 64-jährige Frau. Es wurde bei ihr im Alter von 35 Jahren MS diagnostiziert. Sie wurde kürzlich in ein Akutkrankenhaus wegen einer Verschlimmerung ihrer MS aufgenommen und erhielt intravenöse Steroidbehandlungen. Barbara erhielt auch zwei Ergotherapie- und zwei Physiotherapiesitzungen während der Akutversorgung. Aufgrund einer signifikanten Verschlechterung ihrer Funktionen im Vergleich zum Ausgangsniveau wurde Barbara in eine subakute Rehabilitationseinrichtung mit Ergo- und Physiotherapie entlassen. Ziel der Rehabilitation ist die Steigerung der Sicherheit und Selbstständigkeit in der Mobilität und der Selbstversorgung (ADLs).	Barbaras Betätigungsprofil ergab folgende Ergebnisse: • Barbara lebt gemeinsam mit ihrem Ehemann und einem erwachsenen Sohn. • Barbara ist im Ruhestand. Zuvor war sie die Leiterin ihrer lokalen MS-Selbsthilfegruppe, trat aber kürzlich von dieser Position zurück. • Vor ihrer Akutaufnahme war Barbara in der Lage, selbstständig ADLs mit erhöhtem Zeitaufwand und mithilfe von adaptiven und medizinischen Hilfsmitteln durchzuführen. Die Ausnahme stellten Transfers in die Badewanne dar, die sie mit minimaler Unterstützung ihres Mannes und mithilfe eines Badewannenbrettes durchführte. • Barbara berichtete seit Beginn des Krankheitsschubes von einem signifikanten Verlust der oberen und unteren Körperkraft, einer stärkeren Fatigue und einer Zunahme der Spastizität der unteren Extremitäten. Dieser Zustand führt zu einer allgemeinen Beeinträchtigung bei der Durchführung der ADLs. Sie beklagte sich auch über einen Rückgang ihres Gedächtnisses in den letzten sechs bis acht Monaten. ADL/IADL-Performanz: • Essen: minimale Unterstützung • Pflege: minimale Unterstützung • Baden: moderate Unterstützung • Ankleiden Oberkörper: minimale Unterstützung • Ankleiden Unterkörper: maximale Hilfe • Blasen-/Darmentleerung (Toileting): moderate Hilfe • Bett, Stuhl, Rollstuhltransfer: maximale Unterstützung • Toilettentransfer: maximale Unterstützung • Transfer Badewanne, Dusche: maximale Unterstützung • Essensvorbereitung: unselbstständig • Haushaltsführung: unselbstständig Funktionelle Mobilität: • Barbara benötigt maximale Unterstützung, um vom Sitzen zum Stehen zu kommen, und moderate Unterstützung, um mit einem Rollator zu gehen.	• Michelle, Barbaras Ergotherapeutin, bot zwei tägliche Sitzungen für den 15-tägigen subakuten Aufenthalt von Barbara an. • Michelle sorgte täglich für ein morgendliches Selbsthilfetraining. Dieses Training verfolgt das Ziel, Barbaras Unabhängigkeit und Sicherheit der grundlegenden ADLs zu verbessern. Das Training umfasste Anweisungen zu modifizierten Vorgehensweisen bei der Durchführung der Selbstversorgung unter Anwendung von adaptiven Hilfsmitteln (zum Beispiel Sockenhilfe), medizinischen Hilfsmitteln (zum Beispiel Haltegriffe an der Toilette) und in Energiespartechniken. • Michelle und Barbaras Physiotherapeutin erstellten gemeinsam ein Heimübungsprogramm mit Aerobic-Widerstandsübungen. Ziel des Übungsprogrammes ist die Verbesserung der Ausdauer und der Muskelkraft für die Mobilität und der ADL-Performanz (Bjarndottir, Konradsdottir, Reynisdottir & Olafsson, 2007; Fragoso, Santana & Pinto, 2008; Freeman & Allison, 2004; Geddes, Costello, Raivel & Wilsohn, 2009; Rietberg, Brooks, Uitdehaag & Kwakkel, 2004; Romberg et al., 2004). • Für Barbaras Beeinträchtigungen der Gedächtnisleistung trainierte Michelle Barbara in der Selbstgenerierung von funktionalen Aufgabenschritten für eine verbesserte Erinnerung und Aufgabenperformanz (Goverover, Chiaravalloti & DeLuca, 2008) und Visualisierung mit intermittierender Übung (Chiaravalloti, DeLuca, Moore & Ricker, 2005). • Nach Barbaras Entlassung aus der subakuten Einrichtung empfahl Michelle ambulante ergotherapeutische Maßnahmen, um die ADL-Performanz weiter zu verbessern und die Auswirkungen der Fatigue auf die ADLs zu reduzieren (Patti et al., 2002, 2003).

Hinweis. ADLs = Aktivitäten des alltäglichen Lebens; IADLs = instrumentelle Aktivitäten des alltäglichen Lebens; MS = Multiple Sklerose

Tabelle 3-4: Fallstudie: Klient mit idiopathischem Parkinsonsyndrom: Hausbesuch

Hintergrund	Ergotherapeutische Evaluation	Ergotherapeutische Intervention

Maurice ist ein 76-jähriger Mann, bei dem vor sieben Jahren IPS diagnostiziert wurde. Er wurde kürzlich von einem fünftägigen stationären Aufenthalt in einem Akutkrankenhaus nach einem Sturz nach Hause entlassen. Er erhält jetzt Ergo- und Physiotherapie als Hausbesuch.	Maurices Betätigungsprofil ergab folgende Ergebnisse:
	• Maurice ist seit Kurzem verwitwet und lebt jetzt bei seiner Tochter, ihrem Ehemann und seinen drei Enkelkindern. Seit seiner Entlassung aus dem Krankenhaus hat er 24 Stunden Betreuung und Unterstützung von Familienangehörigen erhalten. Seine Familie möchte für täglich sechs Stunden eine Pflegekraft einstellen.
	• Maurices Tochter berichtet, dass ihr Vater beim Gehen unruhiger geworden ist und mehrmals gefallen ist. Sie ist auch besorgt, dass ihr Vater nicht „er selbst" zu sein scheint und es ihm an Energie und Motivation fehlt, sich aktiv zu betätigen.
	
	ADL/ IADL-Performanz:
	• Essen: moderate Unterstützung
	• Pflege: moderate Unterstützung
	• Baden: maximale Unterstützung
	• Ankleiden Oberkörper: minimale Unterstützung
	• Ankleiden Unterkörper: maximale Unterstützung
	• Blasen-/Darmentleerung (Toileting): moderate Unterstützung
	• Bett, Stuhl, Rollstuhltransfer: maximale Unterstützung
	• Toilettentransfer: maximale Unterstützung
	• Transfer Badewanne, Dusche: maximale Unterstützung
	• Essensvorbereitung: unselbstständig
	• Haushaltsführung: unselbstständig
	
	Funktionelle Mobilität:
	• Maurice benötigte moderate Hilfe beim Laufen an einem Rollator. Er ging mit kurzen Schritten und einem schlurfenden Gang.
	
	Assessment of Motor and Process Skills (AMPS):
	• Maurice absolvierte zwei AMPS-Aufgaben: Zähneputzen und Ankleiden des Oberkörpers. Er war unsicher und nicht in der Lage, beide Aufgaben ohne ständige körperliche Unterstützung zu erfüllen. Er hatte große Schwierigkeiten, seinen Körper zu stabilisieren, und drohte zu
		• Dawn, Maurices Ergotherapeutin, bot zwei wöchentliche Sitzungen als Hausbesuch für acht Wochen an.
		• Folgende Interventionen hat Dawn zur Reduzierung von Stürzen geplant:
		  – Anleitung von Maurice und seiner Tochter in Sicherheitstechniken für den Transfer und die ADLs
		  – Beratung zu Wohnraumanpassung (zum Beispiel Reduzieren von Unordnung auf dem Boden, Entfernen von Überwurfdecken, Verbesserung der Beleuchtung)
		  – Verwenden von adaptiven Hilfsmitteln und medizinischen Hilfsmitteln (zum Beispiel ein WC-Stuhl für den nächtlichen Toilettengang)
		  – Anleitung von Maurices Tochter in Techniken, wie sie nach einem Sturz des Vaters beim Aufstehen helfen kann.
		• Um die Unabhängigkeit beim Ankleiden zu verbessern, empfahl Dawn, aufgrund der Schwierigkeiten von Maurice mit der Feinmotorik, Klettverschlüsse statt Standardverschlüsse zu verwenden.
		• Dawn arbeitet mit Maurices Physiotherapeut zusammen. Gemeinsam entwickeln sie ein Heimprogramm mit Übungen und Aktivitäten für die Verbesserung der Ausdauer, Kraft und Balance und um Stürze zu verhindern (Crizzle & Newhouse, 2006; Dibble, Addison & Papa, 2009; Goodwin, Richards Taylor, Taylor & Campbell, 2008; Keus et al., 2007; Kwakkel, de Goede & van Wegen, 2007; Mehrholz et al., 2010; Stewart & Crosbie, 2009).
		• Nachdem Maurices Tochter eine Pflegekraft eingestellt hatte, wies Dawn die neue Pflegekraft in körpergerechten Techniken ein, damit diese Maurice helfen und gleichzeitig seine Teilnahme an Aktivitäten unterstützen kann.
		• Dawn beobachtete, dass Maurice Schwierigkeiten beim Essen hatte, und führte ein Dysphagie-Assessment durch. Sie war auch besorgt, dass Maurice depressiv sein könnte und überwies ihn deshalb zu einem Rehabilitationspsychologen.
		• Dawn schlug vor, dass Maurices Tochter in Erwägung ziehen sollte, sich einer Selbsthilfegruppe für pflegende Angehörige anzuschließen.

Hintergrund	Ergotherapeutische Evaluation	Ergotherapeutische Intervention
	stürzen. Er zeigte auch Schwierigkeiten beim Koordinieren und Manipulieren von Objekten und bei grundlegenden Selbsthilfetätigkeiten. Häufig war er nicht in der Lage, die Arbeitsschritte einzuleiten oder sie bis zur Fertigstellung fortzusetzen. Maurice zeigte beim Zähneputzen und beim Anziehen des Oberkörpers Beeinträchtigungen.	

Hinweis. ADLs = Aktivitäten des alltäglichen Lebens; IADLs = instrumentelle Aktivitäten des alltäglichen Lebens; AMPS = Assessment of Motor and Process Skills; IPS = idiopathisches Parkinsonsyndrom

Tabelle 3-5: Fallstudie: Klientin mit amyotropher Lateralsklerose: Akutbehandlung

Hintergrund	Ergotherapeutische Evaluation	Ergotherapeutische Intervention
Susan ist eine 55-jährige Frau, bei der vor zwei Jahren ALS diagnostiziert wurde. Susan wurde in ein Akutkrankenhaus mit Lungenentzündung und Verschlechterung des Mobilitätsstatus aufgenommen. Die Ergotherapie erhielt einen Auftrag, eine Evaluation durchzuführen und den Interventionsfokus auf die Beratung und Unterweisung von Susan und ihrer Familie für adaptive Ansätze zur Durchführung der ADLs zu legen.	Susans Betätigungsprofil ergab folgende Ergebnisse: • Susan lebt in einem zweistöckigen Haus gemeinsam mit ihrem Ehemann in einer ländlichen Gemeinde. Sie hat einen Sohn, der auf dem College ist, und eine Tochter, die Senior in der High School ist. • Sie arbeitete bis letztes Jahr als Lehrerin in einer öffentlichen Grundschule. • Vor dieser Einweisung ins Krankenhaus war Susan bei den ADLs selbstständig, benötigte jedoch Hilfe beim Kochen, Einkaufen und im Haushalt. Zudem war sie wegen der Muskelschwäche und der Fatigue nicht mehr in der Lage, Auto zu fahren. Sie konnte mit einem Vierpunktegehstock gehen. ADL-Performanz: • Essen: eingerichtet • Pflege: minimale Unterstützung • Baden: maximale Unterstützung • Ankleiden Oberkörper: minimale Unterstützung • Ankleiden Unterkörper: maximale Unterstützung • Blasen-/Darmentleerung (Toileting): moderate Unterstützung • Bett, Stuhl, Rollstuhltransfer: maximale Unterstützung • Toilettentransfer: maximale Unterstützung • Transfer Badewanne, Dusche: maximale Unterstützung.	• Arjun, Susans Ergotherapeut, bot zusätzlich zu der Evaluation zwei Interventionen in der Akutversorgung an. • Arjun gab Empfehlungen für adaptive und medizinische Hilfsmittel, um die Unabhängigkeit und Sicherheit von Susan bei den ADLs zu erhöhen. Diese Hilfsmittel umfassen Haltegriffe in der Nähe der Toilette, einen Duschstuhl, einen erhöhten Toilettensitz und ein Rutschbrett (Gruis, Wren & Huggins, 2011). Außerdem schlug Arjun Susan vor, die Verwendung eines Bidets in Betracht zu ziehen. Dies könnte die Selbstständigkeit und den Erhalt der persönlichen Würde unterstützen. • Arjun bot Susans Ehemann eine Angehörigenberatung an. Dies beinhaltet eine Anleitung bei der Unterstützung von Susan beim Baden, Anziehen, Toiletten- und Wannentransfer. Zudem beinhaltet dies die Verwendung der oben genannten Hilfsmittel. • Arjun erstellte ein maßgeschneidertes Programm mit leichten Widerstandsübungen, um Susan bei der Aufrechterhaltung der Kraft und der funktionellen Selbstständigkeit bei den ADLs zu unterstützen. Zudem beinhaltet dieses Programm Bewegungsübungen zur Vermeidung von Kontrakturen (Aksu, Karaduman, Yakut & Tan, 2002; Dal Bello-Haas et al., 2007; Drory Goltsman, Reznik, Mosek & Korczyn, 2001). • Arjun verwies Susan zur klinikinternen Rollstuhlabteilung, um zu ermitteln, ob ein Elektrorollstuhl für Susan angemessen sei. Zudem gab er Informationen über ein Sanitätshaus, falls Susan und ihr Mann größere Modifikationen am Haus vornehmen möchten (zum Beispiel Treppenlift, ebenerdige Dusche; Trail, Nelson, Van, Appel & Lai, 2001; Ward et al., 2010).

Hinweis. ADLs = Aktivitäten des alltäglichen Lebens; ALS = amyotrophe Lateralsklerose

Tabelle 3-6: Fallstudie: Klient mit transverser Myelitis: stationäre Rehabilitationseinrichtung

Hintergrund	Ergotherapeutische Evaluation	Ergotherapeutische Intervention

Joe ist ein 22-jähriger Mann, der sich in der Notaufnahme mit einer plötzlichen Schwäche und einem Gefühlsverlust in beiden Beinen vorgestellt hat. Er wurde in eine Akutabteilung für Neurologie aufgenommen und unterzog sich einer umfangreichen Diagnostik. Er wurde mit TM diagnostiziert. Kurz nach seiner Diagnose wurde Joe in eine stationäre Rehabilitationsklinik zur umfassenden multidisziplinären Rehabilitation verlegt.	Joes Betätigungsprofil ergab folgende Ergebnisse:
	• Joe lebt gemeinsam mit seinen Eltern in einem Reihenhaus in einer großen Stadt. Seine Schwester und ihre Familie leben im gleichen Block. Sie sind eine enge, unterstützende Familie. Zu Hause ist Joe dafür verantwortlich, seine eigene Wäsche zu waschen und den Müll rauszubringen. Er macht sein eigenes Frühstück und Mittagessen und isst mit seiner Familie zu Abend.
	• Er hat kürzlich einen Bachelor-Abschluss in Betriebswirtschaft absolviert und sucht derzeit einen Job.
	• Joe hat seit zwei Jahren eine Freundin, der er in den nächsten Monaten einen Heiratsantrag machen wollte. Er und seine Freundin genießen es, neue Restaurants auszuprobieren und ins Kino zu gehen.
	• Vor dem neuen Auftreten von TM war Joe in allen ADLs und IADLs vollständig unabhängig. Er ist ein begeisterter Sportfan und genießt es besonders, Eishockey- und Basketballspiele zu schauen und zu besuchen.
	
	Funktionelle Mobilität:
	• Essen: unabhängig
	• Körperpflege: aufbauend
	• Baden: moderate Hilfe
	• Ankleiden Oberkörper: eingerichtet
	• Ankleiden Unterkörper: maximale Unterstützung
	• Kontinenz: moderate Hilfe
	• Bett, Stuhl, Rollstuhltransfer: maximale Unterstützung
	• Toilettentransfer: maximale Unterstützung
	• Transfer Badewanne, Dusche: totale Unterstützung
	
	IADLS: Derzeit abhängig in allen IADLs
	Kraft, Bewegungsausmaß und Koordination: Joes obere Extremitäten zeigten beidseitig Beeinträchtigungen mit funktionellen Grenzen in der Kraft, Bewegungsausmaß und Koordination. Seine Beinstärke reicht von 2/5 bis 3/5. Er ist aufgrund der Schwäche in den unteren Extremitäten nicht in der Lage, Gewicht zu übernehmen, wenn er versucht zu stehen.
		Amy, Joes Ergotherapeutin, arbeitete mit Joe 90 Minuten täglich, um Joe zu helfen, seine Unabhängigkeit, Sicherheit und Zufriedenheit mit ADLs, IADLs und der Teilhabe an der Gemeinschaft zu maximieren:
		• Amy führte jeden Morgen ADL-Sitzungen mit Joe in der Reha-Abteilung durch. Diese Sitzungen beinhalteten Schulungen zum Einsatz adaptiver Hilfsmittel und modifizierte Ansätze für solche ADLs:
		  – Verwendung eines Rutschbretts für den Transfer von Bett zu Rollstuhl
		  – Durchführung des Ankleidens des Unterkörpers im Bett im Langsitz
		  – Badewannentransfer und Baden mithilfe einer Badewannentransferbank, eines Rutschbretts und einem Duschschwamm mit Stiel
		  – WC-Transfers mit einem erhöhten WC-Sitz und Haltegriffen.
		• Amy wies Joe in Strategien ein, wie er die Wäsche und die Essenszubereitung vom Rollstuhl aus durchführen kann.
		• Joe und Amy planten einen Gemeinschaftsausflug zu einem Restaurant in der Nähe des Krankenhauses. Joe benutzte das Internet, um ein nahe gelegenes Restaurant zu finden. Er rief dort an, um die Rollstuhlzugänglichkeit zu erfragen. Ein anderer Klient aus der Reha-Abteilung begleitete Joe und Amy auf dem Ausflug. Danach diskutierten Joe und Amy die Herausforderungen und Erfolge des Ausflugs. Mit Amys Anleitung nutzte Joe seine neuen Fähigkeiten, um nach seiner Entlassung aus dem Krankenhaus zwei Wochen später mit seiner Freundin einen Date-Abend (Abendessen und einen Film) zu planen.
		• Amy und der Physiotherapeut, der ebenfalls mit Joe arbeitet, führten vor Joes Entlassung eine Hausuntersuchung durch. Sie gaben Empfehlungen für eine Rampe im hinteren Teil des Hauses und Änderungen vor allem im Bad und in der Küche, um diese Räume für ihn als Rollstuhlfahrer zugänglich zu machen.
		• Amy schlug Joe eine weiterführende ambulante Ergotherapie vor, um seinen Fortschritt in der Selbstständigkeit, Sicherheit und Zufriedenheit mit ADLs, IADLs und der Teilhabe an der Gemeinschaft weiter zu verbessern.

Hinweis. ADLs = Aktivitäten des alltäglichen Lebens; IADLs = instrumentelle Aktivitäten des alltäglichen Lebens; TM = transverse Myelitis

und Prioritäten setzen, sodass Evaluierungen und Interventionen zu den Klientenzielen passen. Manchmal kann es nötig sein, Klienten an weitere Berufsgruppen des Gesundheitswesens oder Quellen zu verweisen, um ihnen zu helfen, erfolgreiche Ergebnisse zu erzielen.

3.5.2 Analyse der Betätigungsperformanz

Die Ergotherapeuten nutzen die Informationen aus dem Betätigungsprofil, um spezifische Betätigungsbereiche sowie den Kontext und die Umwelt zu identifizieren, in der die Klienten leben und aktiv sein werden. *Betätigungsperformanz* bezeichnet die Bewältigung ausgewählter Betätigungen, die sich aus der dynamischen Interaktion zwischen Klient, Kontext und Umwelt und der Aktivität oder Betätigung ergibt (AOTA, 2014; S. S14).

Bei der Analyse der Betätigungsperformanz führen Ergotherapeuten normalerweise die folgenden Schritte aus:

- Die Klientin während der Ausführung einer Betätigung in der möglichst normalen und am wenigsten einschränkenden Umwelt (wenn möglich) beobachten und die Effektivität der Performanzfertigkeiten (zum Beispiel motorische, prozesshafte und soziale Interaktionsfertigkeiten) und die Performanzmuster (zum Beispiel Gewohnheiten, Routinen, Rituale, Rollen) dokumentieren.
- Spezifische Assessments und Evaluierungsmethoden (siehe **Tabelle 3-1**) auswählen, um die Faktoren zu ermitteln und zu messen, die mit den verschiedenen Gegenstandsbereichen zusammenhängen und die Performanz der Klienten beeinflussen können. Diese Assessments können sich auf Körperfunktionen und -stukturen, Aktivitäten oder Partizipation richten.
- Die Daten der Assessments analysieren, um zu ermitteln, was die Performanz unterstützt oder beeinträchtigt.
- Eine Hypothese bezüglich der Performanz eines Klienten entwickeln oder verfeinern (zum Beispiel die zugrunde liegenden Schädigungen oder Beeinträchtigungen der Performanzfertigkeiten ermitteln, die die Betätigungsperformanz in verschiedenen Bereichen beeinflussen könnten, zum Beispiel Gleichgewichtsprobleme, die sich auf die Körperpflege am Morgen, Haushaltsaktivitäten, die außerhäusliche Mobilität und die soziale Interaktion auswirken können).

- In Zusammenarbeit mit Klienten und Angehörigen Ziele entwickeln, die auf gewünschte Ergebnisse der Klienten zielen.
- Mögliche, durch Best Practice und die vorhandene Evidenz hergeleitete Interventionsansätze ermitteln und diese mit Klienten und allen Angehörigen und Betreuern besprechen, die einbezogen werden.
- Den Evaluierungsprozess dokumentieren und die entsprechenden Teammitglieder und Dienstleistungsanbieter informieren.

3.5.3 Betätigungsbereiche

Klienten mit NDK erleben Probleme der Betätigungsperformanz in einer oder mehreren Betätigungsbereichen. Die Symptome der NDK können jeden der acht Betätigungsbereiche betreffen. Die durch Klienten mit NDK erlebten Probleme in der Betätigungsperformanz können sich aufgrund der spezifischen Krankheit unterscheiden. **Tabelle 3-1** fasst Betätigungen zusammen, an denen sich die Klienten beteiligen, und bietet Beispiele spezifischer Assessments, die genutzt werden können, wenn Betätigungen von Klienten mit NDK evaluiert werden.

Ergotherapeuten können einen Evaluierungsansatz wählen, der mit der Analyse der Rollen des Klienten mit NDK beginnt und den Betätigungen, die einen für sie typischen Tag definieren (wird auch als *Top-Down-Evaluierung* bezeichnet). Sie können aber auch einen Evaluierungsansatz verwenden, der sich auf mögliche Schädigungen richtet, die die Performanz und die Aufgaben beeinflussen (wird auch als *Bottom-Up-Evaluierung* bezeichnet). Im Top-Down-Ansatz wird eine weiterführende Analyse der zugrunde liegenden Beeinträchtigungen von Aktivität und Partizipation nur durchgeführt, wenn sich Schwierigkeiten bei der Betätigungsperformanz zeigen. Im Bottom-Up-Ansatz richtet sich die Ergotherapeutin auf die Beeinträchtigungen und allgemeinen Fähigkeiten der Klienten und zieht Schlussfolgerungen, wie diese die Performanz in heutigen und künftigen Betätigungen beeinflussen könnten.

Die Wahl des Evaluierungsansatzes ist teilweise durch die Fähigkeit der Klienten beeinflusst, sich aktiv am Evaluierungsprozess zu beteiligen. Während dieses Prozesses können Ergotherapeuten abhängig von der Erholungsphase und den gewünschten Ergebnissen zwischen dem Top-Down- und dem Bottom-Up-Ansatz wechseln.

3.5.4 Performanzfertigkeiten

Die Evaluierung von Klienten mit NDK schließt offensichtliche und subtile Faktoren ein, die ihre Performanz beeinflussen könnten. Performanzfertigkeiten sind zielgerichtete Aktionen, die als kleine Elemente der Beteiligung an Alltagsbetätigungen beobachtbar sind. Sie sind über einen Zeitraum hinweg erlernt und entwickelt und sind verbunden mit bestimmten Kontexten und Umgebungen (Fisher & Griswold, 2014). Performanzfertigkeiten können in motorische, prozesshafte und soziale Interaktionsfertigkeiten unterteilt werden.

Klienten mit NDK können mit Beeinträchtigungen in mehreren Performanzbereichen konfrontiert sein. Zum Beispiel können Beeinträchtigungen in den motorischen Fertigkeiten das Gleichgewicht während des Duschens erschweren. Arbeitet ein Klient beispielsweise als Mechaniker, können Schwierigkeiten auftreten, die Körperteile zu koordinieren. Zeigen sich bei Klienten Probleme mit den prozesshaften Fertigkeiten, ist die Visualisierung von Gegenständen beeinträchtigt, was sich beispielsweise beim Sortieren der Wäsche zeigt oder bei (un)koordinierten Bewegungen beim Einsteigen in einen Bus. Viele Klienten mit NDK erleben kognitive Veränderungen. Sie können sich auf Aufgaben des täglichen beruflichen Lebens auswirken, wie eine Reihenfolge der Planungsschritte eines Langzeitprojekts festlegen. NDK kann auch Herausforderungen bei den sozialen Interaktionsfertigkeiten verursachen und sie können den emotionalen Ausdruck oder die Frustrationstoleranz beeinflussen. Auch soziale Interaktionsfertigkeiten sind möglicherweise betroffen; zum Beispiel der Wechsel in der Konversation zwischen verschiedenen Partnern auf einem sozialen Event.

3.5.5 Performanzmuster

Performanzmuster sind Gewohnheiten, Routinen, Rollen und Rituale, die im Prozess der Beteiligung an Betätigungen oder Aktivitäten benutzt werden. Diese Muster können die Betätigungsperformanz entweder unterstützen oder behindern (AOTA, 2014). Klienten mit NDK verändern manchmal ihre Performanzmuster als Folge ihrer Krankheitssymptome. Zum Beispiel kann es für einen Klienten mit MS mit Fatigue nötig sein, zusätzliche Pausen in die tägliche Routine einzubauen, um sich von stark erschöpfenden Aktivitäten wie Einkaufen oder Gartenarbeit zu erholen. Ergotherapeuten können Empfehlungen zur Organisation der Gewohnheiten und Routinen der Klienten geben, um den Einfluss von Fatigue und anderen Symptomen zu minimieren.

3.5.6 Klientenfaktoren

Klientenfaktoren sind die zugrunde liegenden Fähigkeiten, Werte, Überzeugungen und Spiritualität sowie Körperfunktionen und -strukturen, die sich auf die individuelle Betätigungsperformanz auswirken. Diese Klientenfaktoren werden durch die An- oder Abwesenheit von Krankheit, Deprivation und Beeinträchtigung beeinflusst (AOTA, 2014). Werte, Überzeugungen und Spiritualität beeinflussen die Motivation der Klienten, sich an Betätigungen zu beteiligen, und geben ihrem Leben Bedeutung. Körperfunktionen verweisen auf die physiologischen Funktionen des Körpers (einschließlich der psychologischen Funktionen; World Health Organization [WHO], 2001). Klienten mit NDK können zum Beispiel Veränderungen in sensorischen, mentalen oder atembezogenen Körperfunktionen erfahren. Körperstrukturen sind die anatomischen Teile des Körpers wie Organe, Gliedmaßen und ihre Teile (WHO, 2001). Körperstrukturen und -funktionen stehen in Beziehung zueinander.

3.5.7 Kontext und Umwelt

Ergotherapeuten anerkennen den Einfluss kultureller, klientenbezogener, zeitlicher, virtueller, physischer und sozialer Kontextfaktoren auf Betätigungen und Aktivitäten. Umweltfaktoren (physische und soziale), die die Betätigungsperformanz von Klienten mit NDK unterstützen oder beeinträchtigen, sollten während der Evaluierungs- und Interventionsprozesse festgestellt werden. Kontextfaktoren (kulturelle, klientenbezogene, zeitliche und virtuelle) verweisen auf die Vielfalt zusammenhängender Bedingungen in und um die Klienten (AOTA, 2014). Ergotherapeuten nutzen bei der Evaluierung des Kontextes und der Umwelt von Klienten mit NDK sowohl informelle als auch formelle Evaluierungsprozesse.

Kulturell

Der kulturelle Kontext umfasst die Gewohnheiten, Überzeugungen, Aktivitätsmuster, Verhaltensstandards und Erwartungen der Gesellschaft der Klienten. Manche dieser Performanzmuster (zum Beispiel Händeschütteln zur Begrüßung oder Augenkontakt beim Gespräch) können für Klienten mit NDK schwierig sein. Ergotherapeuten zeigen Bewusstheit und Gefühl für die kulturellen Überzeugungen einer

Klientin. Sie verantworten eine Betreuung, die auf die typischen Aktivitätsmuster und Betätigungen aufgrund der kulturellen Überzeugungen der Klienten ausgerichtet ist, welche die Gesundheit und Betätigungen beeinflussen. Ergotherapeuten schließen die Werte der Klienten, ihre Überzeugungen und Angewohnheiten und ihre Art zu leben in einen Interventionsplan ein, der dann von beiden Seiten akzeptiert ist.

Klientenbezogen

Klientenbezogene Merkmale wie Gender, sozioökonomischer Status, Alter und Ausbildungsniveau fließen in die Evaluierungs- und Interventionsprozesse ein. Muster der Rollenperformanz, die auf kulturellen und persönlichen Erwartungen aufbauen, sowie Vorlieben der Klienten sollten während der Evaluierung und Intervention berücksichtigt werden. Diese Merkmale können sich auch auf den Zugang zu Ressourcen und Angeboten, einschließlich der Ergotherapie, auswirken. Deshalb muss die Ergotherapeutin diese Merkmale berücksichtigen. Zum Beispiel empfehlen Ergotherapeuten Klienten mit NDK üblicherweise angepasste Ausrüstung, Hilfsmittel, widerstandsfähige medizinische Geräte oder umfangreiche Wohnraumanpassungen. Aber oft werden die Kosten dieser Maßnahmen nicht durch Dritte abgedeckt und die Klienten müssten diese selbst bezahlen, was sie sich möglicherweise nicht leisten können. Es ist wichtig, potenzielle Barrieren bezogen auf den Zugang zu Angeboten und empfohlenen Hilfsmitteln zu verstehen, Alternativen anzubieten oder sich für die Klienten einzusetzen, sodass diese die benötigten Angebote und Geräte erhalten.

Zeitlich

Im größeren Rahmen verweist der zeitliche Kontext auf die Lebenszeit des Menschen. Er schließt Lebensphasen, Tages- oder Jahreszeit, Dauer, Aktivitätenrhythmus und Biografie ein. Ein wichtiger zeitlicher Aspekt für Menschen mit NDK ist das Procedere ihrer Krankheit. Da NDK normalerweise fortschreitende Beeinträchtigungen am Nervensystem verursachen, erleben diese Klienten im Verlauf der Zeit unterschiedliche Niveaus und Rhythmen der Beeinträchtigungen. Darum müssen Menschen mit NDK lernen, mit ihrer wechselnden Beeinträchtigung umzugehen und diese zu managen. Ihr Bedarf an Ergotherapie und anderen rehabilitativen Angeboten kann sich deshalb im Laufe ihres Lebens verändern. Des Weiteren müssen spezielle Überlegungen für alternde Menschen mit NDK angestellt werden. Auch wenn die Erstdiagnose in jungen Jahren erfolgte, kommen mit zunehmendem Alter andere Herausforderungen hinzu, verursacht zum Beispiel von Arthritis oder Diabetes, die das Management der Erkrankung beeinflussen. Zusätzlich kann die Fähigkeit einer Klientin mit NDK, eine solche zusätzliche Herausforderung zu bewältigen, im Laufe der Zeit abnehmen.

Ein anderes zeitbezogenes Thema für Ergotherapeuten während des Evaluierungs- und Interventionsprozessess ist das Alter bei Ausbruch der Krankheit. Manche NDK treten mit größerer Wahrscheinlichkeit in gewissen Lebensphasen auf. Zum Beispiel wird IPS oft im höheren Klientenalter diagnostiziert, wenn Individuen bereits pensioniert sind und sich an Betätigungen wie Teilzeitarbeit, Freizeitaktivitäten oder Zeit mit den Enkeln beteiligen. Im Gegensatz dazu wird MS und TM oft im frühen Klientenalter diagnostiziert, wenn sich viele Individuen auf Lebensaufgaben wie Karriere, Aus- und Weiterbildung oder Familiengründung ausrichten.

Physisch

Die physische Umwelt schließt natürliche (zum Beispiel geografisches Gebiet, Pflanzen) und erbaute (zum Beispiel Gebäude, Möbel) Umgebungen ein, in denen Alltagsbetätigungen stattfinden (AOTA, 2014). Ergotherapeuten evaluieren die materielle Umwelt auf Förderfaktoren und Barrieren, die sich auf die Betätigungsperformanz der Klienten auswirken könnten. Evaluierung der physischen Umwelt zu Hause, auf der Arbeit und an viel genutzten öffentlichen Orten ist ein wichtiger Teil, um die Beteiligung an Betätigungsperformanz zu unterstützen. Da MS, IPS, ALS und TM das Potenzial haben, Körperfunktionen zu beeinträchtigen (zum Beispiel mentale, sensorische, bewegungsbezogene) ist das Assessment der physischen Umwelt eine unerlässliche Komponente der Evaluierung von Klienten mit NDK. Aspekte der physischen Umwelt, die evaluiert werden müssen, können die Anordnung und Organisation fester Strukturen und beweglicher Objekte, Beleuchtung und visueller Kontrast, Temperatur (im Speziellen für Menschen mit MS) und Lärm sein.

Sozial

Die soziale Umwelt umfasst das individuelle Netzwerk von Freunden, Familie, sozialen Gruppen und bestimmten Bevölkerungsgruppen, mit denen die Klienten Kontakt haben. Klienten mit NDK können Beeinträchtigungen in funktioneller Mobilität, Mobilität im öffentlichen Raum (zum Beispiel Auto fahren, öffentlichen Verkehr benutzen) oder in der körperlichen Ausdauer erfahren, was die soziale Partizipation beeinträchtigen kann. Zudem können Klienten mit NDK in der sozialen Umwelt aufgrund der kognitiven Anforderungen in solchen Situationen oder wegen Problemen in der verbalen und nonverbalen Kommunikation bei den Gepflogenheiten oder Regeln sozialer Interaktion oder bei Fragen des Selbstbildes (bezogen auf ihre Beeinträchtigungen) gefordert sein.

Virtuell
Die virtuelle Umwelt ist die, in der Kommunikation durch den Äther oder über Computer stattfindet ohne körperlichen Kontakt. Ergotherapeuten müssen die vorherige Erfahrung der Klienten im Gebrauch von Technologien zur Interaktion in der virtuellen Umwelt ermitteln (zum Beispiel E-Mail und SMS schreiben und versenden, sich in Chatrooms und auf Diskussionsforen beteiligen). Die Vertrautheit der Klienten mit Technologien der virtuellen Umwelt können die Ergotherapeuten durch die Auswahl geeigneter Medien zur Unterstützung der sozialen Partizipation (zum Beispiel mit Familie oder Freunden kommunizieren über E-Mail, SMS, soziale Netzwerke), der Arbeit (zum Beispiel an einer Sitzung über virtuelle persönliche Kommunikation teilnehmen), von Bildungsaktivitäten (zum Beispiel einen Onlinekurs besuchen), von IADLs (zum Beispiel Onlinebanking oder Einkaufen) und der Freizeit (zum Beispiel E-Books lesen, Onlinespiele) lenken.

3.5.8 Überlegungen zu Assessments

Ergotherapeuten vertrauen auf ihr Wissen über Assessments und ihr klinisches Beurteilungsvermögen, wenn sie entscheiden, welche standardisierten oder nichtstandardisierten Assessments sie bei einem bestimmten Individuum in einem bestimmten Moment einsetzen. Zusätzlich ist es notwendig, dass sie mit aktuell publizierten Forschungsergebnissen über relevante Assessments zur jeweiligen Klientengruppe vertraut sind sowie die aktuelle Literatur über spezifische Assessments kennen, die sie für ihre Arbeit ausgewählt haben. Die Ergotherapeutin verwendet die Informationen aus den Assessments, um die Faktoren zu ermitteln, welche die Betätigungsperformanz und soziale Partizipation unterstützen und einschränken. Diese Informationen werden anschließend benutzt, um über Interventionen zu entscheiden.

Bei der Evaluierung von Klienten mit NDK müssen spezielle Überlegungen angestellt werden. Falls angebracht, werden Anpassungen während der Dokumentation des Assessments durchgeführt, sodass Beeinträchtigungen von Körperfunktionen (zum Beispiel mentale, sensorische, neuromuskoloskelettale, bewegungsbezogene, stimmliche und sprachliche) nicht unnötig die Ergebnisse des Assessments stören. Als Beispiel: Wenn eine Ergotherapeutin bei einer Klientin mit ALS mit Stimm- oder Sprechproblemen ein Assessment durchführt, kann sie das Assessment so anpassen, dass die Klientin nonverbal antworten kann (mitschreiben, unterstützte Kommunikation). Auf eine ähnliche Art kann ein Klient mit IPS mit Schreibschwierigkeiten trotzdem an einem Assessment teilnehmen, wenn er mündlich antworten kann.

Ergotherapeuten passen die Assessments im Prozess nur an, wenn sie sich zuvor im Handbuch des Assessments informiert haben, ob eine solche Anpassung erlaubt ist und die Integrität der Resultate dadurch nicht beeinflusst wird. Zusätzlich können Ergotherapeuten den Zeitpunkt der Medikationseinnahme (zum Beispiel bei Schmerz oder Fatigue) bedenken und die Assessments demzufolge einplanen.

Zeitliche und umweltbezogene Überlegungen spielen ebenfalls bei den Assessments mit Klienten mit NDK eine Rolle. Der Tageszeitpunkt kann die Ergebnisse beeinflussen, im Besonderen bei den Klienten, deren NDK-Symptome auch körperliche oder kognitive Fatigue beinhalten. So können auch erweiterte Assessments die Assessmentresultate negativ beeinflussen. Es kann unterstützen, Pausen während der Assessments einzubauen, oder dieses aufzuteilen im Tagesverlauf oder über mehrere Tage. Zu guter Letzt sollte die Umwelt, in der Assessments durchgeführt werden, bedacht werden. Im Speziellen sind gute Beleuchtung und Kontraste, minimale Ablenkungen und Unordnung sowie eine angenehme Raumtemperatur zuträglich.

3.6 Intervention

Ergotherapeutische Interventionen bei Klienten mit NDK können im gesamten Verlauf der Krankheit eingesetzt werden. Der Bedarf an Ergotherapie und der Fokus des Angebots verändern sich aufgrund der degenerativen Verläufe von NDK. Eine ergotherapeutische Intervention wird durch die Informationen über die Klienten gelenkt, die während der Evaluierung erhoben wurden, sowie durch das Wissen der Therapeutin über Theorien, Modelle, Bezugsrahmen und Evidenzen (AOTA, 2014). Eine Intervention besteht aus einem dreischrittigen Prozess:
(1) Interventionsplan
(2) Implementierung der Intervention und
(3) Überprüfung der Intervention.

Im Folgenden ist jeder Schritt beschrieben und es wird eine Übersicht über evidenzbasierte Interventionen bei Klienten mit NDK zur Verfügung gestellt.

3.6.1 Interventionsplan

Als einen Teil des ergotherapeutischen Prozesses entwickeln Ergotherapeuten einen Interventionsplan, der folgende Aspekte der Klienten berücksichtigt:
- deren Ziele, Werte, Überzeugungen, Betätigungsbedürfnisse, Gesundheit, Wohlbefinden
- Performanzfertigkeiten und -muster
- den Einfluss des Kontextes, der Umwelt, der Betätigungsanforderungen und der Klientenfaktoren auf die Performanz
- den Kontext der ergotherapeutischen Dienstleistung, in dem die Intervention angeboten wird, um die festgelegten Ergebnisse zu erreichen (zum Beispiel Erwartungen der Betreuer, organisatorische Zwecke, Anforderungen des Kostenträgers, relevante Verordnungen und die beste vorhandene Evidenz; AOTA, 2014).

Bei der Planung bestimmt die Ergotherapeutin objektive und messbare Ziele, wählt angemessene Interventionsansätze aus, bestimmt die Methoden (zum Beispiel Interventionsarten und Anbieter), berücksichtigt Entlassungsbedürfnisse und -pläne und empfiehlt oder verweist die Klienten, falls notwendig, an andere Berufsgruppen. Manche ergotherapeutischen Ansätze können zu gewissen Zeiten angemessener sein als andere. Ergotherapeutische Ansätze sind:
- *Prävention:* ein Ansatz, der für Klienten mit oder ohne Beeinträchtigungen entwickelt wurde, die ein Risiko auf Probleme der Betätigungsperformanz haben (Dunn, McClain, Brown & Youngstrom, 1998); zum Beispiel Sturzprävention.
- *Wiederherstellung von klientenbezogenen Faktoren:* ein Ansatz, der entwickelt wurde, um die Variablen der Klienten zu verändern, eine neue Fertigkeit oder Fähigkeit zu entwickeln oder eine, die beeinträchtigt ist, wiederherzustellen (Dunn et al., 1998); zum Beispiel Kräftigung einer Hand eingebettet in die Aktivität Brotbacken.
- *Anpassung der Umwelt, des Kontextes oder der Anforderung einer Aktivität,* um die sichere, unabhängige Ausführung wertvoller Aktivitäten trotz motorischer, kognitiver oder wahrnehmungsbedingter Beeinträchtigungen zu unterstützen; zum Beispiel den Wohnraum anpassen.
- *Förderung eines gesunden Lebensstils,* was zuverlässige Medikamentenroutinen, angemessene Ernährung und körperliche Betätigung sowie zufriedenstellende Beteiligung an sozialen Beziehungen und Aktivitäten einschließt, indem bereichernde und erweiternde Erfahrungen angeboten werden, die die Performanz aller Klienten im natürlichen Lebenskontext verbessern (Dunn et al., 1998); zum Beispiel ein Kurs in Krankheitsbewältigung und Selbstmanagement.
- *Erhalt von Performanz und Gesundheit,* um die Unterstützung zu bieten, die es Klienten erlaubt, ihre Performanzfähigkeiten zu erhalten, die sie wiedererlangt haben, oder Fähigkeiten aufrechtzuerhalten, die ihren Betätigungsbedürfnissen entsprechen, oder beides; zum Beispiel Kraftverlust verhindern durch die Teilnahme an einem Aquatraining.

3.6.2 Implementierung der Intervention

Hat eine Ergotherapeutin einen Interventionsplan erstellt, dann wendet sie ihn an (AOTA, 2014). Interventionstypen schließen Betätigungen und Aktivitäten, vorbereitende Methoden und Aufgaben, Edukation und Training, Fürsprache und Gruppeninterventionen ein. The *use of the therapeutic self* (der Einsatz der eigenen Persönlichkeit, Wahrnehmung und Beurteilung der Therapeutin; AOTA, 2014) ist ein übergreifendes Konzept, das während jeder therapeutischen Interaktion berücksichtigt werden sollte, einschließlich des Interventionsprozesses. Es unterstützt Ergotherapeuten, eine wirksame therapeutische Beziehung aufzubauen und zu unterhalten. The *use of the therapeutic self* ist eine lebenswichtige Verantwortlichkeit der Ergotherapeuten und von allen Mitgliedern des Interventionsteams.

3.6.3 Überprüfung der Intervention

Die Überprüfung der Intervention ist ein fortlaufender Prozess aus: Re-Evaluierung und Überprüfung des Interventionsplans, der Wirksamkeit des Angebotes, des Fortschritts hinsichtlich des angestrebten Ergebnisses und des Bedarfs an weiterführender Ergotherapie. Möglicherweise wird der Klient auch auf andere Angebote oder Gesundheitsberufe (AOTA, 2014) verwiesen. Re-Evaluierung kann Folgendes einschließen: Assessments der ersten Evaluierung erneut ausführen, eine Befragung zur Zufriedenheit der Klienten erheben oder Fragen stellen zur Evaluierung jedes Ziels. Zum Beispiel könnte eine Ergotherapeutin, die mit Klienten mit NDK arbeitet, das COPM nochmals durchführen (Law et al., 2005), um die

Wirksamkeit der Interventionen zu untersuchen, den Fortschritt hinsichtlich der Klientenziele zu dokumentieren und um zu bestimmen, ob die Fortsetzung oder der Abschluss von Ergotherapie angemessen ist. Re-Evaluieren untermauert normalerweise den Fortschritt in der Zielerreichung, zeigt Veränderungen im funktionellen Status an und lenkt mögliche Änderungen am Interventionsplan (Moyers & Dale, 2007).

3.7 Ergebnis und Ergebniskontrolle

Ergotherapeuten und ihre Assistenten dokumentieren die Ergebnisse in Abschlussevaluierungen oder -berichten (AOTA, 2013a). Diese Dokumentation sollte innerhalb des zeitlichen Rahmens und der formalen Vorgaben und Standards ausgeführt werden, die in diesem Praxissetting durch Regierungsbehörden, externe Akkreditierungsprogramme, Kostenträger und Dokumente des Berufsverbandes AOTA eingeführt sind (AOTA, 2010b). Der Fokus auf die Ergebnisse zieht sich durch den gesamten ergotherapeutischen Prozess (AOTA, 2014). Ergotherapeuten sollten ihre Klientendaten und Perspektiven zu umfassenden, teambasierten Assessments beitragen. Viele der Assessments, die im Evaluierungskapitel dieser Leitlinie aufgezählt sind (*Assessment of Motor and Process Skills*, *COPM*, *Model of Human Occupation Screening Tool*) können nochmals durchgeführt werden, um die Ergebnisse der Ergotherapie festzulegen und zu dokumentieren.

3.8 Abschluss, Entlassungsplanung und Nachsorge

Die Planung des Abschlusses beginnt während des Evaluierungsprozesses durch die Berücksichtigung der Bedürfnisse und Wünsche der Klienten und der Angehörigen. Der Abschluss der Intervention sollte erfolgen, wenn:
(1) die Klienten ihre Ziele erreicht haben
(2) ein Fortschrittsplateau erreicht wurde
(3) die Klienten nicht mehr am Rehabilitationsprozess teilnehmen können oder möchten oder
(4) Ergotherapie nicht mehr länger benötigt wird.

Überlegungen zum Abschluss bei Klienten mit NDK sollten auch die Überweisung an Gemeinschaftsangebote (zum Beispiel Selbsthilfegruppen), stetiges Follow-up durch andere Gesundheitsberufe (zum Beispiel Neurologen, Ärzte, Physiotherapeuten) und die Möglichkeit für weiterführende Ergotherapie einschließen, falls sich am Befinden oder den individuellen Berdürfnissen etwas ändert.

4 Best Practice und Zusammenfassung der Evidenz

Die folgenden Abschnitte beinhalten eine Übersicht über spezielle Interventionen sowie Ergebnisse systematischer Reviews der ergotherapeutischen Interventionen von Klienten mit NDK. Ein Standardverfahren zur Suche nach und Durchsicht von Literatur über die Arbeit mit Klienten NDK fand Anwendung und wurde im **Anhang C** zusammengefasst. Die hier präsentierten Forschungsstudien beinhalten vor allem Level-I randomisierte kontrollierte Untersuchungen (RCTs); Level-II-Studien ohne randomisierte Zuordnungen zu einer Intervention oder Kontrollgruppe (Kohortenstudie) und Level-III-Studien ohne Kontrollgruppen. Sofern es allerdings an höher gelevelten Evidenzen mangelte und die beste Evidenz für Ergotherapie in speziellen Fällen mit einem Level von IV und V bewertet wurden, wurden auch solche Studien eingeschlossen. Unter Level-IV-Studien werden experimentelle Einzel-Fallstudien verstanden und Level-V Evidenzen umfassen beschreibende Fallberichte. Alle im Review erfassten Studien, einschließlich derer, welche in diesem Abschnitt nicht beschrieben werden, sind zusammengefasst in den Evidenztabellen im **Anhang D**. Für weiterführende Informationen sind Leser dazu angehalten, die vollständigen Artikel zu lesen. Die Summe der Ergebnisse der Evidenz sind das Ergebnis von drei Fragen bezüglich der Interventionen von Klienten mit MS, IPS und ALS. Obwohl diese Praxisleitlinie einen Überblick über den Prozess der ergotherapeutischen Intervention, Hintergrundinformationen darüber und Fallstudien für Klienten mit vier NDK (MS, IPS, ALS und TM) umfasst, ergab die literarische Suche, welche für einen systematischen Review über TM durchgeführt wurde, im Rahmen von ergotherapeutischer Praxis keine Ergebnisse (siehe **Tabelle 3-6** für eine Fallstudie einer Intervention eines Klienten mit TM.) Daher wurden nur die Ergebnisse betreffend der drei Fragen zur Intervention von Klienten mit NDK in den Praxisleitlinien zusammengefasst.

Fragestellungen
Folgende Fragen wurden bearbeitet:
- Was macht die Wirksamkeit der Interventionen im Rahmen ergotherapeutischer Interventionen bei MS aus?
- Was macht die Wirksamkeit der Interventionen im Rahmen ergotherapeutischer Interventionen bei IPS aus?
- Was macht die Wirksamkeit der Interventionen im Rahmen ergotherapeutischer Interventionen bei ALS aus?

4.1 Interventionen für Klienten mit MS

Insgesamt wurden 70 Studien in den systematischen Review einbezogen, mit dem Ziel, die Wirksamkeit der Interventionen im Rahmen ergotherapeutischer Interventionen bei MS zu ermitteln. Alle Studien sind in den Evidenztabellen (**Anhang D**) gelistet.

Die Artikel sind in zwei übergeordnete Kategorien unterteilt:
(1) Interventionen mit dem Fokus auf Aktivitäten und Partizipation und
(2) Interventionen mit dem Fokus auf klientenbezogene Kontextfaktoren und Performanzfertigkeiten.

Die folgenden Abschnitte sind in diese übergeordneten Kategorien und schließlich in spezifische Interventionstypen aufgeteilt. Jede Unterkategorie beinhaltet eine Beschreibung der Interventionen, gefolgt von einem Überblick über die Evidenz für diese Intervention.

4.1.1 Interventionen mit Fokus auf Aktivität und Partizipation

Von 70 Studien des systematischen Reviews untersuchten 28 die Wirksamkeit der Interventionen auf der Aktivitäts- oder Partizipationsebene.

Fatigue-Management

Eine der vorrangigen Aufgaben von Ergotherapeuten im MS-Behandlerteam ist es, Fatigue-Management-Schulungen (Radomski & Latham, 2008) anzubieten. Das Ziel von Fatigue-Management ist es, „MS-Klienten zu befähigen, ihre begrenzte Energie für bedeutungsvolle Aktivitäten ihrer Wahl zu nutzen, sodass sie diese in einer anderen Weise durchführen und organisieren können" (Multiple Sclerosis Council for Clinical Practice Guidelines, 1998). Fatigue-Management-Schulung beinhaltet das Erlernen von Energieeffizienzstrategien. Sie sind definiert als: „identifizieren und entwickeln von Modifikationen der Aktivität durch eine systematische Analyse von täglicher Arbeit, des Kontextes zu Hause und von Freizeitaktivitäten, um Fatigue zu reduzieren" (Multiple Sclerosis Council for Clinical Practice Guidelines, 1998). Energie-Effizienz-Strategien basieren auf einer von zwei Energie-Management-Prinzipien: *banking* oder *budgeting* (Packer, Brink & Sauriol, 1995). *Banking* verweist darauf, tägliche Aktivitäten in einer energieeffizienten Weise durchzuführen, um Energie für andere wichtige Aktivitäten zu erhalten. Ein erstes Beispiel: Ein Klient mit MS könnte sich dafür entscheiden, während des Kochens oder Duschens zu sitzen, sodass diese tägliche Aktivität nicht allzuviel Energie erfordert. *Budgeting* verweist darauf, seine Energie klug einzuteilen. In der Energie-Management-Schulung wird Energie als knappes Gut betrachtet. Daher ist es wichtig, dass Energie in einer überlegten und behutsamen Weise aufgewendet wird. Das ermöglicht es Klienten mit Fatigue, Energie für die ihnen wichtigeren und bedeutungsvolleren Aktivitäten frei zu haben. Ein zweites Beispiel: Ein Klient mit MS entscheidet sich dafür, den Rasen nur jedes zweite Wochenende zu mähen anstatt wöchentlich, um Energie zu haben, sich an den freien Wochenenden mit Freunden zum Abendessen oder ins Kino zu verabreden. Obwohl Ergotherapeuten die Fatigue-Management-Schulungen in der Einzeltherapie oder im Gruppensetting anbieten, hat sich die Fatigue-Manegemant-Forschung auf Gruppeninterventionen fokussiert. Es gibt eine hohe Evidenz von hoch qualitativen Studien, die die Effektivität von Face-to-Face-Gruppen in Fatigue-Management-Programmen unterstützen (Yu & Mathiowetz, 2014a). Zwei verschiedene Face-to-Face-Programme wurden untersucht: *Umgang mit Fatigue: Ein Sechs-Wochen-Kurs zum Erhalt von Energie* (Packer et al., 1995), welches in der originalen englischen Version wie auch der deutschen Version getestet wurde, sowie *Fatigue: Kontrolle übernehmen* (Hugos et al., 2010).

Für beide Programme gibt es ein Handbuch über sechs Wochen gruppenbasierter Fatigue-Management-Kurse, welche Unterrichtseinheiten, Gruppendiskussionen und Hausaufgaben enthalten. Sie umfassen Inhalte wie:
- Hintergrundinformationen über Fatigue
- Umweltanpassung und Aktivitäten zum Umgang mit Fatigue
- Identifizieren von Prioritäten und Setzen von Zielen.

Face-to-Face-Gruppen in Fatigue-Management-Programmen reduzieren nachweislich die Auswirkungen von Fatigue, verbessern die Lebensqualität sowie die Selbstwirksamkeit in der Nutzung von Fatigue-Management-Strategien (Blikman et al., 2013 [Level-I]; Hugos et al., 2010 [Level-II]; Kos, Duportail, D'hooghe, Nagel & Kerckhofs, 2007 [Level-I]; Mathiowetz, Finlayson, Matuska, Chen & Luo 2005 [Level-I]; Sauter, Zebenholzer, Hisakawa, Zeitlhofer & Vass, 2008 [Level-II]). Die Effekte des Fatigue-Management-Programms bleiben ein Jahr nach der Anwendung erhalten (Mathiowetz, Matuska, Finlayson, Luo, & Chen, 2007 [Level-I]). Es gibt jedoch widersprüchliche Beweise darüber, ob diese Programme die Schwere der Fatigue mildern (siehe **Tabelle 3-2** für eine Fallstudie). Die Ergebnisse, die in allen Untersuchungen von länger andauernden Fatigue-Management-Programmen ermittelt wurden, sind eine geänderte Version des *Packer's Managing Fatigue Program*. Die getesteten Programme dieser Studie wurden entweder online (Ghahari, Packer & Passmore, 2010 [Level-I]) oder per Telefonkonferenz geliefert (Finlayson, 2005 [Level-III]; Finlayson, Preissner, Cho & Plow, 2011 [Level-I]; Holberg & Finlayson, 2007). Trotz einer Studie (Ghahari et al., 2010) über nicht signifikante Unterschiede zwischen den Onlineprogrammen, einem Informationsprogramm und einem Kontrollprogramm, gibt es eine starke Unterstützung für Fatigue-Management-Programme über eine Telefonkonferenz. Diese sind nachweislich effektiver und wirksamer als das Kontrollprogramm: Der Einfluss der Fatigue auf das tägliche Leben konnte reduziert werden, Vorher-Nachher-Vergleiche mit den Mischproben wiesen die

Effektivität und Wirksamkeit nach, den Einfluss und die Schwere der Fatigue zu reduzieren und einige Aspekte der Lebensqualität zu verbessern (Finlayson et al., 2011 [Level-I]).

Gesundheitsförderung

Gesundheitsförderung ist von der WHO (1986) definiert als ein Prozess, Menschen zu befähigen, ihre Gesundheit stärker selbst zu steuern und zu verbessern. Um einen Zustand kompletten körperlichen, mentalen und sozialen Wohlbefindens zu erreichen, muss eine Person oder eine Gruppe fähig sein, das eigene Streben zu erkennen und zu erfassen, Bedürfnisse zu befriedigen und die Umwelt zu verändern oder mit ihr zurechtzukommen. Gesundheit ist ein Zustand des vollständigen physischen, geistig-seelischen und sozialen Wohlbefindens und nicht nur das Freisein von Krankheit und Gebrechen. Das Konzept der Gesundheitsförderung zeigt sich als passend zur Domäne und den Überzeugungen der Ergotherapie (AOTA, 2013b). Ergotherapeuten sind aufgrund ihres Fokus auf „die Gesundheitseffekte aus zielgerichteten, produktiven und bedeutungsvollen Betätigungen" für die Gesundheitsförderung gut geeignet. Wenn Ergotherapeuten bei der Gesundheitsförderung involviert sind, können sie zum Beispiel Schulungen für Klienten über ihre Rollenperformanz anbieten, Klienten unterstützen, Fähigkeiten zu entwickeln, um ihre täglichen Betätigungen durchzuführen, Selbstmanagement-Schulungen zur Prävention und Gesunderhaltung sowie zur Modifikation der Umwelt anbieten, um eine Betätigungsperformanz zu fördern. Zum jetzigen Zeitpunkt sind die Studien, die die Effektivität von Ergotherapie in der Gesundheitsförderung bei Menschen mit MS unterstützen, nur limitiert vorhanden, aber von hoher Qualität (Yu & Mathiowetz, 2014a). Drei Level-I-RCTs Studien wurden während des systematischen Reviews gefunden (Bombardier et al., 2008; Ennis, Thain, Boggild, Baker & Young, 2006; Plow, Mathiowetz & Lowe, 2009). Das Format der Gesundheitsförderungsprogramme in diesen Studien variiert signifikant und beinhaltet Aktionen wie Diskussionen, Hausaufgaben und motivierend befragende telefonische Beratungsgespräche. Die Ergebnisse dieser Programme beinhalten Verbesserungen der Gesundheit, der körperlichen Aktivität, spirituelles Wachstum, Stressmanagement und Gesundheitsverantwortung.

Rehabilitationsprogramme

Ambulante Interventionsprogramme

Ergotherapeuten bieten Interventionen für ambulante Klienten in Krankenhäusern, Privatpraxen, Arztpraxen und freien ambulanten Einrichtungen an (Schultz-Krohn & Pendleton, 2013). Drei Studien – zwei Level-I- (Patti et al., 2002, 2003) und eine Level-II nichtrandomisierte kontrollierte Studie (Brittle et al., 2008) – untersuchten die Effektivität ambulanter Rehabilitation für Klienten mit MS. Gemeinsam betrachtet, bieten diese Studien eine moderate Evidenz von mittlerer Qualität für die Effektivität von ambulanten Rehabilitationsprogrammen für Klienten mit MS (Yu & Mathiowetz, 2014a). Die Interventionen beinhalten Übungen und Schulungen. Die positiven Outcomes einer individuellen, multidisziplinären ambulanten Rehabilitation, welche in diesen Studien gefunden wurden, beziehen sich auf eine erhöhte Selbsteinschätzung zu einer verbesserten gesundheitsbezogenen Lebensqualität, einen reduzierten Einfluss durch Fatigue und verbesserte soziale Leistungsfähigkeit. Eine Studie kann keine Verbesserungen in den ADLs oder IADLs nachweisen (Brittle et al., 2008); die anderen zwei Studien beschreiben signifikante Verbesserungen im *FIM*™, einschließlich im Bereich der Selbstversorgung (Patti et al., 2002, 2003).

Stationäre Interventionsprogramme

Stationäre Rehabilitationsprogramme bieten eine multidisziplinäre Rehabilitation für medikamentös gut eingestellte Klienten, die mehrere Stunden Therapie am Tag tolerieren (Schultz-Krohn & Pendleton, 2013). Diese beinhalten akute und subakute Rehabilitationsprogramme. Der systematische Review erhob zwei Level-I-RCTs (Craig, Young, Ennis, Baker & Boggild, 2003; Storr, Sørensen & Ravnborg, 2006) und drei Level-III-Vortest-Nachtest-Studien (Grasso, Troisi, Rizzi, Morelli & Paolucci, 2005; Maitra et al., 2010; Vikman, Fielding, Lindmark & Fredrikson, 2008). Diese Studien liefern eine moderate Evidenz mittlerer Qualität zur Unterstützung der Effektivität von individuellen multidisziplinären Rehabilitationsprogrammen im stationären Setting (Yu & Mathiowetz, 2014a). Die Interventionen, die in diesen Rahmen Anwendung fanden, variieren je nach Studie und beinhalten Interventionen diverser Gesundheitsprofessionen (zum Beispiel Ergotherapeuten, Physiotherapeuten, Sozialarbeiter und Pflegekräfte). Diese Interventionen beinhalten therapeutische Übungen (zum Beispiel Dehnung, Gelenkmobilisation, Hydrotherapie, Gleichgewichtstraining, Training zum Umgang mit Hilfsmitteln); Fatigue- und Stressmanagement; ADL-Training und Maßnahmen zur Verbesserung der motorischen Funktionen der oberen Extremitäten, der Kommunikationsfähigkeiten und der Kognition für die ADLs. Die Verminderung der Krankheitsschwere und die Verbesserungen im ADL-Status sind zwei Vorteile, die quer durch die Studien dargelegt werden. Da die Interventionen multidisziplinär angelegt waren, war es nicht möglich, die Ergebnisse der Ergotherapie von denen der anderen Gesundheitsprofessionen zu trennen.

Programme für Interventionen zu Hause
Ergotherapeuten bieten Interventionen in der Gemeinde und im Wohnraum der Klienten an. Der Wohnraum als natürliche Umwelt erweist sich als idealer Rahmen für die Leistungen der Ergotherapie. In einem systematischen Review wurden zwei Level-I-Studien (Huijgen et al., 2008; Ward et al., 2004) und eine Level-III-Studie (Finkelstein, Lapshin, Castro, Cha & Provance, 2008) einbezogen, die eine moderate Evidenz mittlerer Qualität für die Effekte der Interventionen im Wohnraum von Klienten mit MS aufzeigen (Yu & Mathiowetz, 2014a). Spezielle Interventionen dieser Studien beinhalten ein einmonatiges häusliches Telerehabilitationssystem für Arm-Hand-Funktionen mit einem portablen computergestützten Trainingsgerät und Telekonferenzen mit einem Therapeuten (Huijgen et al., 2008); ein 12-wöchiges häusliches Telerehabilitationsprogramm mit einem benutzerdefinierten Übungsprotokoll (zum Beispiel Kräftigungsübungen, Dehnung, Gleichgewichtsübungen; Finkelstein et al., 2008) und einer 12-monatigen Schulung zu Sturzgefahr und Dekubitus mit Empfehlungen einer multidisziplinären Expertengruppe, Informationen für eine persönliche Beratung vom Ergotherapeuten, schriftlichen Informationen (zum Beispiel Krankheit, Status des Klienten und Selbsthilfegruppen), Interventionsplanung und Follow-up-Telefonaten (Ward et al., 2004).

Programme in einer Vielzahl von Settings
Zwei Level-I-Studien (Khan, Pallant, Brand & Kilpatrick, 2008; Khan, Turner-Stokes, Ng & Kilpatrick, 2008) des systematischen Reviews befassen sich mit der Rehabilitation in einer Vielzahl von Settings (zum Beispiel stationär, ambulant, im eigenen Wohnraum oder in der Gemeinde). Diese Studien hoher Qualität liefern eine starke Evidenz für die Effektivität einer multidisziplinären Rehabilitation in vielfältigen Settings (Yu & Mathiowetz, 2014a). Die Ergebnisse suggerieren, dass eine multidisziplinäre Rehabilitation die Bereiche von Aktivität und Partizipation sowie die gesundheitsbezogene Lebensqualität verbessern, auch wenn es, wie bei den Studien zur stationären Rehabilitation, nicht möglich war, den Einfluss der ergotherapeutischen Interventionen von denen der anderen Professionen des therapeutischen Teams zu differenzieren.

Berufliche Rehabilitation
Eine Level-I-Studie (Khan, Ng & Turner-Stokes, 2009), welche in den systematischen Review eingeschlossen wurde, befasst sich mit der Effektivität und den Kosten eines beruflichen Rehabilitationsprogramms für Menschen mit MS. Diese Studie ist selbst ein systematischer Review und schließt eine RCT und eine kontrollierte klinische Studie ein. Sowohl Einzel- als auch Gruppeninterventionen werden in diese Studien einbezogen. Die Interventionen dieser Studien sind auf Probleme wie Offenlegung und Anpassungsplanung, Arbeitsplatzanpassung und weitere Wege zum Erhalt der Arbeitstätigkeit ausgelegt (zum Beispiel Beratung). Aufgrund der limitierten Anzahl von Untersuchungen, der Breite der Zielgruppe und den unstimmigen Ergebnismessungen kann keine abschließende Aussage über die Effektivität einer beruflichen Rehabilitation für Menschen mit MS getroffen werden (Yu & Mathiowetz, 2014a).

Funktionelle Mobilität
Zwei Level-I-Studien (Esnouf, Taylor, Mann & Barrett, 2010; Souza et al., 2010) und eine Level-II nichtrandomisierte kontrollierte Studie (Cattaneo, Marazzini, Crippa & Cardini, 2002) im systematischen Review konzentrieren sich auf die Effektivität der Interventionen zum Erhalt der funktionellen Mobilität im Rahmen der ergotherapeutischen Praxis. In einer dieser Studien (Souza et al., 2010) wurde systematisch die Evidenz bezüglich der Nutzung von Mobilitäts- und Unterstützungstechnologien durch Menschen mit MS untersucht. Die anderen beiden Studien (Cattaneo et al., 2002; Esnouf et al., 2010) verglichen die Effektivität von Fußorthesen. Aufgrund der limitierten Anzahl der Nachweise und der kleinen Mischprobe (Yu & Mathiowetz, 2014a) kann keine abschließende Aussage über die Effektivität der Interventionen zur Förderung der funktionellen Mobilität getroffen werden.

4.1.2 Interventionen mit Fokus auf Performanzfertigkeiten

Von den 70 Studien des systematischen Reviews untersuchten 42 die Effektivität von Interventionen, die auf den Klienten und seine Fertigkeiten ausgerichtet sind. Alle diese Studien sind in der Evidenztabelle gelistet (Anhang D). Die Artikel sind in drei übergeordnete Kategorien gegliedert:
(1) Prozessbezogene Fertigkeiten (einschließlich Interventionen für Kognition und Emotionsregulation)
(2) Soziale Fertigkeiten (einschließlich Emotionsregulation) und
(3) Motorische Fertigkeiten (einschließlich Übungsinterventionen und motorischem Training).

Die folgenden Bereiche sind nach diesen übergeordneten Kategorien geordnet. Jeder Unterbereich enthält eine kurze Beschreibung der Intervention, gefolgt von einem Überblick bezüglich der Evidenz der jeweiligen Intervention.

Prozessbezogene Fertigkeiten

Kognitive Beeinträchtigungen sind ein häufiges Symptom bei MS und betreffen annähernd die Hälfte aller Erkrankten (National Multiple Sclerosis Society, 2013a). Zu den üblichen kognitiven Symptomen zählen Gedächtnis-, Aufmerksamkeits- und Konzentrationseinschränkungen sowie Probleme mit den exekutiven Fähigkeiten.

Computergestütztes kognitives Training

Kognitive Rehabilitation bei MS beinhaltet computergestützte Kognitionstrainingsprogramme, welche die Technologie nutzen, um spezielle kognitive Fähigkeiten (zum Beispiel Aufmerksamkeit, Gedächtnis) zu verbessern. Meistens ist das computergestützte Kognitionstraining vorgesehen, um spezifische kognitive Fähigkeiten wiederherzustellen. Solche Trainingsprogramme können sowohl in der Klinik als auch als häusliche Intervention genutzt werden. Für die Effektivität eines häuslichen, individualisierten und computergestützten Kognitionstrainingsprogramms bei MS besteht eine moderate Evidenz mit einer hohen qualitativen Untermauerung (Yu & Mathiowetz, 2014b). Die Studien des systematischen Reviews (Flavia, Stampatori, Zanotti, Parrinello & Capra, 2010 [Level-II]; Solari et al., 2004 [Level-I]; Shatil, Metzer, Horvitz & Miller, 2010 [Level-II]) bezogen sich auf häusliche Kognitionstrainingsprogramme (zum Beispiel *RehabCom*™ und *CogniFit Kliental Coach*™).

Gesamt betrachtet, zeigen die Studien bezüglich der Kognition unmittelbare und/oder kurzfristige Verbesserungen. Zu den spezifischen kognitiven Fähigkeiten, die sich verbessern, zählen Aufmerksamkeit, Gedächtnis, Informationsverarbeitung und exekutive Funktionen. Um die Langzeiteffekte zu beurteilen, bedarf es jedoch einer erweiterten Forschung. Viele Studien befassen sich mit der Wiederherstellung von Klientenfaktoren und es bedarf noch weiterer Ergebnisse, um den Zusammenhang zwischen verbesserten kognitiven Fähigkeiten und der Betätigungsperformanz zu ermitteln.

Gedächtnistraining

Ergotherapeutische Interventionen zielen entweder darauf ab, das Gedächtnis wiederherzustellen oder die Aktivitäten und den Kontext für Klienten mit MS zu modifizieren, um sie beim Prozess der Anpassung und Kompensation der Gedächtnisdefizite zu unterstützen.

Die Ergebnisse des systematischen Reviews liefern bezüglich des Gedächtnistrainings bei MS eine moderate Evidenz von mittlerer Qualität, dennoch können aufgrund der Vielfalt der Trainings keine Schlussfolgerungen gezogen werden (Yu & Mathiowetz, 2014b). Der systematische Review schloss eine Level-I-Studie mit ein (Chiaravalloti, DeLuca, Moore & Ricker, 2005) sowie vier Level-II-Studien (Brenk, Laun & Haase, 2008; Chiaravalloti, Demaree, Gaudino & DeLuca, 2003; Goverover, Chiaravalloti & DeLuca, 2008; Goverover, Hillary, Chiaravalloti, Arango-Lasprilla & DeLuca, 2009; siehe **Tabelle 3-3** für eine Fallstudie). Die in diesen Studien verwendeten Interventionen bewegen sich in einem Feld zwischen vorbereitenden Methoden hin zu handlungsbasierten Interventionen (zum Beispiel kochen, Umgang mit Finanzen). Ein Beispiel: Die Teilnehmer einer Studie lernten Techniken wie Visualisierung (zum Beispiel Bildsprache/Symbolik), um neue Informationen abzuspeichern. Wenn auch vorliegende Evidenzen nahelegen, dass Gedächtnistraining kurzfristig das Gedächtnis verbessern kann, ist eine ergänzende Forschung notwendig, um die Langzeiteffekte dieser Interventionen und ebenso ihre Beziehung zu der Betätigungsperformanz aufzuzeigen.

Soziale Fertigkeiten

Die Fähigkeiten, die eigenen Emotionen zu regulieren, erlauben den Klienten, wirksam den Betätigungsanforderungen zu begegnen und dort mit einer Auswahl an geeigneten Emotionen zu reagieren. Auch können sie diese beeinflussen (AOTA, 2014).

Interventionen, die darauf abzielen, die emotionale Regulierung zu unterstützen oder zu verstärken, werden oftmals in Gruppen angeboten. Sie können auf speziellen Theorien oder Ansätzen basieren (zum Beispiel Verhaltenstheorie, Psychoedukation) und Aktivitäten wie Gruppendiskussionen, Zielsetzung, Übungsaufträge oder Hausaufgaben beinhalten. Es besteht eine hohe Evidenz durch hoch qualitative Studien, die die Effektivität der Interventionen für die emotionale Regulierung unterstützen (Yu & Mathiowetz, 2014b). Fünf Level-I-Studien (Forman & Lincoln, 2010; Hughes, Robinson-Whelen, Taylor & Hall, 2006; Malcomson, Dunwoody & Lowe-Strong, 2007; Rigby, Thornton & Young, 2008; Thomas, Thomas, Hillier, Galvin & Baker, 2006) und eine Level-II nichtrandomisierte kontrollierte Studie (Mohr, Hart & Goldberg, 2003) über Interventionen zur Förderung der emotionalen Regulation wurden in den systematischen Review eingeschlossen. Eine verbesserte Stimmung, ein reduziertes Depressionsniveau, reduzierter Stress und eine größere Selbstwirksamkeit sind einige Ergebnisse der Interventionen. Zusätzlich untersuchte eine Studie die Beziehung zwischen Fatigue und Depression und fand eine Verbindung zwischen Depression und Fatigue allgemein, der Schwere der Fatigue sowie den Konsequenzen (Mohr et al., 2003).

Motorische und prozessbezogene Übungen
Übung ist eine vorbereitende Methode, die von Ergotherapeuten genutzt wird. Übungsarten, die bei Klienten mit MS angewendet werden, beinhalten Widerstandstraining, passive Bewegungsübungen, um den Bewegungsumfang zu erweitern, Stretching, Yoga und Pilates. Die angestrebten Ergebnisse der Übungen für MS-Klienten variieren, dazu gehören aber verbesserte klientenbezogene Faktoren (zum Beispiel gesteigerte Kraft, verbessertes Gleichgewicht, größere Ausdauer), Reduzierung der Symptome der MS (verminderte Fatigue, verminderter Schmerz) und eine verbesserte Lebensqualität. Es besteht eine starke Evidenz von hoher Qualität für die Effektivität eines auf körperliche Aktivitäten orientierten Programms für Klienten mit leichter bis moderater MS (Yu & Mathiowetz, 2014b), welches den Nutzen von physischen Aktivitäten unterstützt, um Muskelkraft (Bjarnadottir, Konradsdottir, Reynisdottir & Olafsson, 2007; Fragoso, Santana & Pinto, 2008; Rietberg, Brooks, Uitdehaag & Kwakkel, 2004) und Beweglichkeit (Costello, Raivel & Wilson, 2009; Freeman & Allison, 2004; Romberg et al., 2004) zu verbessern (siehe **Tabelle 3-3** für eine Fallstudie). Die Artikel des Reviews liefern eine starke Evidenz mittlerer Qualität und stützen den Nutzen aeroben Trainings für MS-Klienten (Yu & Mathiowetz, 2014b). Die spezifischen aeroben Interventionen variierten dabei in jeder Studie, eingeschlossen waren dabei Ausdauerübungen (Dettmers, Sulzmann, Ruchay-Plossl, Gutler & Vieten, 2009), die Verwendung von Trainingsgeräten (zum Beispiel Laufband, Stepper; McCullagh, Fitzgerald, Murphy & Cooke, 2008) und Wassergymnastik (Roehrs & Karst, 2004). Eine gesteigerte Gehstrecke und Ausdauer (Dettmers et al., 2009) weniger Einfluss von Fatigue (McCullagh et al., 2008; Roehrs & Karst, 2004) und eine verbesserte Lebensqualität (McCullagh et al., 2008; Roehrs & Karst, 2004) zählen mit zu den positiven Ergebnissen. Der systematische Review zeigt sich als Ergebnis von sechs Studien – zwei Level-I-RCTs (Dettmers et al., 2009; Romberg et al., 2004); eine Level-II nichtrandomisierte kontrollierte Studie (DeBolt & McCubbin, 2004); und drei Level-III-Vortest-Nachtest-Studien (Ayan-Perez, Martin Sanchez, de Souza-Teixeira & de Paz Fernandez, 2007; de Souza-Teixeira et al., 2009; White et al., 2004), welche die Auswirkungen von Widerstandstraining an Klienten mit MS untersuchten. Zusammen betrachtet, liefern diese Studien eine moderate Evidenz mittlerer Qualität (Yu & Mathiowetz, 2014b). In einer Level-I-RCT fanden Cakit et al. (2010) heraus, dass Widerstandstraining auf dem Ergometer die Ausdauer, die Gehgeschwindigkeit und das Gleichgewicht fördern, gleichzeitig Sturzangst und den Schweregrad der Fatigue sowie Depression reduzieren sowie die körperliche Leistungsfähigkeit verstärken. Andere Studien fanden heraus, dass Widerstandstraining nützlich ist, um die Kraft spezifischer Gruppen (Ayan-Perez et al., 2007; DeBolt & McCubbin, 2004), die Gehgeschwindigkeit und -ausdauer zu verbessern (Romberg et al., 2004). Zwei Level-II-RCTstudien des systematischen Reviews untersuchten die Effekte von Yoga auf Menschen mit MS (Oken et al., 2004; Velikonja, Curic, Ozura & Jazbec, 2010), und eine Level-III-Vortest-Nachtest-Studie überprüfte die Effekte eines auf Pilates ausgerichteten Gruppen-Übungsprogramms (Freeman & Allison, 2004). Velikonja et al. (2010) fanden heraus, dass Klienten mit MS, die an 10 wöchentlich durchgeführten Stunden Hatha Yoga teilnahmen, signifikante Verbesserungen in der selektiven Aufmerksamkeit erreichen. Allerdings fanden Oken et al. (2004) keine signifikanten Auswirkungen auf kognitive Funktionen oder Aufmerksamkeit, Stimmung, Fatigue oder die Lebensqualität für Klienten mit MS, die sechs Monate am Iyengar Yoga teilnahmen. Signifikante Verbesserungen bezüglich des

Gleichgewichts, des Gangbilds und des Einflusses von Fatigue kann dahingegen eine Studie über Pilates belegen (Freeman & Allison, 2004).

Motorisches Fertigkeitstraining
Ziel des motorischen Trainings ist es, neuromuskoloskelettale und bewegungsbezogene Funktionen sowie motorische und praktische Fertigkeiten wiederherzustellen oder zu entwickeln. Diese Interventionen zielen bei Menschen mit MS auf Bereiche wie Gleichgewicht, Koordination oder Kraft ab. Die verfügbare Evidenz für ein motorisches Training für Menschen mit MS beinhalten eine weite Bandbreite an Interventionen wie Gleichgewichtsförderung (Cattaneo, Jonsdottir, Zocchi & Regola, 2007; Widener, Allen & Gibson-Horn, 2009); robotikbasierte Rehabilitation (Carpinella, Cattaneo, Abuarqub & Ferrarin, 2009) und *Constraint-Induced Movement Therapy* (CIMT; Mark et al., 2008). Der Bandbreite an Interventionen stehen vergleichbar wenige Studien gegenüber. Daher können keine Schlussfolgerungen für die Effektivität eines motorischen Trainings bei Menschen mit MS ermittelt werden.

4.2 Interventionen für Klienten mit IPS

Aus dem systematischen Review sind drei Kategorien von Interventionen aus den Studien über IPS hervorgegangen:
(1) Übung oder körperliche Aktivität
(2) Umweltbedingte Reize, Stimuli und Objekte und
(3) Selbstmanagement und kognitive Verhaltensstrategien.

Alle Kategorien können in einer einzelnen Studie vorliegen, aber ein oder zwei Studien können durch ihren Interventionsansatz oder die Auswahl von Ergebnismessungen hervorgehoben werden. Das Design der Studien wurde entlang einer zeitlichen Dimension untergliedert: synchron oder diachron (Rosenthal & Rosnow, 2008). Im Kontext der Rehabilitationsforschung richten diachrone Studien ihren Fokus auf Veränderungen, die über einen längeren Zeitraum und über eine einzelne Sitzung hinaus auftreten, um die Beständigkeit therapeutischer Effekte über die Zeit hinweg zu testen. Synchrone Studien fokussieren sich auf Veränderungen während einer Interventionssitzung, welche vielleicht für kurzfristige oder längerfristige Auswirkungen verantwortlich sind.

4.2.1 Übung und körperliche Aktivität

Performanzfertigkeiten
Interventionen zur Verbesserung von Performanzfertigkeiten umfassen eindimensionales Training wie progressives Widerstandstraining, Gelenkmobilisation, posturales Stabilitäts- und Gleichgewichtstraining, Gangtraining und aerobe Fitnessaktivitäten (zum Beispiel Laufband, Walking, Fahrrad fahren). Sieben systematische Reviews mit überwiegend diachronen Ergebnissen lieferten eine moderate bis starke Level-I-Evidenz dafür, dass motorische und sensorisch-perzeptive Performanzfertigkeiten durch mehrmalige Einheiten, repetitives körperliches Üben und Aktivität unterstützt werden (die letzteren Fertigkeiten hängen mit posturaler Stabilität und Gleichgewicht zusammen; Crizzle & Newhouse, 2006; Dibble, Addison & Papa, 2009; Goodwin, Richards, Taylor, Taylor & Campbell, 2008; Keus et al., 2007; Kwakkel, de Goede & van Wegen, 2007; Mehrholz et al., 2010; Stewart & Crosbie, 2009). Für kurzfristige Effekte erweist sich die Evidenz stärker als für langfristige Effekte (siehe **Tabelle 3-4** für eine Fallstudie). Im Zusammenhang damit legen die Synthesen nahe, dass Performanzfertigkeiten mehr auf ein aufgabenspezifisches Training als auf ein nichtspezifisches Training ansprechen (Kwakkel et al., 2007). Ein Beispiel: Muskelkraft spricht mehr auf ein Training an, welches direkt auf den Mechanismus der Muskelkräftigung abzielt (zum Beispiel progressive Widerstandsübungen), wohingegen das Gleichgewicht mehr auf ein Training anspricht, das auf die posturalen, kinästhetischen und vestibulären Mechanismen des Gleichgewichts abzielt. Ergänzend scheint es, dass ein direktes Training der Performanzfertigkeiten nicht verallgemeinert werden darf, ebenso wie es der Fall ist bei komplexerer Betätigungsperformanz oder Outcomes zur Lebensqualität bei spezifischen Performanzfertigkeiten.

Es wurden 12 einzelne primäre Studien mit einem diachronen Design gefunden, welche die Effekte von Übung und Fähigkeitstraining auf motorische und sensorisch-perzeptive Performanzfertigkeiten untersuchten, aber nicht in systematische Reviews eingeschlossen wurden: Fünf Studien zeigen eine Level-I-Evidenz (Allen et al., 2010; Qutubuddin et al., 2007; Sage & Almeida, 2010; Smania et al., 2010; Yousefi, Tadibi, Khoei & Montazeri, 2009); drei eine Level-II-Evidenz (Dereli & Yaliman, 2010; Dibble, Hale, Marcus, Gerber & LaStayo, 2009; Nocera, Horvat & Ray, 2009) und vier eine Level-III-Evidenz (Brittle et al., 2008; Gobbi et al., 2009; Jobges et al., 2004; Rossi-

Izquierdo et al., 2009). Diese primären Studien liefern zusätzliche moderate Evidenz, dass Übungsprogramme die motorische Performanz, die posturale Stabilität und das Gleichgewicht verbessern, jeweils bezogen auf Pretest-Baseline-Werte und den Kontrollbedingungen ohne Übung. Eine begrenzte Evidenz deutet darauf hin, dass ein Training der posturalen Kontrolle einen allgemeinen oder nachhaltigen Effekt auf die Angst vor dem Fallen oder die Sturzreduktion hat. Ebenso wurde eine begrenzte Evidenz dafür gefunden, dass spezialisierte körperliche Aktivitäten und intensive aufgabenspezifische Übungen vorteilhafter sind als lockere oder weniger intensive Formen von Übungen. Zwei Studien mit synchronem Design, die die Effekte einfacher Übungen oder körperlicher Aktivität auf Performanzfertigkeiten während einer einzelnen Intervention testeten, liefern eine begrenzte Evidenz, dass Single-Task-Interventionen unmittelbare Wirkungen haben, die für die Entwicklung von Performanzfertigkeiten förderlich sind. Müller und Muhlack (2010) belegen eine Level-I-Evidenz, dass die positiven Effekte der Parkinson-Medikation auf motorische Performanzfertigkeiten (Reaktionszeit, Finger tippen, dübeln) besser durch körperliche Übung unterstützt werden als durch Ruhe. Elkis-Abuhoff, Goldblatt, Gaydos und Corrato (2008) stellten mit einer Studie mit Level-III-Evidenz vor, dass einfache Tonmanipulationsaufgaben die Stimmung verbessern.

Betätigungsperformanz
An dieser Stelle geht es um Dual-Task-, Multitask oder multimodale Aufgaben und Aktivitätstraining (zum Beispiel Transfertraining, funktionelles Mobilitätstraining und Freizeit-Bewegungs-Aktivitäten wie Tanzen und Tai-Chi). Systematische Reviews über Interventionen für Betätigungsperformanz vom Level-I sind selten (Dixon et al., 2007; Gage & Storey, 2004; Rao, 2010) und müssen auf wenige schwache Studien mit diversen Interventionen und Ergebnismessungen bauen, die nur schwer zusammengefasst werden können. Folglich ist es unklar, ob die aufgabenspezifischen Effekte der Trainingsinterventionen für Performanzfertigkeiten durch komplexe (Dual-Task-, Multitask- oder multimodale) Trainingsinterventionen der Betätigungsperformanz für Klienten mit IPS erreicht werden können. Es gibt eine kleine rigorose primäre Effektivitätsstudie, die beispielsweise den Effekt des Selbstpflegetrainings auf die Selbstpflege untersuchte und die Ergebnisse des Trainings zur Essenszubereitung bei IPS darlegte (Kwakkel et al., 2007). Ein systematischer Review über die Ergebnisse der Anwendung von Tai-Chi-Übungen liefert eine limitierte Evidenz, dass Thai-Chi motorische und posturale Performanzfertigkeiten bei IPS verbessert (Lee, Lam & Ernst, 2008). Insgesamt wurden 10 einzelne primäre Studien mit einem diachronen Design gefunden, welche auf komplexe funktionelle Trainingsinterventionen ausgerichtet waren und nicht in einem systematischen Review zusammengefasst wurden. Diese schlossen funktionelle Mobilität, nichtspezifisches ADL-Training und Sport oder der Erholung dienende Aktivitäten (vorrangig Tanz) ein. Von diesen Studien zeigen drei eine Level-I-Evidenz (Hackney & Earhart, 2009a, 2009c; Morris, Iansek & Kirkwood, 2009), eine Studie eine Level-II-Evidenz (Tanaka et al., 2009) und sechs Studien eine Level-III-Evidenz (Batson, 2010; Canning, Ada & Woodhouse, 2008; Hackney & Earhart, 2009b; Stankovic, 2004; Tassorelli et al., 2009; van Eijkeren et al., 2008). Im Gesamten liefern diese Studien eine geringe bis moderate Evidenz, dass ein komplexes und multimodales Aktivitätstraining kurzfristige Verbesserungen der funktionellen Bewegungsaktivitäten unterstützt. Dual-Task-Performanz, insbesondere verbunden mit dem Gleichgewicht (zum Beispiel Objekte beim Gehen zu transportieren), spricht auf ein Training an, welches kognitive sowie motorische Performanzfertigkeiten innerhalb der Aktivitätsperformanz einschließt (Morris et al., 2009). Die Integration eines motorischen und sozialen Trainings der Performanzfertigkeiten beim Tangotanzen, welches eng aufeinander abgestimmte zwischenmenschliche Bewegungen mit einem Partner einschließen, verspricht mehr positive Ergebnisse zu funktioneller Mobilität und zum Gleichgewicht als Übungen ohne Partner oder weniger eng aufeinander abgestimmte zwischenmenschliche Tanzformen (Batson, 2010; Hackney & Earhart, 2009a, 2009b, 2009c). Es gibt nur eine beschränkte Evidenz dafür, dass Interventionen zu multimodaler körperlicher Aktivität positive Auswirkungen auf die Kognition haben, vor allem auf die exekutiven Funktionen (Tanaka et al., 2009). Langzeitverbesserungen wurden bis jetzt noch nicht mit Bestimmtheit nachgewiesen. Zudem wurden die Spezifität sowie Allgemeingültigkeit der Effekte der Interventionen bei diesem Level komplexer Aufgaben und Aktivitäten momentan nicht über einen niedrigen Level der Evidenz dokumentiert. Keine synchrone Studie über Interventionen zur Betätigungsperformanz erfüllt die Einschlusskriterien. Die wenigen der durchgeführten synchronen Studien deuten aber auf die Vermutung hin, dass erkennbare Effekte bei Interventionen zu

komplexeren Aktivitäten sich erst bei Wiederholungen einstellen oder eine Entwicklung brauchen, die sich erst im Verlauf von mehreren Einheiten einstellt, im Gegensatz zu einzelnen Sitzungen.

4.2.2 Umweltbedingte Reize, Stimuli und Objekte

Es erscheinen systematische Reviews vom Level-I über Interventionen bei Klienten mit IPS, welche die Performanz in der Umwelt anreichern oder adaptieren. Sie ermöglichen ein größeres Verständnis über die Ansprechbarkeit des Gehirns auf umgebende Stimuli und dem Zusammenhang, der besteht (Keus et al., 2007; Kwakkel et al., 2007; Lim et al., 2005; Rao, 2010). Es gibt die Hypothese, dass externe Taktung/Zeitplanung von Bewegungen hilft, Defizite des internen zeitlich-motorischen Mechanismus zu kompensieren, welcher mit den Funktionen der Basalganglien verbunden ist (zum Beispiel Ma, Trombly, Tickle-Degnen & Wagenaar, 2004). Lim et al. (2005) führten einen systematischen Review über die Evidenz von rhythmischen externen Cues (Ton, Video und somatosensorisch) durch und schlussfolgern daraus, dass auditive rhythmische Cues eine stärkere Evidenz haben, Menschen mit IPS beim Gehen zu unterstützen, als visuelle, taktile oder andere Formen von Cues. Sie schlussfolgern ebenso, dass diese Art von Cues unmittelbare (synchrone) und multisession (diachrone) Effekte zu haben scheinen. Zum Zeitpunkt des systematischen Reviews war die Evidenz zu begrenzt, um zu ermitteln, ob ein Training unter Versuchsbedingungen auf die Umgebung des Wohnraums verallgemeinert werden kann oder Ergebnisse zum Walking auf die Ergebnisse zu komplexerer Betätigungsperformanz übertragen werden können. Es wurden sieben einzelne primäre Studien mit einem synchronen Design gefunden, die nicht in einem systematischen Review zusammengefasst wurden. Zwei von ihnen liefern eine Level-I-Evidenz über die Effekte von einfachen und komplexen, rhythmischen und unrhythmischen auditiven Cues auf die funktionelle Performanz der oberen Extremitäten (Ma, Hwang & Lin, 2009; Ma et al., 2004). Vier zeigen eine Level-II- (Rochester et al., 2005; Rochester, Burn, Woods, Godwin & Nieuwboer, 2009) oder Level-III-Evidenz (Bachlin et al., 2010; Bryant, Rintala, Lai, Raines & Protas, 2009) über die Effekte von Interventionen, die externes rhythmisches Cueing, Cueing gepaart mit kognitiven Strategien für Bewegung, Cueing bei Freezing und adaptive Hilfsmittel zur Sturzprophylaxe einbeziehen. Eine Studie zeigte eine Level-II-Evidenz über den Effekt von zwei verschiedenen Typen von Interviewfragen (positive versus negative Thematik) über Mimik und emotionalen Ausdruck bei Klienten mit IPS (Takahashi, Tickle-Degnen, Coster & Latham, 2010). Diese Studien liefern einen moderaten Level der Evidenz, dass der umweltbedingte Kontext und die Struktur der Cues wichtig sind, wenn Klienten mit IPS einfache funktionelle Aufgaben durchführen. Performanzfertigkeiten während einfacher und Dual-Task-Aufgaben scheinen am meisten durch einen Kontext unterstützt, der durch auditive rhythmische Stimuli angereichert ist und eine sichere Umgebung bietet, um sich auf die funktionelle Aufgabe zu konzentrieren, gepaart mit Supervision von kognitiven Strategien für eine Einschätzung, wie groß eine Bewegung durchgeführt werden muss als Rückmeldung zu dem Cue oder dem Auslösen von positiven Emotionen. Umgebungsbezogene Cues, die die Aufmerksamkeit oder fokussierte Aufmerksamkeit weg von der primären Aufgabe lenken oder negative Emotionen hervorrufen, scheinen die Performanz zu beeinträchtigen. Vier Studien mit einem diachronen Design, alle mit Level-I-Evidenz, testeten, ob die in synchronen Studien erhobenen umgebungsbedingten Regulationsfaktoren anhaltende Effekte auf die Bewegungsperformanz haben (Elston, Honan, Powell, Gormley & Stein, 2010; Mak & Hui-Chan, 2008; Nieuwboer et al., 2007; Rochester et al., 2010). Diese Studien befassten sich mit den Lücken des systematischen Reviews von Lim et al. (2005). Deren Ergebnisse liefern eine moderate Evidenz, dass das Verwenden externer Cues, die von Klienten bevorzugt werden, während der Performanz von ADLs positive Effekte auf die motorische Kontrolle hat. Die Intervention erfolgte über einige Wochen im Wohnraum, und die Ergebnisse hielten über einige Wochen nach dieser Intervention an. Es ist immer noch unklar, wie lange diese Effekte anhalten, welche Intensität die Intervention benötigt, um andauernde Effekte über wenige Wochen zu erreichen, und zu welchem Grad komplexe ADLs und die Lebensqualität durch ausgestaltete oder adaptierte Kontexte der Performanz beeinflusst werden.

4.2.3 Selbstmanagement und kognitive Verhaltensstrategien

Sieben primäre Studien mit einem diachronen Design befassten sich mit der Integration von Performanzmustern, von Selbstmanagement, von Gesundheit und Wellness in das tägliche Leben von Klienten mit IPS: vier Studien mit Level-I-Evidenz (Guo, Jiang,

Yatsuya, Yoshida & Sakamoto, 2009; Tickle-Degnen, Ellis, Saint-Hilaire, Thomas & Wagenaar, 2010; Ward et al., 2004; White, Wagenaar, Ellis & Tickle-Degnen, 2009), eine Studie mit Level-II-Evidenz (Ghahari & Packer, 2012) und zwei Studien mit Level-III-Evidenz (A'Campo, Spliethoff-Kamminga, Macht & Roos, 2010; Carne et al., 2005). Diese Studien fokussierten sich auf individualisierte Interventionen zur Verbesserung der Gesundheitsförderung und der persönlichen Kontrolle und halfen den Klienten, den Lebensstil zu modifizieren und die Lebensqualität zu verbessern. Die Studien nutzten häufig eine kognitiv-behaviorale Intervention aus Schulung, Zielsetzung, Training der Performanzfertigkeit, Praxis und Feedback und deren Integration in die Gewohnheiten des täglichen Lebens. Die Ergebnisse liefern eine moderate Evidenz dafür, dass diese Formen von Interventionen zielgerichtet die Bereiche der Lebensqualität verbessern. Wenn sich das Ziel auf eine funktionelle körperliche Aktivität und auf Bereiche der Partizipation bezieht, sind die Effekte auf diese Bereiche am größten. Effektive Ergebnisse traten in den Studien auf, welche Interventionen über sechs bis acht Wochen mit über 20 Einheiten einbezogen. Es gibt eine eingeschränkte Evidenz, dass die Ergebnisse der Lebensqualität für einige Wochen bis zu sechs Monaten anhalten können. Es wurden jedoch keine synchronen Studien gefunden. Interventionen für Selbstmanagement, gerichtet auf den Wohnraum und die Teilhabe an der Gesellschaft, sind abhängig vom Nachweis, dass es Zeit benötigt, persönliche Initiative und Praxis, um neue Performanzmuster in das tägliche Leben zu integrieren.

4.3 Interventionen für Klienten mit ALS

Fünf programmatische Themen ergaben sich aus dem Review der Literatur über ALS:
(1) Übung
(2) Hilfsmittel und Rollstühle
(3) Multidisziplinäre Programme
(4) Palliativpflege und
(5) Vorbereitende Methoden.

4.3.1 Übung

Es liegt eine moderate Evidenz einer Level-I-Studie vor, dass sich Teilnehmer eines Eigenübungsprogramms mit täglichem Stretching und Widerstandsübungen auf der *Amyotrophic Lateral Sclerosis Functional Rating Scale* (ALSFRS) und der *SF-36 physical functional scale* ohne negative Effekte verbessern (Dal Bello-Haas et al., 2007). Eine Level-I-Studie zeigte eine begrenzte Evidenz dafür, dass diejenigen, die ein individuelles Übungsprogramm zweimal am Tag durchführen, um die Muskelausdauer zu verbessern, eine bessere funktionelle Fähigkeit und weniger Spastizität aufweisen als die Teilnehmer der Kontrollgruppe ohne Übungen. Allerdings verschlechterten sich diese Ergebnisse mit der Zeit bei der Interventions- sowie der Kontrollgruppe (Drory, Goltsman, Reznik, Mosek & Korczyn, 2001). Es besteht eine begrenzte Evidenz einer Level-II nichtrandomisierten kontrollierten Studie (Aksu, Karaduman, Yakut & Tan, 2002), dass ein betreutes Übungsprogramm die individuelle funktionale Kapazität besser erhält als ein Eigenübungsprogramm. Eine Level-V-Fallstudie über eine Therapie im Bewegungsbad zeigte auf, dass die Teilnehmer nach der Therapieeinheit gesteigerte Energie aufweisen und weniger Hilfe bei den Transfers benötigen (Johnson, 1988; siehe **Tabelle 3-5** für eine Fallstudie).

4.3.2 Hilfsmittel und Rollstühle

Es besteht eine begrenzte Evidenz zweier Level-III-Studien hinsichtlich der Nutzung und der Zufriedenheit mit Rollstühlen. In einer Studie mit Nutzern von Elektrorollstühlen (PWC) waren 77 % der Umfrageteilnehmer zufrieden mit dem Gesamtkomfort ihres Elektrorollstuhls, und 72 % waren mit der Einfachheit der Bedienung zufrieden (Ward et al., 2010). Häufig genutzte Zusätze für den Elektrorollstuhl sind in Neigung und Kippung verstellbare Kopf-, Nacken-, Rumpf- und Armstützen, elektrisch verstellbare Beinstützen, verstellbare Geschwindigkeit durch einen Joystick, Luft- oder Gelkissen, weiche Kopfstütze, Sicherheitsgurt, höhenverstellbare flache Lehnen, Gellehnen oder geformte Armlehnen. Es besteht eine begrenzte Evidenz durch eine Umfrage an Nutzern von Elektrorollstühlen und handbetriebenen Rollstühlen, die aussagte, dass Rollstühle, insbesondere Elektrorollstühle, eine verstärkte Interaktion in der Gemeinschaft ermöglichen (Trail, Nelson, Van, Appel & Lai, 2001). Teilnehmer, die einen Elektrorollstuhl nutzen, berichteten von einer stärkeren Zufriedenheit in Bezug auf ihre Fähigkeit, an Aktivitäten teilzunehmen, im Vergleich zu Nutzern eines handbetriebenen Rollstuhls. Allerdings berichteten Teilnehmer in Bezug auf die Transportierbarkeit eine größere Zufriedenheit bei handbetriebenen Rollstühlen. Es gibt jedoch keinen Unterschied zwischen dem wahrgenommenen Komfort oder der Einfachheit der Lenkung. Die Teilnehmer berichteten des Weiteren, dass eine Unterstützung des Kopfes, des Halses, des Rumpfes und der Extremitäten hilfreich ist, aber gaben dies nicht für Rückengurte (*sling back*) und Schlingenauflagen (*sling seats*) an (siehe **Tabelle 3-5** für eine Fallstudie). Eine Level-III-Studie lieferte eine begrenzte Evidenz dafür, dass einige Hilfsmittel mehr nutzen als andere (Gruis, Wren & Huggins, 2011). Teilnehmer berichteten, dass die folgenden oft oder immer verwendeten Hilfsmittel sehr nützlich sind und eine größere Zufriedenheit liefern: erhöhter Toilettensitz, Griffe/Stangen neben der Toilette, Duschsitz, Duschhocker, Slipper (Schuhe), Sprunggelenksorthesen und Rutschbrett. Die folgenden Hilfsmittel werden eher weniger häufig genutzt, verschaffen aber eine hohe Zufriedenheit: ton- oder stimmenaktivierte Umweltkontroll- und Kommunikationsboards. Die Teilnehmer berichteten darüber hinaus, dass die folgenden Hilfsmittel nicht nützlich sind und somit nur zu einer begrenzten Zufriedenheit führen: Knopflochhilfen, Ankleidehilfen und verlängerte Greifwerkzeuge (siehe **Tabelle 3-5** für eine Fallstudie). Ein Level-I systematischer Review (Foley, Timonen & Hardiman, 2012) lieferte eine begrenzte Evidenz dafür, dass die Informationen der Telemedizin mit einem hohen Maß an Zufriedenheit in Verbindung gebracht werden können. Auch wenn die Teilnehmer mit der Telemedizin zufrieden waren, berichteten sie, dass ein direkter persönlicher Kontakt höher geschätzt wurde, um über psychische und emotionale Anliegen zu sprechen. Eine Level-IV-Studie untersuchte die Effektivität eines Computerprogramms zum Schreiben von Nachrichten sowie Aussuchen von Liedern und Videos mittels einer virtuellen Tastatur und eines Mikroschalters. Nach einem Training mit diesem Computerprogramm waren die Teilnehmer in der Lage, zwei Nachrichten innerhalb einer 20-minütigen Einheit zu schreiben sowie Lieder und Videos selbstständig auszusuchen (Lancioni et al., 2012).

4.3.3 Multidisziplinäre Programme

Eine Level-II-Studie zeigte eine limitierte bis moderate Evidenz, dass diejenigen, die an einem multidisziplinären Programm teilnehmen, eine ca. 30 % höhere Überlebensrate haben als diejenigen mit einer allgemeinen Versorgung (Traynor, Alexander, Corr, Frost & Hardiman, 2003). Multidisziplinäre Programme können mehrere Disziplinen umfassen, wie Neurologie, Pflege, Ergotherapie, Physiotherapie, Logopädie, Pneumologie, Ernährung, Psychologie und Sozialarbeit. Es existiert eine limitierte Evidenz aus einer Level-III-Studie, dass diejenigen, die an einem multidisziplinären Programm teilnehmen, auch zu einem höheren Anteil mit geeigneten Hilfsmitteln versorgt werden. Zudem ist eine höhere Lebensqualität bei sozialen Funktionen und psychischer Gesundheit zu verzeichnen (Van den Berg et al., 2005). Es gibt jedoch keine Unterschiede zwischen den Gruppen für die körperliche Funktionsfähigkeit oder die Lebensqualität der pflegebedürftigen Klienten.

4.3.4 Palliativpflege

Es existiert eine limitierte Evidenz aus einer Level-II-Studie, dass Ergotherapeuten bei Klienten mit ALS unmittelbar vor ihrem Tod als ein Teil des Betreuungsteams einbezogen werden (Albert, Murphy, Del Bene & Rowland, 1999). Ein systematischer Level-I-Review (Foley et al., 2012) ergab, dass die Beibehaltung der Kontrolle bei Entscheidungen über die Sterbebegleitung von ALS-Klienten sehr geschätzt wurde. Die Kontrolle bei der Entscheidungsfindung umfasst sowohl die unabhängige Entscheidungsfindung als auch die gemeinsame Entscheidungsfindung mit Familien und Dienstleistungsanbietern.

4.3.5 Vorbereitende Methoden

Aus einer Level-IV-Studie geht mit einer minimalen Evidenz hervor, dass die elektrische Stimulation die bilaterale Handfunktion und die Knieextension über einen Zeitraum von drei Monaten verbessert (Handa et al., 1995).

4.4 Zusammenfassung

Eine zunehmende Evidenz unterstützt die Wirksamkeit von ergotherapeutischen Interventionen für Menschen mit NDK. Obwohl mehr evidenzbasierte Forschung benötigt wird, unterstützt die Literatur die Rolle der Ergotherapie für diese Bevölkerungsgruppe und belegt den Nutzen vieler häufig angewandter ergotherapeutischer Interventionen. Darüber hinaus schlägt die Literatur innovative Interventionen vor, die Ergotherapeuten berücksichtigen und in ihre Praxis integrieren können. Der Schwerpunkt der Ergotherapie liegt darauf, anderen zu helfen, am täglichen Leben teilzunehmen (AOTA, 2014). Durch den Einsatz klientenzentrierter, betätigungsfokussierter und evidenzbasierter Dienstleistungen sind praktisch tätige Ergotherapeuten bei der Förderung von Gesundheit und Teilhabe für Klienten mit NDK von entscheidender Bedeutung.

Erläuterungen zu der Tabelle 4-1

A – Starke Empfehlung, die Intervention routinemäßig in der Ergotherapie für geeignete Klienten anzuwenden. Der Literaturreview stellte eine gute Evidenzlage fest, dass die Intervention wichtige Ergebnisse verbessert, und kam zu dem Schluss, dass die Vorteile im Vergleich zu den Nachteilen überwiegen.

B – Empfehlung, die Intervention routinemäßig in der Ergotherapie für geeignete Klienten anzuwenden. Der Literaturreview stellte mindestens eine gute Evidenz fest, dass die Intervention wichtige Ergebnisse verbessert, und kam zu dem Schluss, dass die Vorteile im Vergleich zu den Nachteilen überwiegen.

C – Keine Empfehlung für oder gegen Anwendung dieser Intervention in der Ergotherapie. Der Literaturreview stellte mindestens einen ordentlichen Beweis fest, dass durch die Intervention gewünschte Ergebnisse verbessert wurden, und kam zu dem Schluss, dass ähnlich viele Vorteile und Nachteile existieren, sodass keine Empfehlung ausgesprochen werden kann.

D – Die Anwendung dieser Intervention von Ergotherapeuten an ihre Klienten ist nicht empfohlen. Der Literaturreview stellte mindestens einen anständigen Beweis fest, dass die Intervention uneffektiv ist oder die Nachteile die Vorteilen überwiegen.

I – Ungenügende Beweislage, um eine Empfehlung für oder gegen den Einsatz dieser Intervention in der Ergotherapie auszusprechen. Beweise für die Wirksamkeit dieser Intervention fehlen, haben eine schlechte Qualität oder sind widersprüchlich. Es kann das Verhältnis zwischen den Vor- und Nachteilen nicht ermittelt werden.

Anmerkung: Die Empfehlungskriterien basieren auf der *Standard Recommendation Language by the Agency of Healthcare Research and Quality* (o.d.). Empfehlungen in dieser Tabelle basieren auf den Ergebnissen des evidenzbasierten Reviews, kombiniert mit Expertenmeinungen.

Tabelle 4-1: Empfehlungen für ergotherapeutische Interventionen für Klienten mit neurodegenerativen Erkrankungen

Multiple Sklerose

Interventionen mit dem Fokus auf Partizipation und Teilhabe
- Face-to-Face-Fatigue-Management-Programme zur Verringerung der Auswirkungen von Fatigue, zur Verbesserung der Lebensqualität und zur Verbesserung der Selbstwirksamkeit bei der Nutzung von Fatigue-Management-Strategien (A)
- Durch Telekonferenz durchgeführte Fatigue-Management-Programme, um die Auswirkungen von Fatigue auf das tägliche Leben zu reduzieren und die Lebensqualität zu verbessern (A)
- Multidisziplinäre Rehabilitation in einer Variation von Interventionsumgebungen zur Verbesserung der Aktivitäten und der Teilhabe sowie der gesundheitsbezogenen Lebensqualität (A)
- Ambulante Rehabilitationsprogramme für Menschen mit MS zur Verbesserung der Gesundheit und der Lebensqualität, Verringerung der Auswirkungen von Fatigue und Verbesserung der sozialen Funktionen (B)
- Stationäre Rehabilitation zur Verringerung der Schwere der Erkrankung und Verbesserung des ADL-Status (B)
- Ein heimbasiertes Programm zur Verbesserung der Performanz (B)
- Ambulante Rehabilitation zur Verbesserung der ADL-Performanz (B)
- Gesundheitsförderungsprogramme zur Verbesserung der Gesundheit, zur Steigerung der körperlichen Aktivität und der spirituellen Entwicklung sowie zur Reduzierung von Stress (C)
- Berufliche Rehabilitation (I)
- Programm zur Verbesserung der funktionellen Mobilität (I)

Interventionen mit dem Fokus auf Performanzfertigkeiten
Soziale Interaktionsfertigkeiten
- Interventionen zur Emotionsregulation zur Verbesserung der Stimmung, Verringerung der Depression, Stressabbau und Verbesserung der Selbstwirksamkeit (A)

Prozessfertigkeiten
- Heimbasiertes, individualisiertes und computergestütztes kognitives Training zur Verbesserung von Aufmerksamkeit, Gedächtnis, Informationsverarbeitung und Exekutivfunktionen (B)
- Gedächtnistraining zur kurzfristigen Verbesserung des Gedächtnisses (B)

Motorische Fähigkeiten
- Körperliche Aktivitätsprogramme zur Verbesserung der Muskelkraft und Beweglichkeit (A)
- Aerobic-Aktivitätsprogramme zur Verbesserung der Gehstrecke, der Ausdauer und der Lebensqualität (A)
- Widerstandstraining zur Verbesserung von Geschwindigkeit und Ausdauer (B)
- Motorisches Training, um neuromuskuloskelettale und bewegungsbezogene Funktionen sowie motorische und planerische Fertigkeiten wiederherzustellen (I)

Idiopathisches Parkinsonsyndrom

Beteiligung an Übungen und körperlicher Aktivität zur Verbesserung der Performanzfertigkeiten und der Betätigungsperformanz
- Mehrere Sitzungen, repetitive körperliche Übungen (diachron) zur Verbesserung motorischer und sensorisch-perzeptiver Performanzfertigkeiten (A oder B)
- Spezialisiert gestaltete Übungen oder intensivere aufgabenspezifische Übungen (diachron), um die Performanz mehr als bei gewöhnlichen gestalteten Übungen oder weniger intensivem Training zu verbessern (C)
- Single-Task-Interventionen in einer Sitzung zur Unterstützung der Entwicklung von Fertigkeiten (C)

Betätigungsperformanz
- Umweltreize (Hinweise aus der Umgebung), Stimuli und unterstützende Objekte zur Verbesserung der Aufgaben- und Betätigungsperformanz (B)
- Auditorische rhythmische externe Hinweise (Cues), die dabei helfen, das Gehen bei IPS zu regulieren. Visuelle, taktile oder andere Formen von Hinweisen sind weniger effektiv (B)
- Vom Klienten bevorzugte externe Hinweise während ADLs, um die motorische Kontrolle zu verbessern (B)
- Individualisierte Interventionen, die sich auf Wellness, Lebensstilmodifikation und persönliche Kontrolle konzentrieren, um die Lebensqualität zu verbessern (B)
- Komplexe und multimodale Aktivitäten (zum Beispiel Tango tanzen) zur Verbesserung der funktionellen Bewegung auf kurzfristiger Basis (B)
- Tai-Chi zur Verbesserung der motorischen und posturalen Performanzfertigkeiten bei IPS (C)
- Multimodale körperliche Aktivität zur Verbesserung der kognitiven Performanz, insbesondere der exekutiven Funktionen (C)
- Vermeidung von ablenkenden Umwelteinflüssen, welche die Aufmerksamkeit teilen oder von der primären Aufgabe ablenken oder negative Emotionen hervorrufen (D)

Amyotrophe Lateralsklerose
- Heimtrainingsprogramme für tägliches Dehnen und Widerstandsübungen verbessert das funktionelle Outcome ohne Nebenwirkungen (B)
- Die Teilnahme an einem multidisziplinären Programm verbessert das Überleben im Vergleich zur üblichen Versorgung (C bis B)
- Ein überwachtes Trainingsprogramm ist besser als ein Heimtrainingsprogramm für den Erhalt der Funktionsfähigkeit (C)
- Die Teilnahme an einem multidisziplinären Programm führt prozentual zu einer besseren Versorgung mit geeigneten Hilfsmitteln und zu einer höheren Lebensqualität in den Sozialfunktionen und der psychischen Gesundheit als eine allgemeine Versorgung (C)
- Eine einfache Bedienung und der Komfort erhöhen die Zufriedenheit mit dem Elektrorollstuhl; mögliche Ausstattungsmerkmale eines Elektrorollstuhles sind: in Neigung und Kippung verstellbare Kopf-, Nacken-, Rumpf- und Armstützen; Beinstützen elektrisch verstellbar; Geschwindigkeit durch einen Joystick verstellbar; Luft- oder Gelkissen; weiche Kopfstütze; Sicherheitsgurt; höhenverstellbare flache, Gel- oder geformte Armlehnen (C)
- Elektrorollstühle erleichtern die Teilnahme an Aktivitäten im Vergleich zu manuellen Rollstühlen (C)
- Manuelle Rollstühle bieten eine einfachere Portabilität als die PWCs (C)
- Ein hoher Nützlichkeitsgrad und Zufriedenheit werden für erhöhte Toilettensitze, WG-Griffe, Duschsitze, Duschstangen, Slip-on-Schuhe, Knöchelstütze und Rutschbretter berichtet (C)
- Ein hoher Zufriedenheitsgrad, jedoch eine geringe Nutzungsfrequenz werden für schall- oder sprachaktivierte Umweltkontrollen und Kommunikationshilfen berichtet (C)
- Ein geringer Nützlichkeits- und Zufriedenheitsgrad werden für Knopflochhilfen, Ankleidehilfen und verlängerte Greifwerkzeuge berichtet (C)
- Telemedizin wird als nützlich und befriedigend für Klienten mit ALS beschrieben, abgesehen von Diskussionen über psychologische und emotionale Bedenken (C)
- Ein Computerprogramm zum Schreiben von Nachrichten, Auswahl von Liedern und Videos über eine virtuelle Tastatur und einen Mikroschalter werden als nützlich erachtet (I)
- Elektrische Stimulation kann die bilaterale Handfunktion und die Kniestreckung verbessern (I)
- Wassertherapie ist hilfreich, um die Energie zu erhöhen, und reduziert die notwendige Unterstützung für Transfers nach der Therapie (I)
- *Sling back* (Rückengurte) und *sling seats* (Schlingenauflagen) sind für Rollstuhlfahrer nicht hilfreich oder befriedigend (D)

5 Schlussfolgerung für Praxis, Ausbildung und Forschung

5.1 Schlussfolgerung für die Praxis

Ergotherapeutische Ausbildungsprogramme haben in der Vergangenheit dazu geführt, dass Ergotherapeuten und Ergotherapie-Assistenten effektive Therapeuten bei der Arbeit mit Klienten mit NDK geworden sind. Folgende Empfehlungen gelten für die Weiterentwicklung der ergotherapeutischen und ergotherapeutischen Assistenzausbildung:
- Fähigkeiten der Studierenden weiterentwickeln, damit diese die Evidenz nutzen und die Praxis informieren,
- Studierende, die Interesse an der Forschung haben, ermutigen, eine zusätzliche Weiterbildung oder eine Höherqualifizierung in Erwägung zu ziehen (zum Beispiel PhD, Postdoc-Studium),
- Inhalte über das Altern bei chronischen Erkrankungen lehren, einschließlich Fallstudien von Klienten, die mit NDK altern. Diese Inhalte sollten Möglichkeiten für die Studierenden beinhalten, die Rolle der Ergotherapie in Bezug auf Wellness und Habilitation zu verstehen und anzuerkennen.
- Studierenden, die an der Arbeit mit Klienten mit NDK interessiert sind, Möglichkeiten zur Entwicklung von Kenntnissen und Fertigkeiten anbieten, welche sie bei der Arbeit mit dieser Bevölkerungsgruppe unterstützen (zum Beispiel evidenzbasierte Neurorehabilitationskurse, Möglichkeiten der Feldarbeit bei Klienten mit NDK in traditionellen und gemeinschaftsbasierten Einrichtungen oder Organisationen),
- Studierende anleiten, evidenzbasierte Ressourcen wie etwa Praxisleitlinien zu verwenden, um ihre Entscheidungen in der Praxis besser fundieren zu können.

5.2 Schlussfolgerung für die Ausbildung

Die systematischen Reviews zur Klientenforschung mit NDK untersuchten die Wirksamkeit von Interventionen im Rahmen der Ergotherapie. Folgende Empfehlungen gelten für die Weiterentwicklung der bewährten Verfahren (Best Practice):
- Nach Möglichkeit evidenzbasierte, standardisierte Assessments und Erhebungsinstrumente verwenden, um Klienten mit NDK zu evaluieren und die Ergebnisse der ergotherapeutischen Intervention zu bestimmen. Zum Beispiel können Ergotherapeuten das *COPM* (Law et al., 2005) verwenden, um die Bereiche der Betätigung zu beurteilen; das *Assessment of Motor and Process Skills* zur Erhebung der Performanzfertigkeiten; das *OPHI-II* (Kielhofner et al., 2004), um ein Verständnis von einigen Aspekten der Performanzmuster zu erhalten, das *Safety Assessment of Function and the Environment for Rehabilitation* (Oliver, Blathwayt, Brackley & Tamaki, 1993), um Informationen über den Kontext und die Umgebung zu sammeln und Assessments wie der *Nine-Hole Peg Test* (Kellor, Frost, Silberberg, Iversen & Cummings, 1971), manuelle Muskeltests oder die *Berg-Balance-Scale* (Berg, Wood-Dauphinee, Williams & Gayton, 1989) zur Evaluation der Klientenfaktoren. Weitere ausgewählte Assessments für Klienten mit NDK finden Sie in der Tabelle 3-1.
- Nach Möglichkeit evidenzbasierte Interventionen verwenden, um den Nutzen der ergotherapeutischen Dienstleistung für die Klienten zu maximieren. Beispielsweise unterstützt die Evidenz für Interventionen für Klienten mit MS am stärksten:
  - Face-to-Face- und telefonbasierte Fatigue-Management-Programme in Gruppen
  - Multidisziplinäre Rehabilitation in einer Variation von Interventionsumgebungen

- Interventionen zur Emotionsregulation und
- körperliche Aktivitätsprogramme (zum Beispiel Widerstandstraining [resistives Training], Aerobicübungen, Yoga, Pilates) für Klienten mit leichter und moderater MS.
- Die Evidenz für Interventionen für Klienten mit IPS unterstützt am stärksten:
  - Mehrere Sitzungen, repetitive körperliche Übungsaufgaben und Aktivitätslernen
  - Übungsprogramme
  - Komplexes, multimodales Aktivitätentraining
  - Umweltkontext und Cue-Strukturierung
  - Vom Klienten bevorzugte externe Cues und
  - Selbstmanagement von Gesundheit und Wellness.
- Die Evidenz für Interventionen für Klienten mit ALS unterstützt am stärksten:
  - Heimübungsprogramme mit täglichem Dehnen und Widerstandsübungen und
  - Multidisziplinäre Programme (gegenüber üblicher Versorgung).

Weitere Informationen zu diesen und anderen Interventionen finden sich im Unterkapitel *Interventionen* und in den Evidenztabellen für jede NDK.
- Weitere Titel der Reihe *Leitlinien der Ergotherapie* lesen, um in der Praxis über Klienten mit NDK zu informieren. Zum Beispiel kann die *Leitlinie der Ergotherapie* für Klienten mit *Alzheimer-Krankheit* (Schaber, 2010)[5] nützlich für die Verwendung mit Klienten mit IPS-bezogener Demenz sein. Die Inhalte anderer Praxisleitlinien können ebenfalls für Klienten mit NDK relevant sein wie zum Beispiel *Wohnraumanpassung*[6], *Fahr- und Gemeindemobilität*[7] und *Aktives Altern zu Hause*[8].
- Eine Zusammenarbeit mit Forschern erwägen, um klinisch relevante Forschung zu generieren.

Spezifischere Empfehlungen, basierend auf den Ergebnissen der systematischen Reviews zu Klienten mit NDK, befinden sich in der **Tabelle 4-1**.

5.3 Schlussfolgerung für die Forschung

Es existiert eine wachsende Anzahl an Literatur, die den Einsatz von ergotherapeutischen Interventionen für Menschen mit NDK unterstützt. Die Ergebnisse des systematischen Reviews zeigen Bereiche, in denen die Literatur ergotherapeutische Interventionen unterstützt, sowie Bereiche, in denen zusätzliche Forschung benötigt wird. Auf der Grundlage einer Analyse der aktuellen Literatur werden folgende Maßnahmen zur Förderung der besten fachlichen Praxis empfohlen:
- Die Beziehung zwischen den Klientenfaktoren und der Betätigungsperformanz eruieren: Einige Studien zeigten eine Verbesserung der Klientenfaktoren (zum Beispiel Gedächtnis), die Beziehung zwischen den Klientenfaktoren und der Betätigungsperformanz ist jedoch noch nicht gut belegt.
- Mehr zielgerichtete Studien durchführen, um die Aktivitätsperformanz und die Teilhabe zu maximieren.
- Weitere Studien durchführen, die sich auf Wellness, Aufrechterhaltung der Funktion und gesundes Leben mit einer chronischen Erkrankung konzentrieren (zum Beispiel gesundheitliche Selbstmanagementprogramme): Aufgrund bevorstehender Änderungen im Gesundheitssystem wird die Habilitation ein wichtiger Schwerpunkt sein. Mehr Evidenz für Wellness- und Erhaltungsmaßnahmen wird der Ergotherapie in Zukunft helfen, eine wichtige Rolle zu spielen.
- Die langfristigen Auswirkungen von Interventionen untersuchen: Obwohl einige Studien die Teilnehmer über einen längeren Zeitraum begleiten, untersuchten viele Studien nur die kurzfristigen Auswirkungen von Interventionen. Es sind mehr qualitativ hochwertige Studien erforderlich, um festzustellen, wie lange die Effekte von ergotherapeutischen Interventionen anhalten und ob durch eine zusätzliche Therapie (zum Beispiel *Booster*) die Effekte über einen längeren Zeitraum hinweg aufrechterhalten bleiben. Aufgrund von fortschreitenden Verläufen der NDK ist es wichtig, dass Forscher geeignete Ergebnisse für Interventionen in Betracht ziehen, welche die Aufrechterhaltung oder sogar die Verlangsamung des Krankheitsfortschritts einschließen.
- Die Anzahl der Studien erhöhen, die sich auf ergotherapeutische Interventionen konzentrieren: Forschung in multidisziplinären Teams ist wichtig, aber es wäre auch vorteilhaft für den Beruf,

---

5 Diese Leitlinie erscheint in der deutschen Übersetzung ebenfalls im Juni 2018 im Hogrefe Verlag.
6 Diese Leitlinie ist in der deutschen Übersetzung im Oktober 2017 im Hogrefe Verlag erschienen.
7 Diese Leitlinie erscheint in der deutschen Übersetzung wahrscheinlich in 2019 im Hogrefe Verlag.
8 Diese Leitlinie erscheint in der deutschen Übersetzung ebenfalls im Juni 2018 im Hogrefe Verlag.

dass eine stärkere Evidenz für ergotherapeutische Interventionen vorliegt.
- Die Probleme im Zusammenhang mit älteren Menschen mit NDK berücksichtigen: Angesichts einer alternden Gesellschaft in den USA muss sich der Schwerpunkt unseres Gesundheitssystems von einem Modell für die akute Versorgung auf ein Modell für die Langzeitpflege verlagern. Ergotherapeuten können angesichts dieser Schwerpunktverlagerung eine Schlüsselrolle spielen. Wenn eine stärkere Evidenz vorliegt, werden Ergotherapeuten besser in der Lage sein, ihre Rolle und Interventionen zu positionieren.
- In allen Studien konsistente Erhebungsinstrumente verwenden, um bessere Vergleiche zu ermöglichen.
- Die Zusammenarbeit zwischen Forschern und praktisch tätigen Ergotherapeuten berücksichtigen, um klinisch relevante Forschung zu generieren.
- Das Ziel verfolgen, einen hohen Level der Evidenz zu generieren, insbesondere Metaanalysen, systematische Reviews und RCTs.

6 Anhänge

A Vorbereitung und Qualifikationen von Ergotherapeuten und Ergotherapie-Assistenten

Wer sind Ergotherapeuten?
Um als Ergotherapeutin zu praktizieren, hat die Person in den Vereinigten Staaten:
- das vom Accreditation Council for Occupational Therapy Education (ACOTE®) bzw. seinen Vorgängerorganisationen zertifizierte ergotherapeutische Programm absolviert;
- erfolgreich einen Zeit lang Praxiserfahrung unter Begleitung eines erfahrenden Ergotherapeuten gesammelt in einer dafür anerkannten Bildungseinrichtung, die den akademischen Anforderungen an ein Bildungsprogramm für Ergotherapeuten, das durch die ACOTE bzw. Vorgängerorganisationen zertifiziert worden ist, anerkannt wurde;
- hat einen national anerkannten Aufnahmetest für Ergotherapeuten bestanden; und
- erfüllt die staatlichen Anforderungen für die Zulassung, Zertifizierung bzw. Registrierung.

Bildungsprogramme für Ergotherapeuten
Diese beinhalten Folgendes:
- Biologie, Physische-, Sozial- und Verhaltenswissenschaften
- Grundprinzipien der Ergotherapie
- Theoretische Perspektiven der Ergotherapie
- Screening-Erfassung
- Formulierung und Implementierung eines Interventionsplanes
- Kontext von Berufsausübung
- Management der ergotherapeutischen Dienste (Master-Abschluss)
- Mitarbeiterführung und Management (Doktorabschluss)
- Berufsethik, Werte und Verantwortlichkeiten

Die praktische Arbeit als Bestandteil des Programmes wurde dafür entworfen, kompetente und generalistische Berufseinsteiger in der ergotherapeutischen Ausbildung zu entwickeln, indem eine Vielzahl an Erfahrung über Klienten aller Altersgruppen in einer Vielzahl von Behandlungssettings vermittelt wird. Die praktische Arbeit ist ein integraler Bestandteil des Curriculums des Kurses, beinhaltet vertiefte Erfahrung in der Anwendung von ergotherapeutischer Behandlung gegenüber Klienten und fokussiert die Anwendung von zielgerichteter und aussagekräftiger Betätigung beziehungsweise Forschung, Administration und Management von ergotherapeutischen Dienstleistungen. Die Erfahrungen aus der praktischen Arbeit dienen der Förderung des Clinical Reasoning und der reflektierenden Praxis, um die Werte und Vorstellungen, die die ethische Praxis ermöglichen, zu leiten und Professionalismus sowie Kompetenzen in Karrierezuständigkeiten zu entwickeln. Von Doktoranden wird verlangt, eine empirische Untersuchung durchzuführen, die sie in die Lage versetzt, erweiterte Kompetenzen, über das generalistische Niveau hinaus, zu entwickeln.

Wer sind Ergotherapie-Assistenten?
Um als Ergotherapie-Assistent zu arbeiten, hat die Person in den Vereinigten Staaten:
- das vom ACOTE bzw. seinen Vorgängerorganisationen zertifizierte Programm für Ergotherapie-Assistenten absolviert
- erfolgreich einen Zeit lang Praxiserfahrung unter Begleitung eines erfahrenden Ergotherapeuten gesammelt in einer dafür anerkannten Bildungseinrichtung, die den akademischen Anforderungen an ein Bildungsprogramm für Ergotherapeuten, das durch die ACOTE bzw. Vorgängerorganisationen zertifiziert worden ist, anerkannt wurde
- einen national anerkannten Aufnahmetest für Ergotherapeuten bestanden und

- erfüllt die staatlichen Anforderungen für die Zulassung, Zertifizierung bzw. Registrierung.

Bildungsprogramme für den Ergotherapie-Assistenten

Diese beinhalten Folgendes:
- Biologie, Physische-, Sozial- und Verhaltenswissenschaften
- Grundprinzipien der Ergotherapie
- Theoretische Perspektiven der Ergotherapie
- Screening-Erfassung
- Formulierung und Implementierung eines Interventionsplanes
- Kontext von Berufsausübung
- Assistenz im Organisieren von Ergotherapie

Die praktische Arbeit als Bestandteil des Programmes wurde dafür entworfen, kompetente und generalistische Berufseinsteiger in der ergotherapeutischen Ausbildung zu entwickeln, indem eine Vielzahl an Erfahrung über Klienten aller Altersgruppen in einer Vielzahl von Behandlungssettings vermittelt wird. Die praktische Arbeit ist ein integraler Bestandteil des Curriculums von dem Kurs und beinhaltet vertiefte Erfahrung in der Anwendung von ergotherapeutischer Behandlung gegenüber Klienten und fokussiert die Anwendung von zielgerichteter und aussagekräftiger Betätigung. Die Erfahrungen aus der praktischen Arbeit dienen der Förderung des Clinical Reasoning und der reflektierenden Praxis, um die Werte und Vorstellungen, die die ethische Praxis ermöglichen, zu leiten und Professionalismus sowie Kompetenzen in Karrierezuständigkeiten zu entwickeln.

Regulierung der ergotherapeutischen Praxis

Alle Ergotherapeuten und Ergotherapie-Assistenten müssen nach föderalem und staatlichem Gesetz agieren. Derzeit haben 50 Staaten, der District of Columbia, Puerto Rico und Guam Gesetze zur Regulierung der ergotherapeutischen Praxis beschlossen.

B Selected CPT TM Codes ...

The following chart can guide occupational practitioners in making clinically appropriate decisions when selecting the most relevant *CPT*^{TM} code to describe occupational therapy evaluation and intervention for adults with neurodegenerative diseases. Occupational therapy practitioners should use the most appropriate code from the current *CPT* manual, on the basis of specific services provided, individual patient goals, payer coding and billing policy, and common usage.

Examples of Occupational Therapy Evaluation and Intervention	Suggested *CPT* Code
Evaluation	
Encompasses the initial evaluation of patient status and performance in occupations, performance skills, performance patterns, context and environment, and/or client factors. • Initial evaluation includes an occupational profile and use of standardized and nonstandardized assessments. (See Table 2 for examples.)	97003—Occupational therapy evaluation.
Formal reassessment of changes in condition and/or performance in occupations, performance skills, performance patterns, context and environment, and/or client factors in order to determine progress and to identify needed modifications to the intervention plan. • Reevaluation using standardized and/or nonstandardized assessments. (See Table 2 for examples.)	97004—Occupational therapy reevaluation.

(Continued)

Examples of Occupational Therapy Evaluation and Intervention	Suggested *CPT* Code
Specialized testing of neurocognition, including individual mental functions (e.g., attention, memory) and global mental functions (e.g., consciousness, orientation). • Qualified health professional time for administration and interpretation of standardized cognitive assessments and preparation of the report.	**96125**—Standardized cognitive performance testing (e.g., Ross Information Processing Assessment) per hour of a qualified health care professional's time, both face-to-face time administering tests to the patient and time interpreting these test results and preparing the report.
• Participate in a medical team conference as part of a diagnostic-evaluation team that discusses the evaluation findings, diagnoses, and recommendations with a patient and his or her family.	**99366**—Medical team conference with interdisciplinary team of health care professionals, face-to-face with patient and/or family, 30 minutes or more; participation by nonphysician qualified health care professional.
• Participate in a medical team conference as part of a diagnostic-evaluation team that reviews evaluation findings and clarifies diagnostic considerations and recommendations before meeting with a client and his or her family.	**99368**—Medical team conference with interdisciplinary team of health care professionals, patient and/or family not present, for 30 minutes or more; participation by nonphysician qualified health care professional.
• Assess body structure and functions that influence feeding, eating, and environmental positioning; and/or physical and cognitive problems the affect feeding, eating, and swallowing.	**92610–92612**—Clinical evaluation of swallowing function. (See *CPT* for precise descriptions of possible tests.)
Intervention	
Intervene to restore client factors (including strength, endurance, and flexibility and active, assistive, and passive range of motion) using exercises such as progressive resistive; prolonged stretch; isokinetic, isotonic, or isometric strengthening; or close-changed kinetic. • Develop individualized exercise program for physical skill development necessary for returning to work and instruction in a home exercise program to maintain strength and range of motion gained during skilled therapy. • Design and train in an individualized exercise program, for example, to improve strength and range of motion in order to participate in desired occupations (e.g., gardening).	**97110**—Therapeutic procedure, one or more areas, each 15 minutes; therapeutic exercises to develop strength and endurance, range of motion, and flexibility.
Intervene using neuromuscular reeducation and neurorehabilitation approaches. • Use motor relearning principles to design graded tasks to increase coordination and balance that facilitate participation in a desired occupation (e.g., making a meal). • Use motor relearning principles to design graded activities that improve standing balance during upright activities to reduce risk of fall.	**97112**—Therapeutic procedure, one or more areas, each 15 minutes; neuromuscular reeducation of movement, balance, coordination, kinesthetic sense, posture, and/or proprioception for sitting and/or standing activities.
• Design and train in a daily aquatics exercise program to improve function. • Train in an aquatic maintenance program to be completed in the community (e.g., at a public pool or health club).	**97113**—Aquatic therapeutic procedure, one or more areas, each 15 minutes; aquatic therapy with therapeutic exercises.

(Continued)

Examples of Occupational Therapy Evaluation and Intervention	Suggested *CPT* Code
• Use selected individualized therapeutic activities as an intervention to improve performance of specific functional tasks. • Develop and train individual in use of specific activities (e.g., hobbies, guided imagery, relaxation techniques) to reduce stress and increase ability to function in his or her home and community environment.	**97530**—Therapeutic activities, direct (one-on-one) patient contact by the provider (use of dynamic activities to improve functional performance), each 15 minutes.
• Design and train in the use of a computerized cognitive training program to improve attention. • Develop and instruct in the use of smartphone applications to compensate for memory deficits, to facilitate participation in work activities. • Provide strategies that can be used to increase accuracy and efficiency of recall and attention, and compensate for cognitive problems through role-playing instruction in strategies to cope with social interactions.	**97532**—Cognitive development of cognitive skills to improve attention, memory, problem solving (includes compensatory training), direct (one-on-one) patient contact by the provider, each 15 minutes.
• Develop and instruct in compensatory strategies for completion of daily home management activities such as meal preparation and doing laundry. • Train in methods of adapting bathing routine and habits to improve safety and independence for bathing tasks.	**97535**—Self-care and home management training (e.g., activities of daily living [ADLs] and compensatory training; meal preparation; safety procedures; and instructions in use of assistive technology devices and adaptive equipment), direct one-on-one contact by provider, each 15 minutes.
• Teach community mobility skills using public or alternative transportation methods. • Instruct in driving retraining skills to help compensate for visual impairment.	**97537**—Community and work reintegration training (e.g., shopping, transportation, money management, avocational activities, work environment modification analysis, work task analysis, use of assistive technology devices and adaptive equipment), direct one-on-one contact by provider, each 15 minutes.
• Direct group activities for 2 or more clients to support a common goal, such as learning to manage fatigue. • Provide training to small group focusing on disease self-management.	**97150**—Therapeutic procedure(s), group (2 or more individuals). Group therapy procedures involve constant attendance of the physician or therapist, but by definition do not require one-on-one patient contact by the physician or therapist.
• Assess, fit, and train in the use of a wrist splint to compensate for weak wrist extensors and facilitate effective hand positioning during functional tasks.	**97760**—Orthotic(s) management and training (including assessment and fitting when not otherwise reported), upper extremity(ies), lower extremity(ies), and/or trunk, each 15 minutes.
• Assess needs for specialized mobility equipment, such as power wheelchairs or scooters, for community mobility. • Provide recommendations for wheelchair modifications to ensure optimal sitting posture to maintain skin integrity, prevent pressure sores, and facilitate performance in ADLs and IADLs.	**97542**—Wheelchair management (e.g., assessment, fitting, training), each 15 minutes.
• Train in the use of compensatory strategies, appropriate positioning, adaptive equipment, and food textures to maximize oral intake and nutritional status.	**92526**—Treatment of swallowing dysfunction and/or oral function for feeding.

(Continued)

Examples of Occupational Therapy Evaluation and Intervention	Suggested *CPT* Code
• Provide joint mobilization to the wrist and fingers to maintain play and joint integrity to grasp task items such as utensils, pens, and toothbrush.	**97140**—Manual therapy techniques (e.g., mobilization, manipulation, manual lymphatic drainage, manual traction), in one or more regions, each 15 minutes.

Note. Not all payers will reimburse for all codes. For example, medical team conferences are not billable to Medicare but may be useful for reporting productivity. Codes shown refer to *CPT* 2014 (American Medical Association, 2013) and do not represent all of the possible codes that may be used in occupational therapy evaluation and intervention. Refer to *CPT* 2014 for the complete list of available codes. *CPT* codes are updated annually and become effective January 1. *CPT*™ is a trademark of the American Medical Association. *Current Procedural Terminology* five-digit codes, two-digit codes, modifiers, and descriptions only are copyright © 2013 by the American Medical Association. All rights reserved.

C Evidenzbasierte Praxis

Ergotherapeuten und Ergotherapie-Assistenten sehen sich, wie viele andere Gesundheitsberufe auch, zunehmend mit den Anforderungen von Kostenträgern, Regulierungsbehörden und Konsumenten konfrontiert, klinische Wirksamkeit zu beweisen. Zudem sind sie bemüht, Dienstleistungen anzubieten, die klientenzentriert und evidenzbasiert sind und effizient und kosteneffektiv erbracht werden. Seit 25 Jahren gilt die evidenzbasierte Praxis (EBP) als ein Ansatz, die Effektitvität von Gesundheitsdienstleistungen zu gewährleisten.

Seit 1998 hat der amerikanische Ergotherapie-Verband (AOTA) eine Reihe von EBP-Projekten durchgeführt, um die Mitglieder bei der Herausforderung zu unterstützen, Literatur zu finden und zu prüfen, um Wirksamkeitsnachweise ausfindig zu machen, und diese Evidenz im Gegenzug für eine informierte Praxis zu nutzen (Lieberman & Scheer, 2002). Die AOTA-Projekte, die dem Evidenzverständnis von Sackett, Rosenberg, Muir Gray, Haynes und Richardson (1996) folgen, basieren auf dem Grundsatz, dass die EBP in der Ergotherapie auf der Integration von Informationen aus drei Quellen beruht:
- Klinische Erfahrung und Reasoning
- Vorlieben von Klienten und ihren Familien und
- Ergebnisse der besten verfügbaren Forschung.

Ein Schwerpunkt der AOTA-EBP-Projekte ist ein Programm, bei dem fortlaufend und systematisch die multidisziplinäre wissenschaftliche Literatur geprüft wird. Dazu werden gebündelte Fragen und ein standardisiertes Prozedere genutzt, um praxisrelevante Evidenz zu finden, die dann bezüglich ihrer Auswirkungen auf Praxis, Ausbildung und Forschung diskutiert wird. Eine evidenzbasierte Perspektive gründet auf der Annahme, dass wissenschaftliche Nachweise für die Wirksamkeit von ergotherapeutischen Interventionen als mehr oder weniger aussagekräftig und valide bewertet werden können, entsprechend der hierarchischen Einteilung von Forschungsdesigns, einer Bewertung der Studienqualität oder beidem. Die AOTA nutzt einen an der evidenzbasierten Medizin orientierten Evidenzstandard. Dieses Modell standardisiert und ordnet den Wert wissenschaftlicher Belege aus der Biomedizin, nach dem abgestuften System, das auf der Arbeit von Sackett et al. (1996) basiert. In diesem System umfasst das höchste Level der Evidenz, Level-I, systematische Reviews, Meta-Analysen und randomisierte kontrollierte Studien (RCT). In RCT werden die Teilnehmer per Randomisierung (Zufallsprinzip) entweder der Interventionsgruppe oder der Kontrollgruppe zugewiesen. Die Outcomes beider Gruppen werden verglichen. Andere Evidenzlevel umfassen Level-II Studien, bei denen die Zuordnung zur Behandlungs- oder Kontrollgruppe nicht zufällig erfolgt (Kohortenstudie); Level-III Studien, die keine Kontrollgruppe haben; Level-IV Studien mit experimentellem Einzelfall-Design, was manchmal genutzt wird, um über mehrere Teilnehmer zu berichten und Level-V Studien, welche Fallstudien und Expertenmeinungen sind, die narrative Literaturreviews sowie Konsensus-Statements enthalten.

Die systematischen Reviews zu neurodegenerativen Erkrankungen wurden von der AOTA im Rahmen des EBP-Projektes unterstützt. Die AOTA verpflichtet sich, die Rolle der Ergotherapie in diesem wichtigen Bereich der Praxis zu unterstützen. Frühere Reviews wurden für den Zeitraum von 1985-2002 durchgeführt. Die aktuellen systematischen Reviews wurden für den Zeitraum von 2003-2011 aktualisiert. Praktisch tätige Ergotherapeuten benötigen für die Auswahl von ergotherapeutischen Interventionen ei-

Tabelle C-1: Evidenzlevels der Resultate in der ergotherapeutischen Forschung

Evidenzlevel	Definition
I	Systematische Übersichten, Meta-Analysen, randomisierte kontrollierte Versuche
II	Zwei Gruppen, nicht randomisierte Untersuchungen (zum Beispiel Kohorten, Fall-Kontroll-Studien)
III	Eine Gruppe, nicht randomisiert (zum Beispiel vorher-nachher, Prätest und Posttest)
IV	Beschreibende Studien mit Analyse der Resultate (zum Beispiel Einzelfallstudien, Fallserien)
V	Fallbeschreibungen und Meinungen der Experten mit beschreibenden Literaturübersichten und konsensgestützten Empfehlungen

Quelle: Aus „Evidence-Based Medicine: What It Is and What It Isn't," von D.L. Sackett, W.M. Rosenberg, J.A. Muir Gray, R.B. Haynes, & W.S. Richardson, 1996, British Medical Journal, 312, pp. 71–72. Copyright © 1996 durch die British Medical Association. Angepasst mit Erlaubnis.

nen Zugriff auf die Ergebnisse der neusten und besten verfügbaren Literatur. Die vier Fokusfragen welche für die Überarbeitung der Reviews entwickelt wurden, basieren auf den Suchstrategien der vorangegangenen Reviews. Diese Fragen wurden von den Review-Autoren, einer Beratergruppe von Experten auf diesem Gebiet, AOTA Mitarbeitern und dem Berater des AOTA-EBP-Projektes überprüft.

Fokusfragen

Die folgenden vier Fokusfragen aus den Reviews von ergotherapeutischen Interventionen für Klienten mit neurodegenerativen Erkrankungen bilden den Rahmen des Reviews:

- Wie wirksam sind Interventionen im Rahmen der ergotherapeutischen Praxis bei Menschen mit Multipler Sklerose (MS)?
- Wie wirksam sind Interventionen im Rahmen der ergotherapeutischen Praxis bei Menschen mit Parkinson-Krankheit (IPS)?
- Wie wirksam sind Interventionen im Rahmen der ergotherapeutischen Praxis bei Menschen mit amyotropher Lateralsklerose (ALS)?
- Wie wirksam sind Interventionen im Rahmen der ergotherapeutischen Praxis bei Menschen mit transverser Myelitis (TM)?

Methodik

Die Suchbegriffe für die Reviews wurden vom methodischen Berater des AOTA-EBP-Projekts und den AOTA-Mitarbeitern in Absprache mit den Autoren der einzelnen systematischen Reviews entwickelt und von der Beratergruppe überprüft. Die Suchbegriffe wurden nicht nur entwickelt, um relevante Artikel zu erfassen, sondern auch um sicherzustellen, dass die für den spezifischen Thesaurus der jeweiligen Datenbank relevanten Begriffe enthalten sind. Die **Tabelle C-2** listet die in dem jeweiligen Review eingeschlossen Suchbegriffe zu Population und Intervention auf. Ein medizinischer Forschungsbibliothekar mit Erfahrung in der Durchführung systematischer Reviews führte alle Recherchen durch und bestätigte und verbesserte die Suchstrategien. Eingeschlossene Datenbanken und Websites sind Medline, PsycINFO, CINAHL, AgeLine und OTseeker. Darüber hinaus wurden konsolidierte Informationsquellen wie die *Cochrane Database of Systematic Reviews* und die *Campbell Collaboration* in die Suche einbezogen. Diese Datenbanken sind Zusammenfassungen von peer-reviewten Zeitschriftenartikeln. Diese bieten ein System zur Durchführung von evidenzbasierten Reviews zu ausgewählten klinischen Fragen und Themen für Kliniker und Wissenschaftler. Darüber hinaus wurden Referenzlisten von Artikeln, welche in die systematischen Reviews eingeschlossen wurden, auf potenzielle Artikel untersucht. Zudem wurden ausgewählte Zeitschriften von Hand durchsucht, um sicherzustellen, dass alle geeigneten Artikel enthalten waren.

Einschluss- und Ausschlusskriterien sind für den systematischen Reviewprozess von entscheidender Bedeutung, da sie die Struktur für die Qualität, den Typ und die Jahre der Veröffentlichung der Literatur bereitstellen, die in ein Review eingeschlossen sind. Die Reviews der vier Fragen beschränkten sich auf wissenschaftliche peer-reviewte Literatur, die in englischer Sprache veröffentlicht wurde. Die untersuchten Interventionsansätze lagen im Bereich der Ergotherapie. Die in den Reviews enthaltene Literatur wurde zwischen 2003 und 2011 veröffentlicht und umfasste Studienteilnehmer mit neurodegenerativen Erkrankungen (MS, IPS, ALS, TM).

Die vorhergehenden Reviews umfassten Studien, die zwischen 1985 und 2002 veröffentlicht wurden. Die Überprüfung schloss Daten von Präsentationen, Konferenzberichten, nicht peer-reviewter Forschungsliteratur, Dissertationen und Abschlussarbeiten aus. Studien, die in die Reviews eingeschlossen wurden, sind auf den Evidenzlevel-I, II und III. Studien auf dem Evidenzlevel-IV und V wurden nur aufgenommen, wenn zu einem bestimmten Thema keine höheren Evidenz gefunden wurde. Insgesamt wurden 11 672 Zitate und Abstracts in die Reviews eingeschlossen. Für die Frage zu MS gab es 3 484 Referenzen; für die Frage zu IPS gab es 4 061 Referenzen; für die Frage zu ALS gab es 872 Referenzen; und für die Frage zu TM gab es 149 Referenzen.

Der Berater des EBP- Projekts vervollständigte den ersten Schritt der Eliminierung von Referenzen auf der Basis von Zitaten und Abstracts. Alle Artikel wurden aus dem ursprünglichen TM-Review ausgeschlossen, da keine in den Anwendungsbereich der ergotherapeutischen Praxis fiel und die Ergebnisse des Reviews in den Praxisleitlinien nicht behandelt werden. Die systematischen Reviews für IPS und MS wurden als akademische Partnerschaften durchgeführt. Es wurde mit akademischen Fakultäten mit graduierten Studenten zusammengearbeitet, um die Reviews durchzuführen. der systematische Review zu ALS wurde als eine Partnerschaft zwischen dem AOTA-Methodenberater und einem Ergotherapeuten mit Erfahrung in ALS durchgeführt. Die Review-Teams schlossen den nächsten Schritt zur Eliminie-

Tabelle C-2: Suchstrategie für die systematische Reviews zur neurodegenerative Erkrankungen

Kategorie	Suchbegriffe (englisch)	Suchbegriffe (deutsch) Auswahl
Multiple Sklerose		
Population	multiple sclerosis, neurodegenerative	Multiple Sklerose, neurodegenerative Erkrankungen
Intervention	Activities, activities of daily living, assistive devices, assistive equipment, caregiver support, cognitive behavioral therapy, community care, community programs, cognition, disease management, education, emotional regulation, energy conservation, exercise, extended care, fall prevention, fatigue, health maintenance, health promotion, instrumental activities of daily living, intervention, leisure, lifts, mindfulness, mobility, mobility equipment, neurorehabilitation, nonmotor symptoms, occupational therapy, physical therapy, physiotherapy, programs, quality of life, rehabilitation, scooters, self-management, services, sleep, social engagement, therapy, treatment, walkers, wellness programs, wheelchairs, work, yoga.	Aktivitäten, Aktivitäten des täglichen Lebens, Hilfsmittel, Ausrüstung, unterstützende Betreuung, kognitive Verhaltenstherapie, ambulante Pflege, Gemeindepflege, Gemeindeprogramme, Kognition, Disease Management, Krankheitsbewältigung, Bildung, emotionale Regulation, Energieerhalt, Übung, ergänzende Betreuung, Sturzprophylaxe, Fatigue, Gesunderhaltung, Gesundheitsunterstützung, instrumentelle Aktivitäten des täglichen Lebens, Intervention, Freizeit, Lift, Achtsamkeit, Mobilität, Mobilitätsausrüstung, Neurorehabilitation, Begleitsymptome, Ergotherapie, Physiotherapie, Körpertherapie, programme, Lebensqualität, Rehabilitation, Motorroller, Selbstmanagement, Diesntleistungen, Schlaf, soziales Engagement, Therapie, Behandlung, Gehhilfen, Wellness-Programme, Rollstuhl, Arbeit, Yoga
Parkinsonkrankheit		
Population	Parkinson, Parkinsonism, Parkinson's disease, neurodegenerative	Parkinson, Morbus Parkinson, Parkinson Erkrankung, neurodegenerative Erkrankungen
Intervention	Activities, activities of daily living, assistive devices, assistive equipment, caregiver support, cognitive behavioral therapy, community care, community programs, cognition, disease management, education, emotional regulation, exercise, extended care, fall prevention, health maintenance, health promotion, instrumental activities of daily living, intervention, leisure, lifts, mindfulness, mobility, mobility equipment, neurorehabilitation, nonmotor symptoms, occupational therapy, physical therapy, physiotherapy, programs, rhythmic, quality of life, rehabilitation, scooters, self-management, services, sleep, social engagement, therapy, treatment, walkers, wellness programs, wheelchairs, work, yoga.	Aktivitäten, Aktivitäten des täglichen Lebens, Hilfsmittel, Ausrüstung, unterstützende Betreuung, kognitive Verhaltenstherapie, ambulante Pflege, Gemeindepflege, Gemeindeprogramme, Kognition, Disease Management, Krankheitsbewältigung, Bildung, emotionale Regulation, Energieerhalt, Übung, ergänzende Betreuung, Sturzprophylaxe, Fatigue, Gesunderhaltung, Gesundheitsunterstützung, instrumentelle Aktivitäten des täglichen Lebens, Intervention, Freizeit, Lift, Achtsamkeit, Mobilität, Mobilitätsausrüstung, Neurorehabilitation, Begleitsymptome, Ergotherapie, Physiotherapie, Körpertherapie, programme, Lebensqualität, Rehabilitation, Motorroller, Selbstmanagement, Diesntleistungen, Schlaf, soziales Engagement, Therapie, Behandlung, Gehhilfen, Wellness-Programme, Rollstuhl, Arbeit, Yoga
Amyotrophe Lateralsklerose		
Population	amyotrophic lateral sclerosis	Amyotrophe Lateralsklerose
Intervention	Activities, activities of daily living, assistive devices, assistive equipment, caregiver support, cognitive behavioral therapy, community care, community programs, cognition, disease management, education, emotional regulation, exercise, extended care, fall prevention, health maintenance, health promotion, instrumental activities of daily living, intervention, leisure, lifts, mindfulness, mobility, mobility equipment, neurorehabilitation, nonmotor symptoms, occupational therapy, physical therapy, physiotherapy, programs, quality of life, rehabilitation, scooters, self-management, services, sleep, social engagement, therapy, treatment, walkers, wellness programs, wheelchairs, work, yoga.	Aktivitäten, Aktivitäten des täglichen Lebens, Hilfsmittel, Ausrüstung, unterstützende Betreuung, kognitive Verhaltenstherapie, ambulante Pflege, Gemeindepflege, Gemeindeprogramme, Kognition, Disease Management, Krankheitsbewältigung, Bildung, emotionale Regulation, Energieerhalt, Übung, ergänzende Betreuung, Sturzprophylaxe, Fatigue, Gesunderhaltung, Gesundheitsunterstützung, instrumentelle Aktivitäten des täglichen Lebens, Intervention, Freizeit, Lift, Achtsamkeit, Mobilität, Mobilitätsausrüstung, Neurorehabilitation, Begleitsymptome, Ergotherapie, Physiotherapie, Körpertherapie, programme, Lebensqualität, Rehabilitation, Motorroller, Selbstmanagement, Diesntleistungen, Schlaf, soziales Engagement, Therapie, Behandlung, Gehhilfen, Wellness-Programme, Rollstuhl, Arbeit, Yoga

Kategorie	Suchbegriffe (englisch)	Suchbegriffe (deutsch) Auswahl
Transverse Myelitis		
Population	transverse myelitis (myelitis, transverse)	Transverse Myelitis
Intervention (nicht schriftlich fixiert)	Activities, activities of daily living, assistive devices, assistive equipment, caregiver support, cognitive behavioral therapy, community care, community programs, cognition, disease management, education, emotional regulation, exercise, extended care, fall prevention, health maintenance, health promotion, instrumental activities of daily living, intervention, leisure, lifts, mindfulness, mobility, mobility equipment, neurorehabilitation, nonmotor symptoms, occupational therapy, physical therapy, physiotherapy, programs, quality of life, rehabilitation, scooters, self-management, services, sleep, social engagement, therapy, treatment, walkers, wellness programs, wheelchairs, work, yoga.	Aktivitäten, Aktivitäten des täglichen Lebens, Hilfsmittel, Ausrüstung, unterstützende Betreuung, kognitive Verhaltenstherapie, ambulante Pflege, Gemeindepflege, Gemeindeprogramme, Kognition, Disease Management, Krankheitsbewältigung, Bildung, emotionale Regulation, Energieerhalt, Übung, ergänzende Betreuung, Sturzprophylaxe, Fatigue, Gesunderhaltung, Gesundheitsunterstützung, instrumentelle Aktivitäten des täglichen Lebens, Intervention, Freizeit, Lift, Achtsamkeit, Mobilität, Mobilitätsausrüstung, Neurorehabilitation, Begleitsymptome, Ergotherapie, Physiotherapie, Körpertherapie, programme, Lebensqualität, Rehabilitation, Motorroller, Selbstmanagement, Diesntleistungen, Schlaf, soziales Engagement, Therapie, Behandlung, Gehhilfen, Wellness-Programme, Rollstuhl, Arbeit, Yoga

rung von Referenzen auf der Basis von Zitaten und Abstracts ab. Die Volltextversionen potenzieller Artikel wurden überprüft, und die Review-Teams bestimmten die endgültige Aufnahme in das Review auf der Grundlage vorher festgelegter Einschluss- und Ausschlusskriterien.

Insgesamt wurden 140 Artikel in das abschließende Review eingeschlossen. Die **Tabelle C-3** enthält die Anzahl und den Evidenzlevel der jeweiligen Artikel für jede Reviewfrage. Die Teams, die an der jeweiligen Fokusfrage arbeiteten, überprüften die Artikel entsprechend ihrer Qualität (wissenschaftliche Strenge und *Lack of Bias)* und dem Evidenzlevel. Jeder in das Review eingeschlossene Artikel wurde dann anhand einer Nachweistabelle abstrahiert. Diese beinhaltet eine Zusammenfassung der Methoden und Ergebnisse des Artikels sowie eine Bewertung der Stärken und Schwächen der Studie auf der Grundlage von Design und Methodik. Die AOTA-Mitarbeiter und der EBP-Projektberater überprüften die Evidenztabellen zur Sicherung der Qualität. Alle Studien sind vollständig in den Evidenztabellen in Anhang D zusammengefasst. Die Einschränkungen der systematischen Reviews basieren auf dem Design und den Methoden der einzelnen Studien, einschließlich kleiner Stichprobengrößen, hoher Abbrecherquoten und begrenzter Beschreibungen der psychometrischen Eigenschaften der Erhebungsinstrumente. Darüber hinaus beinhalteten viele der Studien, die in das Review eingeschlossen wurden konkurrierende Interventionen und die Trennung von Effekten einer einzelnen Intervention kann schwierig sein.

Tabelle C-3: Anzahl der Artikel im jeweiligen Review sortiert nach dem Level der Evidenz

Evidenzlevel Review	I	II	III	IV	V	Summe für jeden Review
Parkinsonkrankheit	35	7	13	0	0	55
Multiple Sklerose	41	13	16	0	0	70
Amyotrophe Lateralsklerose	3	3	4	3	1	14
Summe	79	23	33	3	1	139

D Übersicht zur Evidenz

Table D1. Evidence on Activity- and Participation-Based Occupational Therapy–Related Interventions for People With Multiple Sclerosis

Author/Year	Study Objectives	Level/Design/Participants	Intervention and Outcome Measures	Results	Study Limitations
		Assistive Technology			
Cattaneo, Marazzini, Crippa, & Cardini (2002) http://dx.doi.org/10.1191/0269215502cr547oa	To compare the effects of a static AFO and a dynamic AFO on standing and walking balance in persons with MS	Level II Nonrandomized, 1-group (3 experimental conditions), posttest only $N = 14$ persons with MS (8 women); M age = 37.2 ± 22.8 (SD) yr; onset of MS = 13.3 ± 12.7 (SD) yr; each participant went through the 3 conditions.	*Intervention* *Static AFO:* Prefabricated with polypropylene. *Dynamic AFO:* Allowed 20° of plantar flexion. *Control group:* Barefoot condition without AFO. *Outcome Measures* • Static balance: CranioCorpoGraphy and Equiscale test • Dynamic balance: PEDro Test and Timed Walking Test without aids.	*Static balance:* Significant improvement was found in participants with static and dynamic AFOs. *Dynamic balance:* Participants with dynamic AFOs had better performance than participants with static AFOs.	Sample size was small. Prefabricated AFOs were used instead of customized AFOs, which may have interfered with the interpretation of the results.
Esnouf, Taylor, Mann, & Barrett (2010) http://dx.doi.org/10.1177/1352458510366013	To examine the effects of the Odstock Dropped Foot Stimulator (ODFS), a single-channel, foot-switch-controlled, external functional electrical stimulation (FES) device, on ADLs in persons with secondary progressive MS	Level I RCT, 2-group, pretest–posttest $N = 64$ persons with secondary progressive MS (34 women); M age = 53 yr for the experimental group, M age = 57 yr for the control group; Expanded Disability Status Scale [EDSS] ranged from 4 to 6.5 (both groups had 13 persons with EDSS scores of 6). Attrition rate = 17% (11/64).	*Intervention* *ODFS group:* Used the ODFS for mobility 1×/day for 18 wk. *Exercise group:* Received strength training focusing on the deep abdominal and lower back muscles to improve core stability and gait for 30 min 1×/day or 2×/day for 18 wk. *Outcome Measures* • Canadian Occupational Performance Measure (COPM).	Participants in the ODFS group improved significantly in both COPM performance and satisfaction. Participants in the exercise group demonstrated significant improvement in only COPM satisfaction.	A relatively few participants reported similar problems in each category.

(Continued)

Table D1. Evidence on Activity- and Participation-Based Occupational Therapy-Related Interventions for People With Multiple Sclerosis (Cont.)

Author/Year	Study Objectives	Level/Design/Participants	Intervention and Outcome Measures	Results	Study Limitations
Souza et al. (2010)	To systematically review the use of mobility assistive technology (MAT) in persons with MS	Level I Systematic review *Article selection:* 50 studies (on types of MAT devices and benefits for persons with MS) that met the criteria of levels of evidence were included. *Databases used:* Ovid MEDLINE, CINAHL, PubMed, and Scopus.	*Intervention* Systematic literature review on the use of MAT such as functional electrical stimulation, orthoses, wheelchairs, canes, and walkers. Studies concerning persons with MS with impaired mobility and service delivery were considered. *Outcome Measures* • Functional mobility • Participation • QoL • Frequency of use.	Fifty articles (Level V = 15, IV = 32, III = 2, and II = 1) were located and categorized. Findings suggest • 50% of persons with MS will require assistance with walking within 15 yr of onset. • Factors such as being seen by an OT and the type of MS were strongest predictors of MAT acquisition. • Current AT prescribed included manual wheelchair (60%), canes and crutches (44%), walkers (39%), and power wheelchairs (8%). • AT is best provided with a team approach. • Psychosocial factors, such as the disease's unpredictability over time, affect use of an AT device, particularly for mobility. • Significantly decreased mobility and self-reported QoL in the MS population indicate important needs for AT.	Insufficient studies with higher levels of evidence were included in the review.

http://dx.doi.org/10.1682/JRRD.2009.07.0096

(Continued)

Table D1. Evidence on Activity- and Participation-Based Occupational Therapy–Related Interventions for People With Multiple Sclerosis (Cont.)

Author/Year	Study Objectives	Level/Design/Participants	Intervention and Outcome Measures	Results	Study Limitations
		Rehabilitation Programs			
Brittle et al. (2008)	To examine the effects of a 10-session Conductive Education Program on mobility, functional independence, and health-related QoL in persons with stroke, Parkinson's disease, and MS.	Level II Nonrandomized, 3-group, pretest–posttest $N = 122$ participants with moderate disability enrolled in the study; 110 completed the intervention; 105 completed the postintervention analyses: 34 patients with stroke (median age = 58.5 yr, median yr since diagnosis = 2), 16 patients with MS (median age = 48 yr, median yr since diagnosis = 14), and 55 patients with Parkinson's disease (median age = 66 yr, median yr since diagnosis = 3).	*Intervention* In advance of the Conductive Educational Program, all participants received a 1-hr individual consultation on perceived problems, motor function assessment, and goal setting. Although advised to attend 1×/day for 2 wk (1.5-hr or 2-hr session), 10 sessions/wk were attended by only 47 persons (45% of the sample). The program was implemented with mixed-ability and diagnosis-specific groups with an average group size of 5. During each session, participants carried out several movement-based tasks, which included a combination of gross and fine motor movements required for daily life, in lying, sitting, and standing positions. Each task series was delivered through use of rhythmical intention. Family members were encouraged to attend the group to promote carry-over to everyday activities in the home.	*MS group:* Although trends of improvements in primary outcomes were noticed, no significant improvements were found on any outcome measure.	Sample size of MS participants was small. There was a lack of a control group. Effect sizes were not reported.

(Continued)

70   6 Anhänge

Table D1. Evidence on Activity- and Participation-Based Occupational Therapy–Related Interventions for People With Multiple Sclerosis (Cont.)

Author/Year	Study Objectives	Level/Design/Participants	Intervention and Outcome Measures	Results	Study Limitations
			Outcome Measures • Modified Barthel Index (BI–10) • Nottingham Extended Activities of Daily Living Index (NEADL) • Multiple Sclerosis Quality of Life–54 questionnaire (MSQoL–54)		
http://dx.doi.org/10.1177/0269215507082334					
Craig, Young, Ennis, Baker, & Boggild (2003)	To compare the effects of comprehensive MDR with standard care on disease severity and motor function	Level I RCT; 3-mo follow-up N = 41 participants with MS (time since onset range = 0–24 yr).	*Intervention* *Intervention group:* MDR focused on goals set during initial assessments; OT included adapted equipment, fatigue and stress management, and referral to social services. *Control group:* Intravenous methylprednisolone management only *Outcome Measures* • Disease severity • Motor impairment	The intervention group showed significant reduction in disease severity and improvement in motor function from baseline to the 3-mo assessment compared with the control group. ADLs, activity profile, and QoL also significantly improved.	The reliability and validity of the primary outcome measure were not provided. Assessors were not blinded.
http://dx.doi.org/10.1136/jnnp.74.9.1225					

(Continued)

Table D1. Evidence on Activity- and Participation-Based Occupational Therapy–Related Interventions for People With Multiple Sclerosis (*Cont.*)

Author/Year	Study Objectives	Level/Design/Participants	Intervention and Outcome Measures	Results	Study Limitations
Finkelstein, Lapshin, Castro, Cha, & Provance (2008)	To evaluate the feasibility, patient acceptance, and magnitude of the clinical impact on persons with MS of a 12-wk home-based physical telerehabilitation program	Level III Nonrandomized, 1-group, baseline, 6 wk of test, and 12 wk of posttest $N = 12$ adults with MS (10 women; M age $= 52 \pm 4$ yr; MS duration: 13 ± 7 yr).	*Intervention* Each participant received a custom 12-wk rehabilitative exercise program and was trained by the therapist during a clinic visit on how to perform the exercises. The exercise protocols were installed in the HAT system, which could be accessed from participants' places. The HAT system consisted of a server and a home unit designed to study how telemedicine practitioners treat and monitor services and help recipients in following individualized self-care plans. Participants received guidance from the server by means of textual, audio, and video prompts for performing each exercise. The HAT can collect self-reported information after completion of each exercise. *Outcome Measures* • Functional status: timed 25-ft walk (T25FW), 6-min walk, Berg Balance Scale (BBS), 12-Item MS Walking Scale (MSWS–12) • MSQOL–54	Participants improved significantly in objective measures (T25FW, 6-min walk, and BBS) from baseline to the 12-wk assessment, but not in self-reported measure (MSWS–12). No significant improvements noticed in disease-specific QoL. Overall, 75% of the participants rated the intervention program as good or excellent.	Sample size was small. There was a lack of a control group and randomization. Description of disease severity of the sample was not clear.

http://dx.doi.org/10.1682/JRRD.2008.01.0001

(*Continued*)

Table D1. Evidence on Activity- and Participation-Based Occupational Therapy–Related Interventions for People With Multiple Sclerosis (Cont.)

Author/Year	Study Objectives	Level/Design/Participants	Intervention and Outcome Measures	Results	Study Limitations
Grasso, Troisi, Rizzi, Morelli, & Paolucci (2005) http://dx.doi.org/10.1191/1352458505ms1226oa	To evaluate the effect of inpatient MDR on, and prognostic factors for, disease severity and functional status	Level III 1-group $N = 230$ participants with MS (M age = 49.42 yr; M disease duration = 16.90 yr, $SD = 9.89$).	*Intervention* Individualized, goal-oriented, inpatient MDR focused on promoting ADL skills, maintaining use of upper limbs for ADLs, and enhancing communication skills and attention span *Outcome Measures* • Disease severity • ADL performance • Mobility.	No change was found in disease severity. Significant improvement in functional status was found at discharge. Participants with mild and moderate MS showed significantly higher effects on ADLs and mobility. Cognitive impairment and longer disease duration were closely and negatively associated with effectiveness in ADLs but not in mobility. Participants without severe sphincteric disturbances had better improvement in ADLs.	No control group or follow-up assessments were used.
Huijgen et al. (2008)	To examine the feasibility of a 1-mo home-based telerehabilitation system compared with the effectiveness of usual care on arm/hand function in persons with stroke, TBI, and MS	Level I RCT, multicenter (Italy, Spain, and Belgium), 2-group, baseline (before intervention), Test 1 (after usual-care intervention), and Test 2 (after Home Care Activity Desk [HCAD] intervention) $N = 81$ adult participants with stroke, MS, or TBI with affected arm/hand function (average age = 48 yr; 24 women; 16 stroke patients, 30 TBI patients, and 35 MS patients); 70 participants who completed the study were analyzed.	*Intervention* The intervention group experienced 1 mo of usual care and 4 training sessions with the HCAD system and 1 mo of actual intervention with the HCAD system at home (at least 1 training session per day, 5 days/wk). The HCAD system comprised a hospital-based server and a portable unit, which summarizes the movements for correct functional activity of the upper extremity, installed at home. The therapists used information that was uploaded to the server for a weekly videoconference with the participants.	*ARAT:* A slight improvement was observed in persons with TBI and MS in the usual-care group. A slight improvement was also observed in persons with MS in the intervention group. *NHPT:* An improvement from baseline to Test 1 for both groups and all 3 diagnosis groups, except for the MS intervention group. There were no clear differences between Test 1 and Test 2, except for the MS group, which showed a slight deterioration in the control group and an improvement in the intervention group.	Sample size in each subgroup was relatively small.

(Continued)

Table D1. Evidence on Activity- and Participation-Based Occupational Therapy–Related Interventions for People With Multiple Sclerosis (*Cont.*)

Author/Year	Study Objectives	Level/Design/Participants	Intervention and Outcome Measures	Results	Study Limitations
Huijgen et al. (2008) (*Cont.*) http://dx.doi.org/10.1258/jtt.2008.080104			The control group received general exercises prescribed by their physicians. Therapists recorded the content of the care. *Outcome Measures* • Action Research Arm Test (ARAT) • Nine-Hole Peg Test (NHPT).	No significant differences were found between Test 1 and Test 2 in stroke, TBI, and MS intervention and control groups.	
Khan, Pallant, Brand, & Kilpatrick (2008) http://dx.doi.org/10.1136/jnnp.2007.133777	To evaluate the effect of an individualized rehabilitation program on activity and participation	Level I Stratified RCT $N = 101$ participants with MS; data from 48 participants in the treatment group and 50 participants in the control group were available for analysis. Inpatient program, $n = 24$; outpatient program, $n = 25$.	*Intervention* Comprehensive MDR over 12 mo; OT included fatigue management and functional retraining in ADLs. *5-day inpatient group:* Therapy 3 hr/day. *Individualized outpatient group:* Therapy 2–3×/wk for ≤6 wk. *Control group:* 8 weekly monitoring phone calls regarding medical and hospital visits in the previous month. *Outcome Measures* • Functional performance • Health–related QoL.	The treatment group showed more improvement in activity and participation and the control group more deterioration over time. No significant results were found for QoL. The 12 control participants required treatment. Significant differences were found between groups on the FIM™ motor scale and FIM domains of self-care, sphincter, transfers, and locomotion.	Data were obtained from a single site.

(*Continued*)

Table D1. Evidence on Activity- and Participation-Based Occupational Therapy–Related Interventions for People With Multiple Sclerosis (Cont.)

Author/Year	Study Objectives	Level/Design/Participants	Intervention and Outcome Measures	Results	Study Limitations
Khan, Ng, & Turner-Stokes (2009); Kahn, Turner-Stokes, Ng, & Kilpatrick (2008) http://dx.doi.org/10.1136/jnnp.2007.127563 http://dx.doi.org/10.1136/jnnp.2007.133777	To evaluate the effect of organized MDR on activity, participation, or both	Level I Systematic review $N = 7$ RCTs, 1 controlled clinical trial.	*Intervention* Trials comparing MDR with routinely available local services, lower levels of intervention, or interventions in different settings or at different levels of intensity. *Outcome Measures* • Levels of evidence • Subgroup analysis—type, setting, and intensity of rehabilitation.	No change was found in impairment level. Inpatient MDR produced short-term effects on levels of activity and participation. For outpatient and home-based MDR, limited evidence was provided for short-term improvement in symptoms and disability with high-intensity programs, and strong evidence was provided for longer term improvement in QoL in low-intensity programs.	Few high-quality studies were found.
Maitra et al. (2010) http://dx.doi.org/10.5014/ajot.2010.090204	To evaluate the effect of OT intervention in an urban inpatient rehabilitation setting	Level III Secondary retrospective analysis of medical charts $N = 193$ charts (148 women; M length of stay = 13.34 days).	*Intervention* OT services, establishment of initial goals, reevaluation of goal status at discharge *Outcome Measures* • Specific OT interventions • Duration of each intervention • FIM scores at initial assessment, goal, and discharge.	Patients received OT on 56% of days. The most common OT interventions were self-care, therapeutic exercise, and occupation-based therapeutic activities. The greatest improvements were found in ADLs. Increasing OT intensity had a positive effect on all FIM scores except feeding. Self-care training was positively associated with independence in all ADL categories, indicating that clients may improve self-care by practicing self-care activities directly.	Data were obtained from a single site. The analysis was retrospective.

(Continued)

Table D1. Evidence on Activity- and Participation-Based Occupational Therapy–Related Interventions for People With Multiple Sclerosis (*Cont.*)

Author/Year	Study Objectives	Level/Design/Participants	Intervention and Outcome Measures	Results	Study Limitations
Patti et al. (2002, 2003) http://dx.doi.org/10.1007/s00415-002-0778-1 http://dx.doi.org/10.1007/s00415-003-1097-x	To evaluate the effect of a 6-wk comprehensive outpatient rehabilitative MDR on QoL, depression, fatigue impact, social experience, impairment, and disability	Level I RCT, 6-wk follow-up $N = 111$ participants with confirmed MS (EDSS score = 4.0–8.0).	*Intervention* *Intervention group:* 6 wk of individualized, goal-directed MDR and 6 wk of home self-exercise *Wait-list control group:* 12 wk of home self-exercise *Outcome Measures* • QoL • Depression • Fatigue impact • Social experience • Impairment • Disability.	The intervention group improved in self-perceived health-related QoL. At follow-up, the intervention group had improved QoL; reduced fatigue impact; and improved social functioning, depression, and motor function. No significant changes were found in impairment.	Little detail was provided about the rehabilitation program.
Storr, Sørensen, & Ravnborg (2006) http://dx.doi.org/10.1191/1352458506ms1250oa	To evaluate the effect of an MDR inpatient program on health-related QoL and level of activity	Level I Double-blinded RCT $N = 106$ participants with MS (EDSS scores < 9.0; median time since diagnosis = 9.0 yr); $n = 41$ intervention (3 withdrew), $n = 65$ control (13 withdrew)	*Intervention* The intervention group had 3–5 wk of MDR based on personal needs and 30-min OT sessions 3×/wk. The wait-list control group had no intervention. *Outcome Measures* • QoL • Impairment • Level of activity.	No significant changes were found between groups on outcome measures. Co-intervention was observed in both the intervention and the control groups.	Co-intervention was not controlled for. Sample sizes were unequal between groups. No information was provided about intervention, except for physical therapy.

(*Continued*)

Table D1. Evidence on Activity- and Participation-Based Occupational Therapy–Related Interventions for People With Multiple Sclerosis (*Cont.*)

Author/Year	Study Objectives	Level/Design/Participants	Intervention and Outcome Measures	Results	Study Limitations
Vikman, Fielding, Lindmark, & Fredrikson (2008)	To evaluate the effects of a 3-wk inpatient MDR program for persons with moderate MS	Level III Nonrandomized, 1-group, pretest–posttest $N = 58$ persons with moderate MS (46 women; M age = 55.8 yr; M disease duration = 19.3 yr; M EDSS = 5.7); $n = 18$ Cohort A (assessment before and after the program), $n = 18$ Cohort B (received a 3-wk, no-treatment control period before the 3-wk rehabilitation program; assessment before and after the control and intervention periods) Cohort B was used because of design change and served as its own control.	*Intervention* Participants in the study received standard inpatient MDR treatment with medical care, PT, OT, and, if necessary, the services of a psychologist, social worker, and/or speech therapist for 3 wk. OT aimed at hand training for 30 min 1×/day, 5×/wk. *Outcome Measures* • SF–36 and Functional Assessment of Multiple Sclerosis (FAMS) for health-related QoL • Fatigue Severity Scale • Beck Depression Inventory (BDI) • Multiple Sclerosis Functional Composite (MSFC) • Grip strength assessment • Box and Block test (B&B) • 9HPT • Clinical Outcome Variables (COVS) • BBS • T25FW • Barthel Index.	In self-reporting, Cohort A demonstrated significant improvement in several subscales of SF–36 (General Health, Vitality, and Mental Health) after intervention. Cohort B had no significant changes in these variables. In physical assessments, Cohort A demonstrated significant improvements in the MSFC, B&B, 9HPT for nondominant hand, COVS, and the BBS. Cohort B improved significantly in the MSFC, B&B, 9HPT for dominant hand, and T25FW after intervention.	Sample size was small for Cohort B. There was a lack of a control group for Cohort A. Effect sizes were unreported.

http://dx.doi.org/10.1080/14038190701288785

(*Continued*)

Table D1. Evidence on Activity- and Participation-Based Occupational Therapy–Related Interventions for People With Multiple Sclerosis (*Cont.*)

Author/Year	Study Objectives	Level/Design/Participants	Intervention and Outcome Measures	Results	Study Limitations
Ward et al. (2004)	To evaluate the effects of a 12-mo home-based educational intervention on the reduction of the incidence and risks of falls and pressure sores in adults with progressive neurological conditions	Level I Stratified (diagnosis), 2-group, pretest–posttest $N = 114$ adults with progressive neurological conditions (53 with PD, 45 with MS, and 16 others; age range = 22–89 yr; 51 women).	*Intervention* Participants were randomly allocated to either an education group or a comparison group within each diagnostic category. Within the first 6 wk, each participant in the education group was given suggestions by the research OT (based on discussion by an expert panel of an OT, PT, speech therapist, general practitioner, social worker, and nurse), ranging from minor changes in the home environment to self-referrals to local services. Participants in the education group received a single follow-through phone call from the OT to confirm and reinforce the educational content. Participants in the comparison group received an information package on generic services and condition-specific self-help organizations 6 wk after baseline assessment. Comparison group participants who had any specific queries were advised to consult routine sources of advice, such as their general physician. *Outcome Measures* • Reports of 1 or more falls or skin sores.	No significant difference in the proportion of people reporting falls at baseline between the education and comparison groups. More first falls were reported in participants in the education group throughout the follow-up period. Participants with PD in the education group reported significantly more falls than those in the comparison group (adjusted odds ratio = 10.89). No significant differences were found within the other 2 diagnostic subgroups.	Co-intervention was not controlled for (consultation with general physician in the comparison group). Assessments were not objective.

http://dx.doi.org/10.1191/0269215504cr792oa

(*Continued*)

Table D1. Evidence on Activity- and Participation-Based Occupational Therapy–Related Interventions for People With Multiple Sclerosis (Cont.)

Author/Year	Study Objectives	Level/Design/Participants	Intervention and Outcome Measures	Results	Study Limitations
Fatigue Management Courses					
Blikman et al. (2013)	To systematically review effects of energy conservation management (ECM) treatment for fatigue in MS and study the effect of ECM on restrictions in participation and quality of life	Level I Systematic review of ECM $N = 4$ RCTs, 2 controlled clinical trials	*Intervention* RCT and controlled clinical trials with people diagnosed with MS that evaluated the effectiveness of ECM or fatigue management on reducing fatigue. *Outcome Measures* • FIS • FSS • Impact on Participation and Autonomy (IPA).	ECM can be more effective than no treatment in reducing the impact of fatigue in the short term and improving 3 aspects of QoL (role physical, social function, mental health).	Results were based on a limited amount of evidence. There was some risk of bias in studies reviewed and the possibility of publication bias.
Cakit et al. (2010)	To evaluate the effects of cycling progressive resistance training combined with balance exercises on walking speed, balance, fatigue, fear of falling, depression, and QoL in persons with MS	Level I RCT, 3-group, pretest–posttest $N = 45$ relapsing–remitting or secondary progressive MS patients with mild to moderate disability level (EDSS scores <6.0) who were capable of standing independently in upright position for more than 3 sec were included in the study; 33 participants completed the study (20 women, 13 men; duration since diagnosis = 3–20 yr; M age = 35.5–43.0 yr).	*Intervention* *Group 1:* 16 training sessions of progressive resistance training on a static bicycle ergometer, with 15 sets of repetitions in each session over 8 wk; each set consisted of 2 min of 40% of the tolerated maximum workload (TMW) and 2 min of low-resistance pedaling on ergometer or 2 min of rest; after cycling training, participants underwent warm-up activities and stretches, balance exercises, and whole-body stretching. *Group 2:* Participated in a home-based exercise program, which was the same exercise program as for Group 1 and aimed at improving lower-limb strength.	Participants in Group 1 demonstrated significant improvement after the intervention in these areas: endurance of exercise, walking speed, static and dynamic balance (TUG, DGI, FR), FES, FSS, and BDI. Participants in Group 2 showed significant improvement in endurance of exercise, tolerated maximum workload, and FES after 8 wk of home-based exercise. No significant improvement was observed in the control group. Improvement in Group 1 was higher than in the other groups, except for the 10-minute walking test.	Sample size was small. There was a lack of a follow-up assessment. Attrition rate was high.

(Continued)

Table D1. Evidence on Activity- and Participation-Based Occupational Therapy–Related Interventions for People With Multiple Sclerosis (Cont.)

Author/Year	Study Objectives	Level/Design/Participants	Intervention and Outcome Measures	Results	Study Limitations
Cakit et al. (2010) (Cont.)			*Group 3 (control group):* No exercise intervention, but participants were asked to continue with their normal living. *Outcome Measures* • 10-min test for walking speed • Timed Up and Go test (TUG) for dynamic balance • Dynamic Gait Index (DGI) for ability to adapt gait to changes in task demands • Functional Reach (FR) for static balance • FES for fear of falling • Fatigue Severity Scale (FSS) • BDI • SF–36.	No significant differences between groups were found in scores on the SF–36. Participants in Group 1 showed significant improvement in physical functioning and Role and Physical Functioning subscales of SF–36. Participants in Group 2 showed significant improvement in Physical Functioning subscale of the SF–36.	
Finlayson (2005); Finlayson & Holberg (2007) http://dx.doi.org/10.1097/PHM.0b013e3181d3e71f	To evaluate the effects of an energy conservation program delivered by teleconference (modified Managing Fatigue program) and to analyze the strengths and limitations of the program for persons with MS	Level III Nonrandomized, 1-group, pretest–posttest *N* = 29 persons with MS (24 women; average age = 47 yr, average postonset = 9.8 yr). Responses of 3 female OTs (program facilitators) who received training on the content and delivery method were used for analyses of the strengths and limitations of the program.	*Intervention* Modified Managing Fatigue course was delivered by teleconference. The adapted content was similar to the original course and consisted of 6 45–60-min sessions for 6 wk, emphasizing information sharing and discussion. Each participant was provided a course manual.	After intervention, study participants demonstrated significant reduction in FSS and FIS: total and all 3 subscales. Participants also demonstrated significant improvement in the SF–36 subscales of Bodily Pain and General Health. Secondary outcomes indicated that most participants used energy conservation strategies (e.g., simplifying activities, adjusting priorities, changing body position, resting, and planning the day to balance work and rest).	Participants mainly had relapsing–remitting MS, which may limit the generalizability of the results. Problems with logistics and time for both participants and therapists and diverse needs of participants.

(Continued)

Table D1. Evidence on Activity- and Participation-Based Occupational Therapy–Related Interventions for People With Multiple Sclerosis (*Cont.*)

Author/Year	Study Objectives	Level/Design/Participants	Intervention and Outcome Measures	Results	Study Limitations
			Feedback on the strengths and limitations of the intervention were sent by mail. Two questions were posed: (1) What did you like about the teleconference energy conservation course? and (2) What did you not like or find challenging about the teleconference energy conservation course? Data from the OTs were collected through individual session notes. *Outcome Measures* • FSS • Fatigue Impact Scale (FIS) • SF–36 for health-related QoL.	Strengths of the intervention for participants included social support and normalization, quality and usefulness of the resources, and comfort and confidence with the format. OTs' strengths included the power of peers and value of repetition.	
http://dx.doi.org/10.2182/cjot.06.0018					
Finlayson, Preissner, Cho, & Plow (2011)	To evaluate efficacy and effectiveness of a group-based, teleconference-delivered fatigue management program on fatigue impact, fatigue severity, health-related QoL, and self-efficacy	Level I RCT, randomly allocated 2-group time series design with a wait-list control group $N = 190$ (M age = 56 yr for intent-to-treat group, M age = 55 yr for protocol group; M FSS score = 5; M PDSS score = 4).	*Intervention* Six-week group-based fatigue management group delivered by teleconference, 70 min/wk. Modified for teleconference delivery from Managing Fatigue course. *Outcome Measures* • FIS • FSS • SF–36 • Self-Efficacy for Energy Conservation Questionnaire.	Intervention was more effective and efficacious than control for reducing fatigue impact but not fatigue severity. Before-and-after comparisons with the pooled sample demonstrated efficacy and effectiveness for fatigue impact, fatigue severity, and 6 of 8 heath-related QoL dimensions. Changes were maintained for 6 mo with small to moderate effect sizes.	Self-report measures were used. Research assistants were not blinded to participants' allocation status. Whether other interventions contributed to the results is unknown.

(*Continued*)

Table D1. Evidence on Activity- and Participation-Based Occupational Therapy–Related Interventions for People With Multiple Sclerosis (*Cont.*)

Author/Year	Study Objectives	Level/Design/Participants	Intervention and Outcome Measures	Results	Study Limitations
Ghahari, Packer, & Passmore (2010) http://dx.doi.org/10.3109/09638288.2011.613518	To evaluate the effects of an online fatigue self-management program on fatigue impact, activity participation, and QoL	Level I RCT, 3-mo follow-up N = 95 participants; 74 with fatigue secondary to MS, 8 with fatigue secondary to PD, and 13 with fatigue secondary to postpolio syndrome Attrition rate = 9% at posttest, 21% at follow-up.	*Intervention* *Fatigue self-management group (FG):* 7-wk online program with content, activities, and discussion. *Information-only group (IP):* Identical content but no access to fatigue group. *Control group:* No intervention *Outcome Measures* • QoL • Activity participation • Fatigue impact • Personal Wellbeing Index (PWI).	No significant differences were found among the 3 groups on the primary outcome measures except for a posttest difference in the PWI between the IP and control group. Significant improvement was found on fatigue impact and activity participation in the FG and IP groups over time. The observed power for the FG group was extremely low.	Diagnoses in the sample were mixed. Subgroups were unequal in size.
Hugos et al. (2010)	To evaluate the effect of the Fatigue: Take Control program on fatigue and self-efficacy	Level I RCT N = 30 participants with MS (M age = 56.87 yr; M EDSS score = 5.2 for Fatigue: Take Control group and 4.0 for control group).	*Intervention* *Fatigue: Take Control group:* 6 2 hr/wk sessions consisting of DVD viewing, topic-focused group discussion, individual goal setting, and homework assignments; topics were identification of treatable or secondary causes of fatigue, priority setting, environmental modifications, management of mobility problems, energy effectiveness strategies, and the importance of exercise.	No significant changes were found in fatigue severity in either group. Participants in the Fatigue: Take Control group had significant improvement in MFIS Total, Physical, and Psychosocial scores. After taking the course, the wait-list control group showed improvement that did not reach significance. A significant effect was observed in overall mean self-efficacy scores for the Fatigue: Take Control group.	Sample size was small. A higher percentage of participants in the experimental group (33.3%) than in the wait-list group (13.3%) received interferon.

(Continued)

Table D1. Evidence on Activity- and Participation-Based Occupational Therapy–Related Interventions for People With Multiple Sclerosis (*Cont.*)

Author/Year	Study Objectives	Level/Design/Participants	Intervention and Outcome Measures	Results	Study Limitations
Hugos et al. (2010) (*Cont.*) http://dx.doi.org/10.1177/1352458510364536			*Wait-list control group:* 20–30 min biweekly meeting to complete study documents. *Outcome Measures* • Modified Fatigue Impact Scale (MFIS) • FSS • Self-efficacy.		
Kos, Duportail, D'hooghe, Nagel, & Kerckhofs (2007)	To determine the efficacy of multidisciplinary fatigue management programs (MFMP) in MS	Level I RCT, single-blind randomized placebo controlled design with matched pairs $N = 51$ (M age = 42.9 yr for Group A, M age = 44.5 yr for Group B; Modified FIS = 46).	*Intervention* MFMP was provided for 4 2-hr sessions over 4 wk. Information provided included possible strategies to manage fatigue and reduced energy levels (i.e., pharmacological treatment, diet, informing and involving the social environment, regular sleep, exercise, relaxation, cooling, assistive devices, adaptation of home or work environment and energy saving methods). *Outcome Measures* • MFIS • FSS • MS Self-Efficacy Scale • Mental Health Inventory • IPA.	No efficacy in reducing the impact of fatigue compared with a placebo intervention program. Significant changes in fatigue impact in both intervention and placebo groups. A clinically relevant reduction in fatigue impact was found in 17% of individuals after the intervention compared with 44% after the placebo intervention program.	Sample size was small. Intervention and placebo were possibly too similar.

(*Continued*)

Table D1. Evidence on Activity- and Participation-Based Occupational Therapy–Related Interventions for People With Multiple Sclerosis (*Cont.*)

Author/Year	Study Objectives	Level/Design/Participants	Intervention and Outcome Measures	Results	Study Limitations
Lee, Newell, Ziegler, & Topping (2008) http://dx.doi.org/10.1111/j.1440-172X.2008.00670.x	To systematically review the effects of interventions for fatigue in persons with MS	Level I Systematic review *Article selection*: 15 studies (10 pharmacological studies and 5 psychosocial/psychological interventions), which met the inclusive criteria (published in English, RCTs, open-label trials, cross-over trials, and examining fatigue in MS as an outcome measure) were included. The sources reviewed were the Web of Knowledge, Cochrane Database of Systematic Reviews, Database of Abstracts of Reviews of Effects, PsycINFO, Ingenta, Zetoc, LILACS, Medline, ADOLEC, National Research Register, HMIC, NeLH, and GALE.	*Intervention* Abstracts were printed and examined. Two reviewers read all articles possible for inclusion and determined the appropriateness for inclusion. *Outcome Measures* • Assessment of fatigue • Self-efficacy • QoL.	The included studies were divided into (1) pharmacological and (2) psychosocial/psychological trials. No conclusion could be drawn about pharmacological interventions because of methodological difficulties. No conclusion could be established in findings of psychosocial/psychological studies because of heterogeneous groups, poor quality of methodology, and vague outcome measures in psychosocial/psychological studies.	This study could have included more exploratory studies in the review.

(*Continued*)

Table D1. Evidence on Activity- and Participation-Based Occupational Therapy–Related Interventions for People With Multiple Sclerosis (Cont.)

Author/Year	Study Objectives	Level/Design/Participants	Intervention and Outcome Measures	Results	Study Limitations
Mathiowetz, Finlayson, Matuska, Chen, & Luo (2005); Mathiowetz, Matuska, Finlayson, Luo, & Chen (2007) http://dx.doi.org/10.1191/1352458505ms1198oa http://dx.doi.org/10.1097/MRR.0b013e3282f14434	To evaluate the efficacy and effectiveness of a 6-wk energy conservation course in terms of fatigue impact, QoL, and self-efficacy	Level I RCT, crossover, 1-yr follow-up $N = 169$ participants with MS (M age = 48.34 yr; M time since diagnosis = 9.47 yr). Attrition rate = 23%.	*Intervention* Managing Fatigue course: 6 2-hr/wk sessions on the importance of rest, communication, body mechanics, ergonomic principles, environmental modification, priority setting, activity analysis and modification, and balanced lifestyle. *Control period*: No treatment *Outcome Measures* • FIS • QoL • Self-efficacy.	A significant decrease was found in intervention group scores immediately postcourse, except on the FIS Cognitive subscale (moderate to large effect sizes for all subscales). Significant increases were found in Vitality, Role–Physical, and Mental Health subscale scores (moderate to large effect sizes) for the intervention group postcourse. Self-efficacy improved significantly postcourse. These beneficial effects were maintained at the 1-yr follow-up.	The attrition rate was high. No placebo control group was used.

(Continued)

Table D1. Evidence on Activity- and Participation-Based Occupational Therapy–Related Interventions for People With Multiple Sclerosis (*Cont.*)

Author/Year	Study Objectives	Level/Design/Participants	Intervention and Outcome Measures	Results	Study Limitations
Sauter, Zebenholzer, Hisakawa, Zeitlhofer, & Vass (2008)	To investigate the effects of a 6-wk energy conservation course on fatigue in persons with MS	Level II Nonrandomized, 2-group, pretest–posttest, follow-up (7–9 mo) $N = 26$ persons with MS (53% with relapsing–remitting MS, 13.3% with primary progressive MS, and 33.3% with secondary progressive MS; average yr of diagnosis = 11.8). Attrition rate = 16% (5 dropped out of the study).	*Intervention* Participants in the intervention group received the German version of the Managing Fatigue course by Packer, Brink, & Sauriol (1995) with the same topics, including the importance of rest; communication and body mechanics; environmental adaptations; personal priorities; standards; time management; and balancing self-care, work, and recreational tasks, for 6 wk. Groups of 6–8 participants attended 6 2-hr sessions/wk. Participants in the waitlist control group received the same intervention after termination of the courses of the intervention group. *Outcome Measures* • EDSS for measuring disability level • MSFC • FSS • MS-specific Fatigue Scale • MFIS	Symptom severity did not change significantly (EDSS and MSFC) after participating in the course. Participants demonstrated significant improvement in fatigue severity and fatigue impact after intervention and at the follow-up assessment (per total scores and the Cognitive and Physical subscales of the MFIS). However, the subscale of Psychosocial Impact and the MS-specific Fatigue Scale were not significant. For the secondary outcome measures, participants demonstrated significantly decreased depression and improved sleep quality after intervention and maintained after 7–9 mo.	Sample size was small. More homogeneous participants could have been included.

http://dx.doi.org/10.1177/1352458507084649

(*Continued*)

Table D1. Evidence on Activity- and Participation-Based Occupational Therapy–Related Interventions for People With Multiple Sclerosis (Cont.)

Author/Year	Study Objectives	Level/Design/Participants	Intervention and Outcome Measures	Results	Study Limitations
		Health Promotion Programs			
Bombardier et al. (2008) http://dx.doi.org/10.1016/j.apmr.2008.03.021	To evaluate the effect of a 12-wk motivational interviewing–based telephone counseling program on health promotion activities and other health outcomes	Level I RCT, single-blinded $N = 130$ community-dwelling adults (age range = 19–70 yr) able to walk ≥90 m without assistance.	*Intervention* *Treatment group:* 1 60–90-min motivational interview and goal-setting meeting and 5 follow-up telephone counseling sessions to promote follow-through with the plan. *Wait-list control group:* No treatment *Outcome Measures* • Health-Promoting Lifestyle Profile (HPLP) II.	Six participants in the treatment group and 1 in the wait-list control group did not complete the study. The majority of participants (58.6%) chose exercise promotion activities. The treatment group showed significant improvement in physical activity, spiritual growth, and stress management. Those who chose exercise engaged in more health promotion activities and self-reported minutes of exercise per week, but no significant improvement was found for fatigue.	Reliability and validity of the primary outcome measure were not provided.
Ennis, Thain, Boggild, Baker, & Young (2006) http://dx.doi.org/10.1177/0269215506070805	To evaluate the effect of a health promotion education program (OPTIMIZE) on self-efficacy and health-promoting behaviors	Level I RCT, 3-mo follow-up $N = 62$ adults, most with moderate relapsing–remitting MS (M age = 45 yr in the treatment group, 30 yr in the control group).	*Intervention* *Treatment group:* 8 3-hr sessions/wk of group OPTIMIZE program providing knowledge, skills, and confidence to undertake health-promoting activities; 5 components were (1) exercise and physical activity, (2) lifestyle adjustment and fatigue management, (3) stress management, (4) nutritional awareness, and (5) responsible health practices. *Control group:* Continuation of present level of care *Outcome Measures* • HPLP II.	Significant differences between the groups were observed at the postintervention evaluation (HPLP Total scores and HPLP Health Responsibility, Physical Activity, Spiritual Growth, and Stress Management subscales). The benefit of the program was maintained 3 mo postintervention.	Reliability and validity of the primary outcome measure were not provided.

(Continued)

Table D1. Evidence on Activity- and Participation-Based Occupational Therapy–Related Interventions for People With Multiple Sclerosis (*Cont.*)

Author/Year	Study Objectives	Level/Design/Participants	Intervention and Outcome Measures	Results	Study Limitations
Plow, Mathiowetz, & Lowe (2009)	To compare the efficacy of individualized physical rehabilitation (IPR) with a group wellness intervention (GWI) in promoting physical activity and health	Level I RCT, 8-wk follow-up $N = 42$ participants with MS (M age = 48.5 yr) able to walk with or without an assistive device. $N = 38$ in primary analysis; 4 participants missing at posttest.	*Intervention* *IPR:* 4 PT exercise sessions 1× every other week and phone calls between sessions to emphasize functional limitations or to make exercises more challenging. *GWI:* Discussion of physical activities and incorporation of selected portions of the energy conservation course, 2 hr/wk for 7 wk. *Both groups:* Home exercise program for 45 min 5 days/wk, consisting of indoor bicycling and stretching (3 days/wk) and strength and balance training (2 days/wk). *Outcome Measures* • QoL • MFIS • Mental Health Inventory.	In terms of overall effects postintervention, both groups significantly improved in health and physical activity, but no significant differences were found between the two groups. In terms of immediate effects, the intervention group significantly decreased in QoL Physical Summary but improved on the Mental Health Inventory at posttest. No improvement in MFIS scores was found. At follow-up, significant improvement was found in MFIS scores. No significant improvement was noted in QoL and Mental Health Inventory scores. The IPR had a greater effect in reducing fatigue impact (.66) and impeding the decline of physical health (−.28), whereas the GWI had a greater effect on mental health (.65).	A true control group was not used.

http://dx.doi.org/10.4278/ajhp.071211128

(*Continued*)

Table D1. Evidence on Activity- and Participation-Based Occupational Therapy–Related Interventions for People With Multiple Sclerosis (Cont.)

Author/Year	Study Objectives	Level/Design/Participants	Intervention and Outcome Measures	Results	Study Limitations
			Others		
Khan, Ng, & Turner-Stokes (2009) http://dx.doi.org/10.1002/14651858.CD007256.pub2	To evaluate the effectiveness of vocational rehabilitation programs applied to persons with MS in comparison to alternative programs or care as usual on return to employment To evaluate the cost effectiveness of these programs	Level I Systematic review *Article selection*: 2 studies were included; selection criteria: RCTs and controlled trials that recruited participants with MS and incorporated a clearly defined vocational rehabilitation or work therapy (general rehabilitation program, MS specialized vocational rehabilitation, and pan-disability vocational rehabilitation program). Several electrical databases, including Cochrane Multiple Sclerosis Group's Specialized Register (February 2011), PEDro (1990–2011), Cochrane Occupational Health Field Database, Clinicaltrials.gov, Rehabtrials.org, Controlled-trials.com, and ISI Science Citation Index, and hand searched articles from *Work* and *Journal of Vocational Rehabilitation* were used.	*Intervention* Specialized services geared toward job retention for employed MS participants vs. standard medical care; 2 vocational rehabilitation programs geared toward career reentry for unemployed MS participants. *Outcome Measures* • Change in proportion of persons with MS in competitive and supported employment.	One RCT and 1 CCT with different target populations (aimed respectively at work retention for employed persons with MS and work reentry for unemployed persons with MS) were included in this review. Given the diversity of target population, aim of intervention, and the small number of studies included, no conclusive statements regarding the purposes of the review could be made by the authors.	Only 2 studies were included.

(Continued)

Table D1. Evidence on Activity- and Participation-Based Occupational Therapy–Related Interventions for People With Multiple Sclerosis (Cont.)

Author/Year	Study Objectives	Level/Design/Participants	Intervention and Outcome Measures	Results	Study Limitations
Steultjens, Dekker, Bouter, Leemrijse, & van den Ende (2005)	To summarize the research evidence available from systematic reviews of the efficacy of OT for practitioners, researchers, purchasing organizations, and policymakers	Level I Systematic review *Article selection:* 15 systematic reviews of the efficacy of OT interventions were included from 1966 to 2004, retrieved from the Cochrane Database of Systematic Reviews and the Database of Reviews of Efficacy.	*Intervention* Identified studies were categorized on the basis of the type of target population, then into training of sensory–motor functions, training of cognitive functions, training of skills, counseling instruction on joint protection and energy conservation, advice and instruction on the use of assistive devices, provision of splints, and education of primary caregiver. *Outcome Measures* • Functional ability • Participation • Well-being • Falls.	*Progressive neurological diseases and mental illness category:* No conclusion could be made due to a small number of studies with a small number of participants included. *Stroke category:* The evidence supports the efficacy of OT in improvement of functional ability and participation in persons with stroke; however, the efficacy for outcomes of arm–hand function, decreasing muscle tone, and cognitive functions is not apparent. *Rheumatoid arthritis category:* The evidence supports the efficacy of OT in the improvement of functional ability in persons with rheumatoid arthritis; however, unclear efficacy of OT on other outcomes was noticed. *Elderly people:* Evidence supports the efficacy of OT intervention in the improvement of functional ability, participation, and well-being, and the reduction of the incidence of falls for the elderly people category. *Cerebral palsy category:* No conclusion, as only 1 review was identified and included.	Methodological rigor was not assessed for this review.

http://dx.doi.org/10.11191/0269215505cr870oa

Note. ADL/ADLs = activity/activities of daily living; AFO = ankle-foot orthosis; AT = assistive technology; CCT= controlled clinical trial; hr = hour/hours; HAT = home automated telemanagement; *M* = mean; MDR = multidisciplinary rehabilitation; min = minute/minutes; mo = month/months; MS = multiple sclerosis; OT = occupational therapist/occupational therapy; QoL = quality of life; PT = physical therapist/physical therapy; RCT = randomized controlled trial; sec = second/seconds; *SD* = standard deviation; TBI = traumatic brain injury; wk = week/weeks; yr = year/years.

This revised table is a product of AOTA's Evidence-Based Practice Project and was originally published in the *American Journal of Occupational Therapy*. Copyright © 2014 by the American Therapy Association. It may be freely reproduced for personal use in clinical or educational settings as long as the source is cited. All other uses require written permission from the American Occupational Therapy Association. To apply, visit http://www.copyright.com.

Table D2. Evidence on Occupational Therapy–Related Interventions Focusing on Client Factors and Performance Skills for People With Multiple Sclerosis

Author/Year	Study Objectives	Level/Design/Participants	Intervention and Outcome Measures	Results	Study Limitations
		Cognitive Training			
Bovend'Eerdt, Dawes, Sackley, Izadi, & Wade (2010) http://dx.doi.org/10.1016/j.apmr.2010.03.008	To examine the feasibility of a motor imagery program integrated into physiotherapy and OT	Level I Single-blinded, RCT, 2-group, pretest–posttest, and follow-up (at 6 wk) $N = 30$ adults (11 women; M age = 50.3 yr) with central nervous system dysfunction; 28 with stroke, 1 with traumatic brain injury, and 1 with relapse in MS.	*Intervention* All participants received regular physiotherapy and OT. All therapists received training on motor imagery and were asked to use it with participants in the experimental group at least 3×/wk for the first 3 wk and at least 2×/wk for the last 2 wk of the regular therapy. The experimental group was provided a motor imagery film and asked to use imagery outside. The control group was provided a physical practice film and was encouraged to use physical practice. *Outcome Measures* The Goal Attainment Scale (GAS), which utilized Barthel ADL Index and Nottingham Extended ADL scale; ADL function; Timed Up and Go (TUG) test; Action Research Arm Test; and Rivermead Mobility Index.	Eighty-five percent of therapists used less than the proposed amount of time on imagery, and 72% of participants in the intervention group did not use motor imagery as much outside the therapy sessions. GAS scores improved significantly at postintervention and follow-up assessments, but no significant findings between groups over time were observed. No significant differences were found in other outcome measures between the experimental and control groups.	Only 1 participant with MS included. Small sample size. No robust outcome measures.

(Continued)

Table D2. Evidence on Occupational Therapy–Related Interventions Focusing on Client Factors and Performance Skills for People With Multiple Sclerosis (Cont.)

Author/Year	Study Objectives	Level/Design/Participants	Intervention and Outcome Measures	Results	Study Limitations
Brenk, Laun, & Haase (2008)	To examine the effect of a selected nonspecific, homework-based, short-term (6-wk) cognitive training program on neuropsychological deficits and depression in MS patients and matched healthy controls	Level II Nonrandomized, 2-group, pretest–posttest $N = 27$ relapsing–remitting MS participants (15 women, M age = 43.5 yr, age range = 25–59 yr; Expanded Disability Status Scale [EDSS] ≤5) and 14 healthy participants (7 women, M age = 39.6 yr, age range = 24–55).	*Intervention* Each participant completed the 6-wk home-based cognitive training program aimed at memory, attention function, and verbal performances. *Outcome Measures* • Neuropsychological test battery • *Memory aspects (revised Wechsler Memory Scale [WMS])*: verbal repeating of numbers forward (ZNS–V) and backward (ZNS–R) • *Attention*: Test Battery of Attentional Performance (TAP) • *Executive function*: Regensburger Word Fluency Test (RWT) and Rey-Osterrieth Complex Figure Test (CFT) • *Depression*: Beck Depression Inventory (BDI) and Hamburg Quality of Life Questionnaire in MS (HAQUAMS).	*Baseline comparison:* Significant differences between the 2 groups were found. The control group had better performance in several aspects of cognitive flexibility, attention, depression, and QoL than the intervention group. *After intervention:* Both groups improved significantly in short-term and working memory after training; improvement as a result of pure training, however, was not found. Interaction effect between training effect and main effect of MS group for visuoconstructive performance was noticed; the ability of MS participants increased and that of controls deteriorated. No significant differences between pre- and post-intervention were observed in attention and communication ability.	Small sample size. Insufficient demographic data of study participants. Lack of follow-up assessment.

http://dx.doi.org/10.1159/000157885

(Continued)

Table D2. Evidence on Occupational Therapy–Related Interventions Focusing on Client Factors and Performance Skills for People With Multiple Sclerosis *(Cont.)*

Author/Year	Study Objectives	Level/Design/Participants	Intervention and Outcome Measures	Results	Study Limitations
Chiaravalloti, DeLuca, Moore, & Ricker (2005) http://dx.doi.org/10.1191/0269215503cr586oa	To examine the effect of imagery and context in improving new learning deficits	Level I RCT, 5-wk follow-up *N* = 29 participants with MS and impaired verbal new learning (1 participant dropped out).	*Intervention* *Experimental group:* Story memory technique. *Control group:* Memory exercise. *Outcome Measures* Attention, memory.	The intervention group showed more improvement in learning ability and memory immediately after treatment than the control group. No differences were found between groups in maintenance and long-term efficacy.	Small sample size.
Chiaravalloti, Demaree, Gaudino, & DeLuca (2003)	To evaluate the effect of increased repetition on recall ability in persons with MS	Level II Nonrandomized, 2-group, repeated measures (30 min, 90 min, and 1wk after intervention) *N* = 64 persons with MS (78% women); 21 with relapsing–remitting MS, 18 with primary progressive MS, 25 with secondary progressive MS, and 20 healthy individuals (80% women). Duration of MS from diagnosis range = 1–39 yr; EDSS range available for 57/64 = 0–8.5.	*Intervention* Both the MS and healthy control (HC) groups underwent the same procedure. An open-trial Selective Reminding Test (SRT) procedure was used for participants to learn a list of 10 semantically related words over a maximum of 15 trials. Participants were reminded only of words that were missed during Trials 2–15. But all trials required recalling all words on the list during the next trial. The SRT data from both MS and HC groups were used as a criterion forming low- and high-trial groups. *Outcome Measures* Paced Auditory Serial Addition Test (PASAT) for complex information processing; Auditory	Participants who experienced a larger number of learning trials had poorer recall across learning trials. The number of learning trials experienced (low vs. high) did not influence the decline in recall performance across delay periods. Significant differences in trials between low- and high-trial groups were noticed. The MS and HC groups demonstrated similar recall pattern in both low and high trials. Both the low- and high-trial MS groups demonstrated a decrease in the number of words across delay periods. Both low- and high-trial groups demonstrated a significant forgetting rate across recall periods. The number of learning trials experienced did not affect forgetting rate.	Unequal group size in the sample.

(Continued)

Table D2. Evidence on Occupational Therapy–Related Interventions Focusing on Client Factors and Performance Skills for People With Multiple Sclerosis (*Cont.*)

Author/Year	Study Objectives	Level/Design/Participants	Intervention and Outcome Measures	Results	Study Limitations
			Threshold Serial Addition Test (AT–SAT) for speed of information processing; Visual Threshold Serial Addition (VT–SAT) for speed of information processing in the visual modality; Weschler Adult Intelligence Scale–Revised (WAIS–R), Digit Span subtest for Auditory Attention and Working Memory.		
http://dx.doi.org/10.1191/0269215503cr586oa					
Flavia, Stampatori, Zanotti, Parrinello, & Capra (2010)	To examine the efficacy of a 3-mo computer-based intensive training program for attention, information processing, and executive functions	Level II Two-group $N = 20$ adults with MS; M EDSS score = 2.5 for intervention group, 1.5 for control group; average length of illness = 16.5 yr for intervention group, 18.5 yr for control group.	*Intervention* *Intervention group*: Use of RehaCom package for 3 consecutive mo to organize, plan, and develop solutions for realistic simulations using a small city map. *Control group*: No treatment. *Outcome Measures* Attention, memory.	The intervention group performed better in information processing, attention, and decision making. Younger participants had significantly greater improvement.	Small sample size. No randomization. Questionable appropriateness of outcome measures. No follow-up assessment.
http://dx.doi.org/10.3109/10.1016/j.jns.2009.09.024					

(Continued)

Table D2. Evidence on Occupational Therapy–Related Interventions Focusing on Client Factors and Performance Skills for People With Multiple Sclerosis (*Cont.*)

Author/Year	Study Objectives	Level/Design/Participants	Intervention and Outcome Measures	Results	Study Limitations
Goverover, Chiaravalloti, & DeLuca (2008)	To examine the utility of self-generation strategy in improving recall and performance of actual everyday tasks, specifically meal preparation and managing finances, in persons with MS	Level II Nonrandomized, 2-group (MS patients and healthy persons), pretest–posttest, follow-up (1 wk) *N* = 38 participants (20 persons with MS, 18 healthy persons). 80% (*n* = 16) of the participants were diagnosed with relapsing–remitting MS, 10% with primary progressive MS, and 10% with secondary progressive MS.	*Intervention* All participants performed 4 IADL tasks (2 cooking tasks, 2 managing finance tasks) in 2 conditions (provided vs. generated). Task presentations were followed by immediate recall, and 30 min after task presentation, participants were asked to actually perform the task. *Outcome Measures* Assessments were implemented 1 wk after initial presentations by phone to assess verbal recall of task steps for all 4 tasks. *Neuropsychologic tests:* • Processing speed: Symbol Digit Modalities Test (SDMT) oral version. • Executive control: 3 selected subtests of the Delis–Kaplan Executive Function System (D–KEFS; Trail-Making Test [TMT] for flexibility of thinking, Verbal Fluency Test, Color–Word Interference Test) • Language functions: Boston Naming Test (BNT) • Verbal memory: California Verbal Learning Test (CVLT) • Emotional functioning: State–Trait Anxiety Inventory (STAI) for anxiety and Chicago Multistate Depression Inventory (CMDI) for depression.	Significant differences between the 2 groups were found in executive control (cognitive functioning), but not on other measures. Significant benefit of self-generation over provided presentations across the tasks learned was found. Both groups benefited from the self-generation strategy. The control group demonstrated the greatest benefit from self-generation at immediate recall; however, the MS group benefited most from self-generation at the 1-wk recall.	Small sample size. Unreported disease severity of the participants. Procedure design (counterbalanced conditions and tasks).

http://dx.doi.org/10.1016/j.apmr.2007.11.059

(*Continued*)

Table D2. Evidence on Occupational Therapy–Related Interventions Focusing on Client Factors and Performance Skills for People With Multiple Sclerosis (*Cont.*)

Author/Year	Study Objectives	Level/Design/Participants	Intervention and Outcome Measures	Results	Study Limitations
Goverover, Hillary, Chiaravalloti, Arango-Lasprilla, & DeLuca (2009) http://dx.doi.org/10.1016/j.apmr.2007.11.059	To examine the spacing effects in the acquisition of everyday functional tasks in persons with MS	Level II Nonrandomized, 2-group, pretest–posttest $n = 20$ persons with MS (M age = 48.4 yr; 16 women; 65% of them with relapsing–remitting MS; average disease duration = 10.6 yr), $n = 18$ healthy control participants (M age = 41.4 yr; 12 women).	*Intervention* Participants in both groups underwent the same protocol: paragraph learning (verbal stimulus) and a mapped-route learning task (visual stimulus in nature) for a total of 3 trials per task. For each task, each participant was provided 2 conditions: massed (consecutive presentation of the task) vs. spaced (5-min delay for the next task). The condition and the order of task were counterbalanced to control for systematic order effects. *Outcome Measures* • Neuropsychologic testing for cognitive function: Digit Span subtests of the WAIS–R for working memory. • SDMT–Oral version for processing speed. • CVLT for learning and memory. • D–KEFS for executive functions.	The MS group performed significantly worse than the HC group on all tasks except for the CVLT and Digit Span–Backward. The mean number of elements recalled under the spaced condition was significantly higher than in the massed condition. No significant differences were found between the 2 groups, which suggested that both groups benefited from spaced learning across time during paragraph recall. No interaction was found between time and condition, suggesting that participants benefited similarly from learning new material in the spaced condition. No significant differences between the 2 conditions were found for either the immediate or the 30-min delayed recall of the Map Learning task.	Tasks not relevant to the participants' daily life.
Shatil, Metzer, Horvitz, & Miller (2010) http://dx.doi.org/10.3233/NRE-2010-0546	To explore adherence to a personalized, home-based, computerized cognitive training program and examine the impact of training on cognitive performance	Level II Matched 2-group $N = 107$ participants with MS (M age = 43.78 yr for intervention group, 41.35 yr for control group; M EDSS score = 3.06 for intervention group, 2.66 for control group). Attrition rate = 57%.	*Intervention* Intervention group: 24 sessions of CogniFit Personal Coach. Control group: No treatment during experimental period. *Outcome Measures* Cognitive abilities (memory, attention), eye–hand coordination.	The intervention group had significantly greater improvement in general memory, visual working memory, and verbal–auditory working memory. Cognitive training was shown to be related not only to improved memory but also to increased information retrieval and recall speed.	No randomization. No active control group. High attrition rate.

(*Continued*)

Table D2. Evidence on Occupational Therapy–Related Interventions Focusing on Client Factors and Performance Skills for People With Multiple Sclerosis (*Cont.*)

Author/Year	Study Objectives	Level/Design/Participants	Intervention and Outcome Measures	Results	Study Limitations
Solari et al. (2004) http://dx.doi.org/10.1016/j.jns.2004.04.027	To examine the effect of a computer-aided retraining program (RehaCom) on memory and attention	Level I RCT, double-blinded, 16-wk follow-up $N = 77$ participants with MS (age range = 22–65 yr; EDSS scores = 1.5–7.0).	*Intervention* Intervention group: Memory and attention retraining. Control group: Visuoconstructional and visuomotor coordination retraining. *Outcome Measures* Cognitive function.	No significant differences were found between groups, with one exception: The intervention group showed a greater mean percentage change on the word list generation test of the Brief Repeatable Battery of Neuropsychological Tests (BRB–N; phonemic retrieval) at both 8 and 16 wk.	Diversity of disease severity.
Emotional Regulation					
Forman & Lincoln (2010) http://dx.doi.org/10.1177/0269215509343492	To examine the effectiveness of group CBT in improving mood in persons with MS	Level I RCT, 3-mo follow-up $N = 40$ participants with MS and depression, anxiety, or both (age range = 25–68 yr).	*Intervention* Intervention group: 6 2-hr sessions of CBT over 12 wk. Wait-list control group: No intervention, but access to all other services as usual. *Outcome Measures* Anxiety, depression, MS impact, self-efficacy, QoL.	The intervention group had significantly lower scores on depression but not on anxiety or QoL after intervention. At 3-mo follow-up, the intervention group had improved, whereas the control group had deteriorated.	Small sample size.
Hughes, Robinson-Whelen, Taylor, & Hall (2006)	To evaluate the efficacy of a stress self-management program on stress and health behaviors in women with physical disabilities	Level I RCT, 2-group (wait-list control), pretest–posttest, 3-mo follow-up $N = 105$ women (63 completed the study; M age = 51.22 yr); 49.2% of participants completed college or graduate school; onset of disease range = 1–50 yr; 47.6% of participants had	*Intervention* The workshop, Stress Self-Management for Women with Disabilities Program (SSMWD), was based on CBT and influenced by feminist psychology and the philosophy of the independent living movement. It consisted of 6 weekly 2.5-hr group sessions.	Stress self-management intervention caused a significant decrease in stress and mental health, but not in physical health, compared with the control group at follow-up. Effects of the intervention on proposed mediators: Generalized increase in self-efficacy over time in both groups was observed. The workshop	Less heterogeneous groups used. High attrition rate.

(*Continued*)

Table D2. Evidence on Occupational Therapy–Related Interventions Focusing on Client Factors and Performance Skills for People With Multiple Sclerosis (Cont.)

Author/Year	Study Objectives	Level/Design/Participants	Intervention and Outcome Measures	Results	Study Limitations
		joint and connective tissue diseases (27% with MS, 7.9% with neuromuscular disorders, 6.3% with spinal impairments).	The workshop used 2 peer facilitators and emphasized action planning, problem-solving, peer support, and role modeling with 6 different topics. *Outcome Measures* Perceived Stress Scale (PSS); 2 subscales of the SF–36 (General Mental Health and Role Limitations); Center for Epidemiologic Studies–Depression Scale (CES–D); SF–36 (General Health, Pain and Role Limitation due to physical health) for assessing participants' physical health; Generalized Self-Efficacy Scale (GES); Stress Management Self-Efficacy Scale; Social Connectedness Scale–Revised (SCS–R); Health-Promoting Lifestyle Profile (HPLP II; Stress Management and Interpersonal Support subscale) for assessing health behaviors.	group had significantly greater stress management self-efficacy at posttest and greater social connectedness at follow-up. No significant differences on health-promoting behavior were found.	

http://dx.doi.org/10.1016/j.whi.2006.08.003

(Continued)

Table D2. Evidence on Occupational Therapy–Related Interventions Focusing on Client Factors and Performance Skills for People With Multiple Sclerosis (Cont.)

Author/Year	Study Objectives	Level/Design/Participants	Intervention and Outcome Measures	Results	Study Limitations
Malcomson, Dunwoody, & Lowe-Strong (2007) http://dx.doi.org/10.1007/s00415-006-0349-y	To review the effect of psychosocial interventions on QoL, well-being, or both	Level I Systematic review $N = 33$ articles published in English before January 2006.	*Intervention* CBT for depression (individual and group, led by psychologist and OT), group stress management, horseback riding (group), exercise (group and individual), relaxation (group), wellness and support (group vs. individual). *Outcome Measures* Emotional well-being, QoL.	Limited evidence was found of positive benefits of group CBT in reducing depression and improving vitality. Evidence was found to support use of combined education, multidisciplinary focus, goal setting, homework assignments, and discussion forums. Weak evidence was found for use of exercise training, relaxation, and stress management.	Few studies with high-quality methodology included.
Mohr, Hart, & Goldberg (2003)	To examine the effects of treatment for depression on fatigue in persons with MS	Level II Nonrandomized, 3-group, pretest–posttest $N = 71$ participants (60 completed the assessments used for analysis); $n = 22$ in CBT group, $n = 22$ in supportive–expressive group (SEGP), $n = 16$ in sertraline treatment. M age = 44.6 yr; 43 women; 85% White; M yr since diagnosis = 31; M ambulation index (AI) score = 2.45, with a 0–8 range in the study participants, indicating mild-to-moderate gait impairment.	*Intervention* This study compared 3 16-wk interventions for depression on fatigue: individual CBT, SEGP, and sertraline. The individual CBT involved 16 individual 50-min meetings per week with a PhD-level psychologist, aimed at specific skills for managing MS-related symptoms and problems. The SEGP was conducted in group (5–9 persons) with two PhD-level psychologists for 16 90-min sessions/wk, focusing on enhancing emotional expression. Participants in the sertraline group received	Significant reduction in overall fatigue and fatigue severity was observed over the course of treatment. However, differences among the 3 treatments reached only marginal significance. After removing effects of other variables in the model, depression was found significantly associated with Week 16 total FAI, Global Fatigue Severity subscale, and Fatigue Consequences subscale. No relationship was found between BDI and Responsiveness to Rest/Sleep subscale. The effect	Lack of an active control group. High attrition rate.

(Continued)

Table D2. Evidence on Occupational Therapy–Related Interventions Focusing on Client Factors and Performance Skills for People With Multiple Sclerosis (*Cont.*)

Author/Year	Study Objectives	Level/Design/Participants	Intervention and Outcome Measures	Results	Study Limitations
			sertraline: initially 50 mg/day, increased by 50 mg every 4 wk until a dosage of 200 mg was reached, or until full remission was achieved. *Outcome Measures* • BDI • Fatigue Assessment Instrument (FAI) consisted of 4 subscales: Global Fatigue Severity, Situation-Specific Fatigue, Fatigue Consequences, and Responsiveness to Rest/Sleep).	size for change in overall fatigue accounted for 9% of variance and 12% for global severity of fatigue. The authors reported that the SEGP has the least effects compared with the others.	
http://dx.doi.org/10.1097/01.PSY.0000074757.11682.96					
Rigby, Thornton, & Young (2008)	To examine the effect of group psychological interventions on mood, self-efficacy, and resiliency	Level I RCT, 3-group, repeated measures $N = 147$ adults with MS (age range = 20–65 yr; M duration = 9.0 yr; median EDSS score = 6). Attrition rate = 35%.	*Intervention* *Information booklet group (IBG)*: Suggesting sources of help and coping strategies. *Social discussion group (SDG)*: Booklet and 3 90-min sessions/wk aimed at enabling participants to talk about their condition. *Psychotherapeutic group (PG)*: Booklet and 3 90-min sessions/wk to facilitate sense of perceived control and self-efficacy and to enhance participants' feelings of well-being, led by a clinical health psychologist. *Outcome Measures* Anxiety, depression, self-efficacy.	No differences were found between groups at any time points for depression. For anxiety, PG > IBG and SDG > IBG; for self-efficacy, PG > IBG and SDG > IBG. Significant differences were found between PG and IBG and between SDG and IBG for resiliency.	No active control. Short intervention period. High attrition rate.
http://dx.doi.org/10.1348/135910707X241505					

(*Continued*)

Table D2. Evidence on Occupational Therapy–Related Interventions Focusing on Client Factors and Performance Skills for People With Multiple Sclerosis (*Cont.*)

Author/Year	Study Objectives	Level/Design/Participants	Intervention and Outcome Measures	Results	Study Limitations
Thomas, Thomas, Hillier, Galvin, & Baker (2006) http://dx.doi.org/10.1002/14651858.CD004431.pub2	To review the effectiveness of psychological interventions	Level I Systematic review $N = 16$ RCTs examining psychological theory and practice interventions for persons with MS using disease-specific and general QoL, psychiatric symptoms, psychological functioning, disability, or cognitive outcomes.	*Intervention* Psychological interventions for persons with MS and cognitive impairment, MS and moderate to severe disability, MS alone, and MS with depression *Outcome Measures* QoL, psychiatric symptoms, psychological functioning, cognition.	No significant benefits were found for interventions for people with MS and cognitive impairment. No conclusion could be drawn about interventions for people with MS and moderate to severe disability. Some evidence indicates that CBT provides benefits in stress inoculation, understanding, coping with emotions, and self-efficacy for people with MS alone. CBT was effective for people with MS and mild to moderate depression.	Insufficient studies with higher quality of methodology included.
Exercise					
Asano, Dawes, Arafah, Moriello, & Mayo (2009) http://dx.doi.org/10.1177/1352458508101877	To review research on the role of exercise and provide a guide for exercise prescription	Level I Systematic review $N = 11$ RCT studies published in a scientific journal involving participants with MS, active exercise or physical activity, both intervention and control groups, and quantitative results.	*Intervention* Aerobic exercise, yoga, resistance and strengthening exercise, stretching exercise; range = 3 wk to 6 mo; sessions lasting 30–90 min; frequency range 1×–5×/wk *Outcome Measures* Body function and structure; activity, such as walking test or physiological test; QoL.	Physiotherapy Evidence Database (PEDro) scores for the 11 studies ranged from fair to good. Aerobic exercise with or without additional exercise components was the most common type of exercise intervention. Effect sizes for body function = −0.29 (quadriceps maximum voluntary contraction) to 3.50 (maximal oxygen consumption); effect sizes for activity = −0.06 (body sway) to 0.48 (10-m walk test); effect sizes for QoL = −0.36 to 2.56.	Mixed age and disease severity in the sample.

(*Continued*)

Table D2. Evidence on Occupational Therapy–Related Interventions Focusing on Client Factors and Performance Skills for People With Multiple Sclerosis *(Cont.)*

Author/Year	Study Objectives	Level/Design/Participants	Intervention and Outcome Measures	Results	Study Limitations
Ayán Pérez, Sánchez, Teixeira, & Fernández (2007)	To examine the effects of a 6-wk resistance training program for persons with mild MS on muscle strength, balance, and walking speed	Level III Nonrandomized, 1-group, pretest–posttest $N = 36$ persons with MS (22 women; able to walk; EDSS range = 1–6, M score = 1.5). 12 participants dropped out of the study.	*Intervention* 60-min sessions, 3×/wk for 6 wk. The exercises were strengthening of the lower extremities and the core muscles, based on calisthenic or body-weight exercises, where the participant's body weight is the load to be lifted, without additional equipment. *Outcome Measures* Clapping test (CT) and dynamic flexibility test (DF) for mobility of arms and time–space orientation; zigzag run of 9 m for walking speed; throwing a medicine ball over the head; vertical jump with feet together; abdominal test, back muscle test, leg lifts, and a Kraus–Weber (K–W) test for trunk strength; flamingo balance test for balance.	Significant improvements were noticed in the back muscles, arm strength (medicine ball), leg lifts, and repetitions of sit-ups. Significant increase in walking speed was also observed. In addition, female participants demonstrated significant changes in all tests of strength. However, male participants demonstrated significant changes only in 2 tests (leg lift and sit-up repetitions) and 1 orientation test (DF). Significant improvement in balance was not observed in either men or women.	Small sample size. Lack of a control group. Outcome measures were not robust.

(Continued)

Table D2. Evidence on Occupational Therapy–Related Interventions Focusing on Client Factors and Performance Skills for People With Multiple Sclerosis *(Cont.)*

Author/Year	Study Objectives	Level/Design/Participants	Intervention and Outcome Measures	Results	Study Limitations
Bjarnadottir, Konradsdottir, Reynisdottir, & Olafsson (2007) http://dx.doi.org/10.1177/1352458506073780	To evaluate the effects of aerobic and strength exercise on physical fitness and QoL in persons with mild MS	Level I RCT, 2-group, pretest–posttest $N = 16$ persons with mild relapsing–remitting MS (11 women; M age = 38.7 yr/36.1 yr [treatment/control]); EDSS = 2.1/1.8 (treatment/control). Attrition rate = 30% (7/23 participants).	*Intervention* *Treatment group:* 60-min session, 3×/wk for 5 wk, or a total of 15 hr. Exercise period consisted of (1) aerobic exercise, including 3 min of warm-up and cool-down at 33% of VO_2 peak and 15–20 min of anaerobic threshold (55% of VO_2 peak); (2) resistance exercise, including 13 exercises of major muscle groups; and (3) stretching and relaxation during the last 5 min. *Control group:* Participants recorded a diary of all physical activity that exceeded 20 min and occurring more than 2×/wk. *Outcome Measures* EDSS for disease severity; SF–36 for QoL; VO_2 for physical fitness.	Participants in the treatment group showed increased VO_2 peak (14.7%), peak workload (18.2%), and anaerobic threshold (27.3%). No significant change was found in those in control group. There was a trend toward improvement in SF–36 in the treatment group, but only the Vitality subscale reached statistical significance. One participant in each group developed an MS relapse during the study period and was withdrawn from the study immediately. No changes in disease severity were observed among the 16 participants.	High attrition rate. Small sample size.
Cakit et al. (2010)	To evaluate the effects of cycling progressive resistance training combined with balance exercises on walking speed, balance, fatigue, fear of falling, depression, and QoL in persons with MS	Level I RCT, 3-group, pretest–posttest $N = 45$ relapsing–remitting or secondary progressive MS patients with mild to moderate	*Intervention* *Group 1:* 16 training sessions of progressive resistance training on a static bicycle ergometer, with 15 sets of repetitions in each session over 8 wk. Each set consisted of 2 min of 40%	Participants in Group 1 demonstrated significant improvement after the intervention in these areas: endurance of exercise, walking speed, static and dynamic balance (TUG, DGI, and FR), FES, FSS, and BDI.	Small sample size. Lack of a follow-up assessment. High attrition rate.

(Continued)

Table D2. Evidence on Occupational Therapy-Related Interventions Focusing on Client Factors and Performance Skills for People With Multiple Sclerosis (Cont.)

Author/Year	Study Objectives	Level/Design/Participants	Intervention and Outcome Measures	Results	Study Limitations
		disability level (EDSS scores <6.0) who were capable of standing independently in upright position for more than 3 sec; 33 completed the study (20 women, 13 men; duration since diagnosis = 3–20 yr; *M* age range = 35.5–43 yr).	of the tolerated maximum workload (TMW) and 2 min of low-resistance pedaling on an ergometer or 2 min of rest. After cycling training, participants underwent warm-up activities and stretches, balance exercises, and whole-body stretching. *Group 2*: Home-based exercise program, which was the same exercise program as for Group 1 and aimed at improving lower-limb strength. *Group 3 (control group)*: No exercise intervention but asked to continue with their normal living. *Outcome Measures* • 10-min test for walking speed • TUG for dynamic balance • Dynamic Gait Index (DGI) for ability to adapt gait to changes in task demands • Functional Reach (FR) for static balance • FES for fear of falling • Fatigue Severity Scale (FSS) • BDI • SF–36.	Participants in Group 2 showed significant improvement in endurance of exercise, tolerated maximum workload, and FES after 8 wk of home-based exercise. No significant improvement was observed in the control group. Improvement in Group 1 was higher than in the other groups, except for the 10-min walking test. No significant differences between groups were found in scores on the SF–36. Participants in Group 1 showed significant improvement in Physical Functioning and Role-Physical Functioning scales of SF–36. Participants in Group 2 showed significant improvement in Physical Functioning subscale of the SF–36.	

http://dx.doi.org/10.1097/PHM.0b013e3181d3e71f

(Continued)

Table D2. Evidence on Occupational Therapy–Related Interventions Focusing on Client Factors and Performance Skills for People With Multiple Sclerosis (*Cont.*)

Author/Year	Study Objectives	Level/Design/Participants	Intervention and Outcome Measures	Results	Study Limitations
DeBolt & McCubbin (2004) http://dx.doi.org/10.1016/j.apmr.2003.06.003	To examine the effect of an 8-wk home-based resistance exercise program on balance, power, and mobility	Level II Stratified (age and EDSS score), matched 2-group $N = 29$ women (M age = 50.3 yr) and 8 men (M age = 51.1 yr) with MS, capable of walking ≥20 m without rest (1 participant in the exercise group did not complete the posttest because of symptom exacerbation).	*Intervention* *Exercise group:* 2 wk of instructional sessions and exercise 3×/wk, then 8 wk of home-based resistance training 3×/wk, focusing on increasing strength and power in the lower extremities. *Control group:* No treatment during study period. *Outcome Measures* Balance, leg power, functional ability.	*Exercise adherence:* 95% of sessions were completed. *Balance:* No significant differences were found between groups. *Leg extensor power:* The exercise group showed significant improvement after intervention. No significant difference between groups was found at posttest (effect size = 0.22). No significant findings were found for mobility.	Small sample size.
de Souza-Teixeira et al. (2009) http://dx.doi.org/10.1055/s-0028-1105944	To examine the effects of 8-wk progressive resistance training on strength manifestations, muscle mass, and functionality in persons with MS	Level III Nonrandomized, 1-group, pretest–posttest, self-control $N = 13$ persons with mild to moderate MS (M age = 43 yr, EDSS: 3.4 ± 1.7). Male:female ratio not reported.	*Intervention* After 8-wk control period (no physical training), all participants underwent 8 wk of progressive resistance training 2×/wk. Participants were trained on a leg extension machine used in the evaluation. *Outcome Measures* MRI of the thigh for strength manifestation, MVC and maximal power of knee extensors for strength, maximal number of repetitions a participant could achieve for muscular endurance, and TUG for functionality.	After 8 wk of training, significant improvement in MVC (effect size = 0.43), maximal power (effect size = 0.96), and muscular endurance (effect size = 1.83) and significant reduction in time of completion the TUG. No significant correlations between gain in cross-sectional area and any gain in the strength manifestation and between the increase in power and the decrease in time for TUG after the training.	Small sample size.

(*Continued*)

Table D2. Evidence on Occupational Therapy–Related Interventions Focusing on Client Factors and Performance Skills for People With Multiple Sclerosis *(Cont.)*

Author/Year	Study Objectives	Level/Design/Participants	Intervention and Outcome Measures	Results	Study Limitations
Dettmers, Sulzmann, Ruchay-Plössl, Gütler, & Vieten (2009)	To evaluate the effects of a 3-wk endurance training program on walking ability in persons with mild MS	Level I RCT, 2-group, pretest–posttest *N* = 30 persons with mild MS (21 women); EDSS score <4.5; 15 participants in each group; most had relapsing–remitting MS (10 and 11, respectively, for the intervention and control groups). *M* EDSS = 2.6 and 2.8, respectively, for the groups; *M* duration since diagnosis = 8 and 6/1 yr, respectively.	*Intervention* Participants in the intervention group received 3 45-min weekly group training sessions (with 3–5 persons) directed by a trained PE student, including warming up, mild strength training, and repetitive endurance exercise, followed by relaxation and feedback. The content of training was incorporated with games and other playful elements. Participants in the control group received a training program consisting of warming up, sensory training, stretching, balance, and coordination training and periods of relaxation for 3 wk. *Primary Outcome Measures* Walking ability: walking distance and walking time. *Secondary Outcome Measures* Modified Fatigue Impact Scale (MFIS), Fatigue Scale for Motor and Cognitive Functions (FSMC), BDI, and HAQUAMS.	Participants in the intervention group demonstrated significant improvement in walking ability. The average walking distance increased 650 m in the intervention group and 96 m in the control group. The walking time increased by 11 min in the intervention group, whereas increase of 1 min was observed in the control group. As for the secondary outcome measures, significant improvement was observed in the control group rather than the intervention group.	Lack of a blinded assessor. Small sample size.

http://dx.doi.org/10.1111/j.1600-0404.2008.01152.x

(Continued)

Table D2. Evidence on Occupational Therapy–Related Interventions Focusing on Client Factors and Performance Skills for People With Multiple Sclerosis (*Cont.*)

Author/Year	Study Objectives	Level/Design/Participants	Intervention and Outcome Measures	Results	Study Limitations
Fragoso, Santana, & Pinto (2008)	To examine the effects of a 20-wk physical activity program in MS patients with fatigue	Level III Nonrandomized, 1-group, pretest–posttest $N = 10$ persons with MS who experienced symptoms of fatigue (9 women; age range = 20–49 yr; 4 had mild depression); 1 participant withdrew (due to lack of motivation).	*Intervention* The program included • 4 wk of stretching exercise (60 min per session), 10 wk of a progressive program of stretching exercises for 15 min, followed by 30 min of a repetitive series of exercises with light weights and then another series of stretching exercises for 15 min, and • 6 wk of increased duration, including 30 min of stretching, 30 min of muscle resistance, and 30 min of conditioning exercises, with walks and short running periods. *Outcome Measures* Physiological testing, BMI, percentages of body fat, lean mass, blood pressure, and heart frequency. Chalder Fatigue Scale for assessing severity of fatigue.	The average attendance rate was 80.6% (range = 71%–95%). The study participants demonstrated significant changes in some parameters of physical conditioning, including heart frequency and systolic and diastolic blood pressure after the intervention. Significant improvement in the severity of fatigue after the training program was also observed. No significant differences were found in BMI, percentage of body fat, and lean mass, suggesting that this program did not have an effect on muscle building.	Small sample size. Lack of a control group. No description of Chalder Fatigue Scale (one of the primary outcome measures).

(*Continued*)

Table D2. Evidence on Occupational Therapy–Related Interventions Focusing on Client Factors and Performance Skills for People With Multiple Sclerosis *(Cont.)*

Author/Year	Study Objectives	Level/Design/Participants	Intervention and Outcome Measures	Results	Study Limitations
Freeman & Allison (2004) http://dx.doi.org/10.1002/pri.307	To assess the effects of a group exercise class program on mobility, balance, fatigue, and well-being in ambulant persons with MS	Level III Nonrandomized, 1-group, pretest–posttest, 4-wk follow-up $N = 10$ ambulant persons with MS were included (8 women); age range = 29–69 yr; yr since diagnosis = 1–40. M EDSS = 5.0 (range 3.0–6.5).	*Intervention* All participants experienced 10 1-hr sessions of group exercise. Each session consisted of 30 min of exercise in the standing position and 30 min of floor-based exercises (based on the Pilates principles of core stability), postures, and stretches. A support session was led by the participants after each exercise session without the appearance of the therapist. *Outcome Measures* Berg Balance Scale (BBS); the MS Impact Scale (MSIS) for impact of fatigue related to MS; the 12-Item Multiple Sclerosis Walking Scale (MSWS–12) and the 6-min walking test (6MWT) for mobility; Physiological Cost Index (PCI).	After the intervention, participants demonstrated significant improvements in balance performance, 6MTW (both distance and speed of walking), performance in MSWS–12, Physical component of the MSIS, and Motor component of the MSIS. At the 4-wk postintervention assessment, all scores apart from the PCI remained improved in comparison to the baseline assessment. Both the balance performance and the speed and distance walked in the 6MWT continued to improve at the follow-up assessment.	Small sample size. Lack of a control group.

(Continued)

Table D2. Evidence on Occupational Therapy–Related Interventions Focusing on Client Factors and Performance Skills for People With Multiple Sclerosis (Cont.)

Author/Year	Study Objectives	Level/Design/Participants	Intervention and Outcome Measures	Results	Study Limitations
Geddes, Costello, Raivel, & Wilson (2009)	To assess the effects of a 12-wk home walking program on cardiovascular parameters, fatigue perception, and walking distance in persons with MS	Level I RCT, 2-group, pretest–posttest N = 12 ambulatory persons with MS were included (9 women; age = 22–64 yr; EDSS range = 3.5–6).	*Intervention* Participants in the exercise group received an individualized 20–30 min home walking program, 3×/wk for 12 wk, based on the results of the 6MWT. Walking speeds were adjusted to stay within their prescribed heart rate range. Participants in the control group were asked to refrain from any regular exercise during the experimental period. *Outcome Measures* FSS for self-perceived fatigue level; 6MWT for physical performance; PCI for gait efficiency and energy expenditure; Borg's Rating of perceived exertion (RPE) for exercise intensity; heart rate reserved (HRR) method for prescribed exercise intensity.	Participants in both groups demonstrated improvement in physical performance (mean walking distance) and gait efficiency and energy expenditure (PCI), but no significant differences between the 2 groups were found. Participants in the exercise group reported no incidence of falls, no increase in fatigue level, and no adverse effects related to the exercise program.	Small and unequal sample size. Heterogeneity of sample participants. Unreported effect size.
McAuley et al. (2007)	To evaluate the effects of a 3-mo efficacy enhancement intervention on adherence and perceptions of well-being following an exercise program in persons with MS	Level I RCT, 2-group, pretest–posttest N = 26 adults with MS (M age = 43.46 yr; mo after diagnosis = 106.73;	*Intervention* All participants received a 3-mo, 3×/wk (1-hr sessions) physical activity program of stretching exercise and aerobic exercise. Participants in both groups	Effects on exercise adherence, perceived exertion, and affective responses: Although no significant effect was found on adherence, participants in the efficacy enhancement group	Small sample size. Lack of a control group. High attrition rate (42%).

(Continued)

Table D2. Evidence on Occupational Therapy–Related Interventions Focusing on Client Factors and Performance Skills for People With Multiple Sclerosis *(Cont.)*

Author/Year	Study Objectives	Level/Design/Participants	Intervention and Outcome Measures	Results	Study Limitations
	To examine the effects of the intervention on affective and perceived exertion response to acute exercise across the intervention	23 women; 24 White; 24 relapsing-remitting MS); 15 participants (9 in the intervention group and 6 in the control group) completed the study.	then received biweekly workshops (either efficacy enhancement or standard care) after physical activity. The efficacy enhancement workshop focused on providing efficacy-based information relative to physical activity participation through lectures and discussion and homework assignments. The standard care workshop focused on general health-related topics presentation and discussion. *Outcome Measures* • 6-item Exercise Self-Efficacy (EXSE) scale • Satisfaction With Life Scale (SWLS) • 12-item Short Form Survey (SF-12) for physical and mental health status • Daily attendance logs for exercise adherence • Measures of enjoyment, affect, and ratings of perceived exertion following each exercise session.	tended to attend more exercise sessions than those in the standard care group (effect size: medium). Significant effect on perceptual responses to exercise was observed in participants in the efficacy enhancement group: Participants felt that they worked harder during exercise and felt better after exercise. There was a significant interaction effect between time and intervention group for well-being. Participants in the efficacy enhancement condition maintained levels of satisfaction with life over the intervention period. However, those in the standard care group declined over time. Relationships between self-efficacy, affective responses, and adherence: Participants with a stronger sense of self-efficacy in exercise demonstrated significantly greater adherence with the exercise program. However, no association between feeling better during exercise and exercise adherence was found.	

http://dx.doi.org/10.1177/1352458506072188

(Continued)

Table D2. Evidence on Occupational Therapy–Related Interventions Focusing on Client Factors and Performance Skills for People With Multiple Sclerosis (Cont.)

Author/Year	Study Objectives	Level/Design/Participants	Intervention and Outcome Measures	Results	Study Limitations
McCullagh, Fitzgerald, Murphy, & Cooke (2008) http://dx.doi.org/10.1177/0269215507082283	To determine the immediate and long-term effects of exercise on QoL and fatigue in persons with MS	Level I RCT, 2-group, 3-mo follow-up $N = 30$ people with mild MS who were independently mobile and able to exercise independently at home; $n = 17$ in exercise group, $n = 13$ in control group.	*Intervention* *Exercise group:* 2 50-min weekly sessions, in groups of 4–6, consisting of treadmill exercise, cycling, StairMaster training, arm-strengthening exercises, volleyball, outdoor walking, and 40-min to 60-min/wk home exercise for 12 wk. *Control group:* Normal activity levels and PT 1×/mo. *Outcome Measures* QoL, MFIS, and graded exercise test measured at baseline, 3 mo, and 6 mo.	The exercise group showed significant immediate effects in improved QoL, self-perceived impact of fatigue, and exercise capacity. Participants showed improvements in QoL and impact of fatigue at follow-up but not in exercise capacity. Additionally, all participants completed ≥20 of the 24 hospital-based classes. No one completed more than half of the home sessions.	Small sample size. Randomization process was not followed completely during assignment, as intervention group appeared to be getting too large. Large proportion of dropouts. Low compliance to home program.
Oken et al. (2004)	To compare the effects of yoga and aerobic exercise on cognitive function, fatigue, mood, and QoL in persons with mild MS	Level I RCT, 3-group, pretest–posttest $N = 57$ persons with MS in 2 intervention groups and 1 wait-list control group (53 women; M age range = 48.4–49.8 yr; M scores on EDSS = 2.9–3.1); participants were stratified by age, sex, and baseline EDSS scores. Attrition rate = 17% (12/69).	*Intervention* *Yoga group:* Modified Iyengar yoga for 90-min sessions/week over 6 mo. All poses were adapted to suit individual needs. There was an emphasis on breathing for concentration and relaxation during the session. Daily home practice was encouraged. *Aerobic exercise group:* Bicycling on recumbent or dual-action stationary bicycles with the schedule similar to yoga group.	No significant effects of assigned groups were observed on any of the cognitive function or alertness measures. Participants in yoga and aerobic groups performed better on several self-rated scales than those in the wait-list control group (Vitality subscale of the SF–36). Compared with the control group, both interventions showed similar improvement. No significant improvements on fatigue, mood, and QoL were found.	Small sample size.

(Continued)

Table D2. Evidence on Occupational Therapy–Related Interventions Focusing on Client Factors and Performance Skills for People With Multiple Sclerosis (Cont.)

Author/Year	Study Objectives	Level/Design/Participants	Intervention and Outcome Measures	Results	Study Limitations
			Participants continued bicycling until they were ready to stop due to fatigue, onset of other MS symptoms, or reaching their personal goal. Regular home bicycling was encouraged. *Control group:* No treatment. *Outcome Measures* • Cognition: Stroop Color and Word Test (focusing attention) • Alertness: Stanford Sleepiness Scale, Profile of Mood Status (POMS), and EEG median power frequency analysis • Mood (fatigue and vigor): POMS • Fatigue: Multidimensional Fatigue Inventory (MFI) • Stress: STAI and SF–36.		

http://dx.doi.org/10.1212/01.WNL.0000129534.88602.5C

(Continued)

Table D2. Evidence on Occupational Therapy–Related Interventions Focusing on Client Factors and Performance Skills for People With Multiple Sclerosis (Cont.)

Author/Year	Study Objectives	Level/Design/Participants	Intervention and Outcome Measures	Results	Study Limitations
Ratchford et al. (2010) http://dx.doi.org/10.3233/NRE-2010-0588	To evaluate the safety and preliminary efficacy of home FES cycling for 6 mo in persons with progressive MS	Level III *Design:* Nonrandomized, 1-group, pretest–posttest *Participants:* 5 persons with MS were included (3 men; 3 participants with secondary progressive MS, median age = 50 yr; M duration of disease = 13 yr); EDSS = 6.0–6.5; 1 participant who dislocated a shoulder during a fall unrelated to the intervention was included in the safety analysis.	*Intervention* FES cycling: Installed in home, at least 3×/wk for 1 hr per session. Quadriceps, hamstrings, and gluteals selected for FES. *Outcome Measures* Walking ability: 2-min walk test (2MWT), Timed 25-Foot Walk Test (T25FWT), and TUG.	*FES cycle usage:* The data were captured by the cycle and transmitted to an Internet database. The mean number of sessions per week was 3.8 (range = 3.1–5.1). *Safety analyses:* No serious adverse events were reported. *Walking ability:* In the 2MWT, the mean distance improved by 13%. In the T25FWT, the mean time improved by 36%. In the TUG, the mean time improved by 22%.	Small sample size in most studies may have led to Type 2 error. Lack of a control group.
Rietberg, Brooks, Uitdehaag, & Kwakkel (2004) http://dx.doi.org/10.1002/14651858.CD003980.pub2	To assess the effect of exercise therapy on ADLs and health-related QoL	Level I Systematic review $N = 9$ RCTs with participants not presently experiencing an exacerbation and with outcome measures of activity limitation, health-related QoL, or both.	*Intervention* Outpatient interventions: General exercise, combined arm and leg ergometry, aerobic training, task-oriented training vs. facilitation training. Home exercise interventions: Home mobility exercises, home weighted-leg exercise, resistance exercise. *Outcome Measures* Body function, physiological symptoms, disease severity, ADLs, QoL.	Strong evidence was provided for exercise therapy compared with no exercise therapy in terms of muscle power, exercise endurance, and mobility-related activities. Moderate evidence was found for improvement in mood. No effects of exercise therapy were found for fatigue and self-perceived disability.	Few studies with high-quality methodology.

(Continued)

Table D2. Evidence on Occupational Therapy–Related Interventions Focusing on Client Factors and Performance Skills for People With Multiple Sclerosis (Cont.)

Author/Year	Study Objectives	Level/Design/Participants	Intervention and Outcome Measures	Results	Study Limitations
Roehrs & Karst (2004)	To assess the effects of a 12-wk aquatic exercise program on QoL in persons with MS	Level III Nonrandomized, 1-group, pretest–posttest N = 31 persons with MS were included in the study (12 withdrew); data from the remaining 19 participants were used for analyses (12 women ages 39–71 yr, EDSS range = 3.5–8; 7 men ages 40–65 yr, EDSS range = 1.5–8). Attrition rate = 39%.	*Intervention* Participants received individualized aquatic exercise program (based on the scores of EDSS evaluated by a neurologist or specialized MS nurse) 2×/wk, 1 hr per session, for 12 wk. The pool water temperature was maintained at 83°–85°. However, individual or group exercise was not mentioned. *Outcome Measures* • Two self-reported outcome measures used for measuring health-related QoL: SF–36 and the Multiple Sclerosis Quality of Life Inventory (MSQLI) • MFIS.	After intervention, participants demonstrated significant improvement in the Social Function subscales of the SF–36 and significant changes in MFIS and Medical Outcome Study (MOS) Modified Social Support Survey (MSSS) of the MSQLI. No significant correlation between the change in the QoL measures and the number of classes attended or the initial EDSS score was found. A significant negative correlation between the pre-exercise MSSS score and the change in the MSSS following the exercise was observed, suggesting that participants who perceived lower social support prior to the intervention tended to have greater improvement after the exercise program.	Small sample size. Lack of a control group. High attrition rate.

http://dx.doi.org/10.1097/01.NPT.0000281186.94382.90

(Continued)

Table D2. Evidence on Occupational Therapy–Related Interventions Focusing on Client Factors and Performance Skills for People With Multiple Sclerosis (Cont.)

Author/Year	Study Objectives	Level/Design/Participants	Intervention and Outcome Measures	Results	Study Limitations
Romberg et al. (2004)	To examine the effect of a progressive 6-mo exercise program on walking performance and other aspects of physical function	Level I Stratified (by gender) RCT $N = 114$ participants with mild to moderate MS; 95 included in analysis (M age = 43.8 yr in intervention group, 43.9 yr in control group).	*Intervention* *Intervention group:* 5 supervised strengthening and 5 aerobic exercise sessions in hospital; 3 strengthening sessions per week and 1 aerobic exercise session at home. *Control group:* Avoided great changes in physical activity habits. *Outcome Measures* Walking performance.	Both groups showed significantly improved walking speed at posttest (effect size = 0.50 for exercise, 0.19 for control). Walking endurance improved significantly in the exercise group (effect size = 0.26) but not in the control group.	No long-term follow-up.
http://dx.doi.org/10.1212/01.WNL.0000145761.38400.65					
Schulz et al. (2004)	To examine the effects of an 8-wk aerobic bicycle training on functional domains and physiological factors as well as coordinative function in persons with MS	Level I RCT, 2-group, pretest–posttest $N = 39$ persons with MS; $n = 28$ persons included in the immune–endocrine study (19 women; M EDSS scores = 2.0/2.5 [training/control]), $n = 39$ persons included in the coordinative study (10 women; M EDSS scores = 2.5/2.7 [training/control]).	*Intervention* Participants in the exercise group exercised 2×/wk with an interval-training schedule for 30 min at a maximal intensity of 75% of the maximal watts taken from the ergometry results for 8 wk. Participants in the wait-list control group received no treatment. *Outcome Measures* • *Fitness parameters:* Maximum performance (in watts) and relative VO_2 max • *Coordinative function:* Walking test and Figure 8 test from the *Bewegungs und Koordinationstest fur Kur-Teilnehmer*.	*Fitness parameters:* Significant increased physical fitness in the training group was observed. No significant changes in biochemical assays were observed. No significant effects of the training program were found in the depression and anxiety tests. Results showed an improvement in disease-specific QoL in the training group, while the control group remain stable. No significant changes were found in the walking test.	Small sample size. High attrition rate.

(Continued)

Table D2. Evidence on Occupational Therapy–Related Interventions Focusing on Client Factors and Performance Skills for People With Multiple Sclerosis (Cont.)

Author/Year	Study Objectives	Level/Design/Participants	Intervention and Outcome Measures	Results	Study Limitations
			• *Biochemical assays:* Endocrine assays, neurotropic factors BDNF and NGF, IL–6 and sIL–6R ELISA. • POMS for distinct affective states • Hospital Anxiety and Depression Scale (HADS) for affective symptomatology • HAQUAMS • German version of the generic SF–36 for QoL.	The training group demonstrated improvements in 2 of 3 coordinative tasks.	
http://dx.doi.org/10.1016/j.jns.2004.06.009					
Snook & Motl (2009)	To examine the effect of exercise training interventions on walking mobility	Level I Meta-analysis *N* = 22 studies published in English that measured walking mobility and included only an exercise training intervention or an exercise intervention plus a control condition.	*Intervention* *Intervention setting:* Home, exercise facility, or both. *Mode of exercise:* Aerobic, nonaerobic, resistance, aerobic plus resistance. *Mode of aerobic exercise:* Cycling and treadmill. *Length of intervention:* <3 mo, ≥3 mo. *Outcome Measures* Walking mobility.	The effect of exercise training on walking mobility differed by type of MS. A significant effect for exercise training occurred in a supervised setting. A significant effect was found for intervention of <3 mo. The small number of effect sizes for each level of variable may be attributed to the results of analysis.	Less homogeneous studies with related topics included.
http://dx.doi.org/10.1177/1545968308320641					

(Continued)

Table D2. Evidence on Occupational Therapy–Related Interventions Focusing on Client Factors and Performance Skills for People With Multiple Sclerosis (Cont.)

Author/Year	Study Objectives	Level/Design/Participants	Intervention and Outcome Measures	Results	Study Limitations
Sosnoff, Motl, Snook, & Wynn (2009) http://dx.doi.org/10.3233/NRE-2009-0486	To examine the chronic effect of unloaded leg cycling exercise on spasticity in persons with MS	Level II Nonrandomized, 2-group, pretest–posttest (1 day, 1 wk, and 4 wk after intervention) $N = 22$ persons with relapsing–remitting MS ($n = 19$), primary progressive MS ($n = 2$), or secondary progressive ($n = 1$) MS; EDSS range = 0–6; Modified Ashworth Scale (MAS) score = 1–3.	*Intervention* The exercise program consisted of unloaded leg cycling performed on a stationary cycle ergometer for 30 min/session 3×/wk across a 4-wk period. The control condition accounted for passage of time and instrumentation effects. *Outcome Measures* H-reflex of the soleus muscle of the right leg (an electrophysiological index of spasticity), MAS (clinical index of spasticity), and MS Spasticity Scale (MSSS–88; a self-reported measure of MS-related spasticity).	Significant interaction effect between training and time was found. *H reflex (H_{max}/M_{max} ratio):* A significant reduction in the H_{max}/M_{max} ratio immediately after the 4-wk period in the control group and a significant reduction in the ratio 4 wk after the intervention period in the exercise group were observed. *MAS:* No significant effect was observed in both conditions. *MSSS:* There was a significant reduction in overall MSSS–88 scores immediately after the exercise condition, and the effect persisted for 1 wk and 4 wk after the intervention. There was a significant reduction in pain and discomfort scores immediately after the exercise. The reduction persisted for 1 wk and 4 wk after the intervention.	Lack of an active control group. Small sample size.
Surakka et al. (2004)	To examine the effects of a 6-mo aerobic and strength exercise on multiple types of fatigue in men and women with MS	Level I Stratified (by gender), RCT, 2-group, pretest–posttest $N = 95$ participants; $n = 49$ exercise group (30 women; assessed at the baseline,	*Intervention* Participants in the exercise group received 5 aquatic aerobic training sessions and 5 supervised resistance exercise sessions on alternate days during the first	Ninety-eight percent of women and 85% of men completed the targeted amount of exercise sessions. In the exercise group, no association between motor fatigue (FI) and the amount	Unequal-sized male and female groups.

(Continued)

Table D2. Evidence on Occupational Therapy–Related Interventions Focusing on Client Factors and Performance Skills for People With Multiple Sclerosis (Cont.)

Author/Year	Study Objectives	Level/Design/Participants	Intervention and Outcome Measures	Results	Study Limitations
		3 wk, and 6 mo), *n* = 50 control group (31 women; assessed at baseline and 6 mo); 88 (44 in each group) completed the postintervention assessment. *M* EDSS = 2.0 and 2.9 in women; *M* EDSS = 2.9 and 3.1 in men.	3 wk of intervention. If a participant could not participate in the aquatic exercise, an ergometry exercise session of 30–35 min was used for replacement. The resistance exercise program consisted of circuit type. Participants continued to receive 23 wk of home-based exercise, 4 weekly exercise sessions during Weeks 1–17, and 5 during the last 6 wk (Weeks 18–23). Participants in the control group were asked to continue with their normal living. *Outcome Measures* Maximum value of the muscle torque (Nm), Fatigue Index (FI) for motor fatigue, FSS, and Ambulatory Fatigue Index (AFI).	of aerobic or strength exercise was found. *Knee extension:* The changes after a 26-wk intervention were equivalent in men and women. The exercising men were faster in reaching the maximal torque level than women in knee extension and flexion torques at 6 mo. *Knee flexion:* Statistically significant interaction among gender and time was observed. Less fatigue among female exercisers in knee extension than controls was found. However, no differences were found in the changes in flexion fatigue between male exercisers and controls. Women in the exercise group significantly improved their fatigue resistance in knee extension during the 23-wk home exercise period, but no improvement was found in men. A positive correlation was found at the baseline between the FI in knee extension and EDSS in the male exercise group. The time effect was statistically significant for fatigue in walking in both groups.	

http://dx.doi.org/10.1191/0269215504cr780oa

(Continued)

Table D2. Evidence on Occupational Therapy–Related Interventions Focusing on Client Factors and Performance Skills for People With Multiple Sclerosis (Cont.)

Author/Year	Study Objectives	Level/Design/Participants	Intervention and Outcome Measures	Results	Study Limitations
Velikonja, Čurič, Ozura, & Jazbec (2010)	To examine effects of sports climbing and yoga on spasticity, cognitive impairment, mood change, and fatigue in patients with MS	Level I RCT, 2-group, pretest–posttest $N = 20$ persons with relapsing–remitting, primary progressive, or secondary progressive MS (age = 26–50 yr); EDSS <6; EDSS pyramidal functions score >2.	*Intervention* Both sport climbing and yoga were held 1×/wk for 10 wk. Sport climbing was supervised by 2 sport climbing instructors. The climbing height was adjusted for persons with physical disability by adding numerous and bigger holds. Participants in the yoga group received adjusted Hatha yoga by a MS specialist nurse. *Outcome Measures* EDSS for disease disability; MAS for spasticity; Mazes subtest of Executive module from the Neuropsychological Assessment Battery (NAB) and Tower of London Test (TOL) for cognitive function (executive function); Brickenkamp d2 test for attention span; Center for Epidemiologic Studies Depression Scale (CES–D); MFIS.	*Spasticity*: No significant change in the level of spasticity was observed after intervention of sport climbing or yoga. However, there was a statistically significant reduction in the EDSS pyramidal functions score in the sport climbing group. *Cognitive function*: A significant improvement on the test of selective attention was observed after the yoga intervention. No significant changes in test of executive functions in either group. *Mood*: No significant differences were observed after interventions. *Fatigue*: A significant effect of sport climbing on the self-perceived impact of fatigue was observed (reduced impact of fatigue on physical and cognitive function, but not psychological function).	Lack of a control group. Small sample size.

http://dx.doi.org/10.1016/j.clineuro.2010.03.006

(Continued)

Table D2. Evidence on Occupational Therapy–Related Interventions Focusing on Client Factors and Performance Skills for People With Multiple Sclerosis *(Cont.)*

Author/Year	Study Objectives	Level/Design/Participants	Intervention and Outcome Measures	Results	Study Limitations
White et al. (2004)	To examine the effect of an 8-wk progressive resistance training program on lower-extremity strength, ambulatory function, and self-reported fatigue and disability in persons with MS	Level III Nonrandomized, 1-group, pretest–posttest $N = 8$ persons with MS (7 women; age = 25–55 yr; EDSS range = 1–5); participants who were using MS disease-modifying drugs (interferon beta 1α and 1β, glatiramer acetate) included.	*Intervention* Study participants received 2 supervised resistance training sessions per week for 8 consecutive wk. The training protocol: a warm-up set (40% MVC) at Week 1, one set of 6–10 repetitions at 50% of MVC; at Week 2, one set of 10–15 repetitions at 60% of MVC; at Weeks 3–8, one set of 10–15 repetitions at 70% of maximal predicted force for all lower body exercises. *Outcome Measures* • Dynamometer and MVC for lower-limb muscle strength testing and quadriceps activation. • 3D MRI for muscle cross-sectional area (CSA) and volume of the thigh for quantification of the muscle contractile area. • T25FWT and 3-min step test for ambulatory function • MFIS • Self-reported EDSS.	No MS exacerbations were reported during the intervention phase. Significant increases for strength of knee extension and plantar flexion were observed. After training, unchanged central activation ratio and unchanged CSA of quadriceps and hamstring muscle were found. Steps completed in 3-min step test increased significantly after the intervention. However, no significant change was observed in T25FWT speed. Impact of fatigue was decreased after resistance training; however, level of disability did not change significantly.	Small sample size. Lack of an active control group and a follow-up assessment.

http://dx.doi.org/10.1191/1352458504ms1088oa

(Continued)

Table D2. Evidence on Occupational Therapy–Related Interventions Focusing on Client Factors and Performance Skills for People With Multiple Sclerosis (*Cont.*)

Author/Year	Study Objectives	Level/Design/Participants	Intervention and Outcome Measures	Results	Study Limitations
Motor Training					
Carpinella, Cattaneo, Abuarqub, & Ferrarin (2009) http://dx.doi.org/10.2340/16501977-0401	To make a preliminary evaluation of the feasibility of a robot-based rehabilitation protocol for the improvement of upper-limb motor coordination in a group of patients with MS	Level II Nonrandomized, 2-group, pretest–posttest $N = 16$ persons were included in the study; $n = 7$ persons with MS (4 women; M age = 46 yr; EDSS range = 4.5–6.5), $n = 9$ healthy persons in the control group.	*Intervention* *Experimental group:* Total of 8 training sessions within 2 wk (1×/day, 5 days/wk). The robot can be programmed to design resistive, assistive, or perturbing force fields to help or disturb the execution of upper-limb movements. Each participant performed center-out reaching movements, starting from the same central position toward targets presented in 2 directions. Each session consisted of 200 reaching movements. *Control group:* The same protocol was followed as used in the experimental group. *Outcome Measures* Nine-Hole Peg Test (9HPT), Tremor Severity Scale (TSS).	Participants in the experimental group demonstrated significantly higher duration of reaching movements, more jerky trajectories, and more deviation from linearity at baseline. After training, all participants with MS improved their indicators after training, except for the jerk metric parameter, which was not improved in 1 participant. MS participants significantly reduced the duration of the tracking movement and improved the smoothness of the trajectory.	Small sample size. No random assignment. Lack of a follow-up assessment.

(*Continued*)

Table D2. Evidence on Occupational Therapy–Related Interventions Focusing on Client Factors and Performance Skills for People With Multiple Sclerosis *(Cont.)*

Author/Year	Study Objectives	Level/Design/Participants	Intervention and Outcome Measures	Results	Study Limitations
Cattaneo, Jonsdottir, Zocchi, & Regola (2007) http://dx.doi.org/10.1177/0269215507077602	To examine the effect of 2 types of balance retraining: motor retraining and integrated sensory–motor retraining	Level I RCT, 3-group $N = 50$ participants with MS (4 dropped out; M age $= 46.0$ yr; M duration since onset $= 13.8$ yr) recruited from an inpatient unit.	*Intervention* *Group 1:* Balance retraining aimed at improving motor and sensory strategies. *Group 2:* Balance retraining aimed at motor strategies. *Group 3:* Conventional therapy. *Outcome Measures* Static, dynamic balance.	No significant improvement was found in static balance in balance training groups as compared with conventional therapy. Group 1 showed significant differences in dynamic balance after intervention. No differences were found between Groups 2 and 3. Ceiling effects were found in BBS scores.	Lack of blinded assessors.
Mark et al. (2008) http://dx.doi.org/10.1177/1352458508090223	To evaluate whether constraint-induced movement therapy (CIMT) may benefit chronic upper-extremity hemiparesis in progressive MS	Level III Nonrandomized, 1-group, pretest–posttest, and 4-wk follow-up $N = 5$ persons with mild primary or secondary progressive MS who had an asymmetric upper-extremity motor deficit; eligible participants required to have mild to moderate motor deficit on active movement of the affected upper extremity.	*Intervention* CIMT performed 3 hr weekly over 2–10 consecutive wk, depending on the participants' preferences, for a total of 30 hr. Treatment involved (1) repetitive task practice with more-affected arm on a wide variety of functionally relevant activities; (2) shaping of training tasks gradually; and (3) restraint of the less-affected hand. *Outcome Measures* Motor Activity Log (MAL) and Wolf Motor Function Test (WMFT) for upper-extremity motor function; daily visual analog fatigue rating.	Participants improved significantly on all clinical measures, except for the WMFT performance time. Treatment effect sizes on all measures were > 0.57.	Small sample size. Lack of a control group.

(Continued)

Table D2. Evidence on Occupational Therapy–Related Interventions Focusing on Client Factors and Performance Skills for People With Multiple Sclerosis (Cont.)

Author/Year	Study Objectives	Level/Design/Participants	Intervention and Outcome Measures	Results	Study Limitations
Mills, Yap, & Young (2007) http://dx.doi.org/10.1002/14651858.CD005029.pub2	To systematically review the effects of interventions for ataxia in persons with MS	Level I Systematic review *Article selection:* 10 articles met the inclusion and exclusion criteria: blinded (double-blinded in pharmacological intervention, single-blinded in nonpharmacological intervention), RCTs (either placebo-controlled or compared 2 or more treatments); cross-over trials. *Electronic resources:* Cochrane MS Group trials register, the Cochrane Central Register of Controlled Trials, MEDLINE, EMBASE, and the National Health Service National Research Register. *Manual search:* Bibliographies of relevant articles, pertinent medical and neurology journals, and abstract books of neurology and MS conferences. *Type of participants:* Persons with confirmed MS with symptoms or signs of ataxia	*Intervention* Types of intervention: • *Pharmacological:* Isoniazid and pyridoxine; cannabis-based medicine; baclofen • *Surgical:* Thalamotomy vs. deep brain stimulation • *Orthoses:* Neuromuscular rehabilitation with and without Johnstone pressure splint • *Physiotherapy:* Hospital PT vs. home PT; impairment-based training vs. task-oriented training. *Outcome Measures* Disease severity, tremor, hand function, balance, gait.	Six placebo-controlled (pharmacological intervention) and 4 comparative (1 stereotactic neurosurgery and 3 neurorehabilitation) studies met the criteria. No significant differences were observed in pharmacological intervention vs. placebo. Physiotherapy was safe and showed small amount of improvement. However, treatment effects were not sustained. Surgical intervention demonstrated good short-term effects in MS patients with severe symptoms. However, tremor may return by 6 mo.	Insufficient number of well-designed studies.

(Continued)

Table D2. Evidence on Occupational Therapy–Related Interventions Focusing on Client Factors and Performance Skills for People With Multiple Sclerosis (Cont.)

Author/Year	Study Objectives	Level/Design/Participants	Intervention and Outcome Measures	Results	Study Limitations
Widener, Allen, & Gibson-Horn (2009)	To examine the immediate effect of balance-based torso weighting (BBTW) on upright mobility	Level I Stratified RCT, 2-group (Phases 1 and 2) $N = 38$ people with MS able to walk 30 ft, having difficulty with walking, and afraid of falling; 18 people with MS in the control group for Phase 1.	*Intervention* *Phase 1:* BBTW vs. no treatment; intervention group wore a vest like garment with application of weight to counter the direction of balance loss and asymmetry of resistance *Phase 2:* BBTW vs. standard weight placement (1.5% of participant's body weight). *Outcome Measures* Walking performance.	*Phase 1:* The intervention group showed significant improvement on the TUG, T25FWT, sharpened Romberg, and 360° turns. No significant differences were found in the control group. *Phase 2:* Participants in the BBTW group showed significantly greater improvement on the TUG, whereas the standard weight placement group improved significantly in the T25FWT.	Small sample size. Less homogeneous participants. Lack of follow-up.

http://dx.doi.org/10.1177/1545968309336146

Note. ADL/ADLs = activity/activities of daily living; BMI = body mass index; BDNF = brain-derived neurotropic factor; CBT = cognitive-behavioral therapy; EEG = electroencephalography; ELISA = enzyme-linked immunosorbent assay; IADL/IADLs = instrumental activity/activities of daily living; IL-6 = interleukin-6; M = mean; min = minute/minutes; mo = month/months; MRI = magnetic resonance imaging; MS = multiple sclerosis; MVC = maximal voluntary contraction; NGF = nerve growth factor; OT = occupational therapy/therapist; PE = physical education; PT = physical therapy/therapist; QoL = quality of life; RCT = randomized controlled trial; sec = second/seconds; sIL–6R = soluble interleukin-6 receptor; VO_2 = oxygen consumption; wk = week/weeks; yr = year/years.

This revised table is a product of AOTA's Evidence-Based Practice Project and was originally published in the *American Journal of Occupational Therapy*. Copyright © 2014 by the American Therapy Association. It may be freely reproduced for personal use in clinical or educational settings as long as the source is cited. All other uses require written permission from the American Occupational Therapy Association. To apply, visit http://www.copyright.com.

Table D3. Evidence on Occupational Therapy–Related Interventions for People With Parkinson's Disease

Author/Year	Study Objectives	Level/Design/ Participants	Intervention and Outcome Measures	Results	Study Limitations
Engagement in Exercise and Physical Activity to Improve Performance Skills and Occupational Performance					
Allen et al. (2010) http://dx.doi.org/10.1002/mds.23082	To determine the effect of a 6-mo minimally supervised exercise program on fall risk factors in people with PD	Level I RCT $N = 48$ patients with PD who had fallen or were at risk of falling were randomized into exercise or control group (M age = 67 yr, HY stage not reported).	*Intervention* *Exercise group:* A 40–60-min exercise program of progressive lower-limb strengthening and balance exercises was conducted 3×/wk for 6 mo. This included a monthly exercise class conducted by 1 or 2 therapists, with remaining exercises done at home. *Control group:* Usual care was provided. Both groups received standardized falls prevention advice in a booklet. *Outcome Measures* *Primary:* PD falls risk score *Secondary:* Standing balance, Freezing of Gait Questionnaire (FOG), QoL, fear of falling, and measures of physical ability.	Exercise group had no major adverse events and showed a greater improvement than the control group in the falls risk score, which was not statistically significant. There were statistically significant improvements in the exercise group compared with the control group for 2 secondary outcomes: FOG ($p = .03$) and timed sit-to-stand ($p = .03$). There were statistically nonsignificant trends toward greater improvements in the exercise group for measures of muscle strength, walking, and fear of falling but not for the measures of standing balance.	Sample size was small. Minimal supervision of exercise was provided.

(*Continued*)

Table D3. Evidence on Occupational Therapy-Related Interventions for People With Parkinson's Disease (Cont.)

Author/Year	Study Objectives	Level/Design/Participants	Intervention and Outcome Measures	Results	Study Limitations
Batson (2010)	To assess the feasibility and safety of group delivery of an intensive trial of modern dance on mobility and balance in adults with early- to middle-stage PD. To explore the value of quantitative measures of balance and to examine qualitative data for trends toward physical and behavioral change	Level III Quasi-experimental, single-group, pretest–posttest $N = 11$ persons with early- to middle-stage PD (age range = 50–85 yr, HY Stages 1–2.5).	*Intervention* Group dance classes (modern dance) were conducted over 3 wk by a professionally trained dancer. There were 9 classes, 85 min long, for a total of approximately 11 hr of instruction. *Outcome Measures* Feasibility assessed by attendance, attrition, and responses to participation on feedback questionnaire; Modified Falls Efficacy Scale for perceived balance confidence in daily activities; Timed Up and Go (TUG) test; and Fullerton Advance Balance Scale (FAB).	Modern dance appears to be a feasible alternative to other modes of exercise. Results on the FAB were significant, showing a trend toward balance improvement. Further research is suggested.	Sample size was small. The study did not include a control group. The study did not include long-term follow-up.
http://dx.doi.org/10.1177/1533210110383903					
Brittle et al. (2008)	To evaluate the impact of 10 sessions of Conductive Education on mobility, functional independence, and HRQoL in adults with MS, PD, and stroke	Level III Observational, pretest–posttest $N = 129$ self-referred community-living individuals with moderate disability (MS, PD, and stroke), $n = 55$ patients with PD (median age = 65 yr, HY stage not reported).	*Intervention* 10 sessions of daily/weekly Conductive Education by 2 conductors for diagnostic-specific groups of 5 individuals. Each session lasted 1.5–2 hr. Movement components of functional tasks were performed in sequences of repeating rhythmic exercises, with verbal cueing and reinforcement. Family members were encouraged to attend the groups. *Outcome Measures* Modified Barthel Index (BI–10), Nottingham Extended Activities of Daily Living Index (NEADL), and Parkinson's Disease Questionnaire (PDQ–39). All self-administered.	For the PD group, no statistically significant improvements were observed. However, the mean change in ADL, Stigma, and Social Support dimension scores of the PDQ–39 approached statistical significance. Of the 2 degenerative neurological conditions, PD showed the least improvement.	The study did not include a control group. Sample size was small. Results rely solely on subjective, self-reported assessments of ADLs.
http://dx.doi.org/10.1177/0269215550782334					(Continued)

Table D3. Evidence on Occupational Therapy–Related Interventions for People With Parkinson's Disease (Cont.)

Author/Year	Study Objectives	Level/Design/ Participants	Intervention and Outcome Measures	Results	Study Limitations
Canning, Ada, & Woodhouse (2008)	To evaluate the feasibility of multiple-task walking training as an intervention for people with mild to moderate PD and to determine whether the size of the potential effect is worthwhile	Level III Repeated-measures, baseline-controlled study $N = 5$ persons with idiopathic PD (M age = 61 yr, HY Stages 2–3).	*Intervention* Walking training provided while performing cognitive and manual tasks with increasing complexity. Three phases of training—baseline, training phase, retention phase—were conducted over 10 wk. *Outcome Measures* *Feasibility*: Participants' perception of fatigue, difficulty, anxiety, confidence *Effect of training*: Walking velocity, cadence, stride length as compared with baseline.	Multiple-task training was feasible. It also may be effective (large effect size for an increase in walking velocity) in increasing multiple-task walking velocity in people with mild to moderate PD. Improvements in multiple-task walking performance can also be maintained.	Sample size was small. A RCT would lead to a more definitive conclusion. The study included a short follow-up period.
http://dx.doi.org/10.1177/0269215507082341					
Crizzle & Newhouse (2006)	To review existing studies evaluating the effectiveness of physical exercise on mortality, strength, balance, mobility, and ADLs for people with PD	Level I Systematic review of 7 studies $N = 6–46$ (438 in 1 study) people with early- to middle-stage PD.	*Intervention* Interventions ranged from physical exercise and balance and resistance training to pole striding and body weight–supported treadmill training. Intervention provided by physical therapist for 4–14 wk (4.1 yr in 1 study). Setting not reported. *Outcome Measures* Walking speed, spinal flexibility, functional reach, axial mobility, motor ability, muscle strength, number of falls, Unified Parkinson's Disease Rating Scale (UPDRS), PDQ–39, Columbia University Rating Scale (CURS), Basic Motor Test (BMT), Mini-Mental State Examination (MMSE), Sickness Impact Profile (SIP), and Adjective Mood Questionnaire of Zeersen (AMQZ; disease severity, QoL, mood, mental status).	Physical exercise is beneficial for patients with PD. All exercise modes resulted in improvements, although treadmill training was found to be superior to regular PT, especially as far as short-step gait is concerned. One study showed that functional improvement is most noticeable in the setting in which training occurs. A person who may not show significant improvements in ADLs may still obtain improved QoL based on perceived improvements made during the rehabilitation program.	Limited number of studies included in the review. Methodological shortcomings in included studies. None of the studies included long-term follow-up to at least 1 yr to demonstrate long-term improvements.
http://dx.doi.org/10.1097/01.jsm.0000244612.55550.7d					

(Continued)

Table D3. Evidence on Occupational Therapy-Related Interventions for People With Parkinson's Disease (Cont.)

Author/Year	Study Objectives	Level/Design/Participants	Intervention and Outcome Measures	Results	Study Limitations
Dereli & Yaliman (2010)	To compare the effects of a physiotherapist-supervised exercise program in an exercise unit and self-supervised home exercise program on QoL in patients with PD	Level II Quasi–randomized trial (alternate allocation) $N = 32$ patients with idiopathic PD (13 women, 19 men; M age = 75 yr; HY Stages 1–3). Allocated to 2 groups: Physiotherapist-supervised group, $n = 16$; home group, $n = 16$.	*Intervention* *Physiotherapist-supervised group*: Supervised exercises (strengthening, ranging mobility, balance, gait, breathing) and provided individual education sessions. *Home group*: Self-supervised models of the above exercises were reinforced with an individual education session by physiotherapist. The exercise program was conducted over 10 wk, 3×/wk, for 45 min per session. *Outcome Measures* PD Quality of Life Questionnaire (PDQLQ), Nottingham Health Profile (NHP), UPDRS, and Beck Depression Inventory (BDI).	There were significantly higher improvements in PDQLQ total, Parkinson's symptoms, and emotional functioning scores in the physiotherapist-supervised group vs. the home group. Physiotherapist supervision is more effective in ameliorating motor symptoms, daily living activities, and mental and emotional functions. However, it can be said that both groups have beneficial effects on QoL, as both groups showed an increase from baseline states.	The study did not include a control group with no exercise. The study does not follow the long-term benefits of the program between the 2 groups. Sample size was small. The study design included alternate allocation instead of randomization.

http://dx.doi.org/10.1177/0269215509358933

(Continued)

Table D3. Evidence on Occupational Therapy-Related Interventions for People With Parkinson's Disease (Cont.)

Author/Year	Study Objectives	Level/Design/ Participants	Intervention and Outcome Measures	Results	Study Limitations
Dibble, Addison, & Papa (2009)	To systematically review studies that examine the effects of exercise interventions on balance outcomes for people with PD, within the categories defined by the WHO in the *ICF* model	*Level I* Systematic review of 16 studies Participants with idiopathic PD only. *Body function: Postural instability category* $N = 15-23$ (55% men, range of disease severity = 1.8–2.3 on HY). *Activity: Balance task performance category* $N = 18-142$ (62% men, range of disease severity = 2.2–2.9 on HY). *Participation: QoL* $N = 18-142$ (67% men, disease severity = 1–4 on HY).	*Intervention* *Body function: Postural instability category* Whole-body vibration, imagery, balance training, and traditional PT exercises were provided for 3–12 wk, 2–10×/wk, for a total intervention time of 6–24 hr. *Outcome Measures* Sensory Organization Test (SOT), computerized posturography, and Posterior Pull Test in the UPDRS. *Activity: Balance task performance category* Whole-body vibration, progressive tango training, treadmill training, and lower-extremity strengthening exercises were provided for 3–12 wk, 2–10×/wk, for a total intervention time of 6–20 hr. *Outcome Measures* Functional Reach Test, Tinetti Balance Assessment Tool, Dynamic Gait Index (DGI), Berg Balance Scale (BBS), TUG, and time to turn around a chair.	*Body function: Postural instability category* There was moderate evidence that physical activity and exercise may result in improvements in postural instability outcomes in persons with mild to moderate PD. *Activity: Balance task performance category* There was moderate evidence to support physical activity and exercise as an effective intervention to improve balance performance in persons with mild to moderate PD. *Participation: QoL* There was limited evidence to support an improvement in QoL outcomes with physical activity and exercise in persons with mild to moderate PD.	Search strategy limited to evidence ranked as Level I, II, or III (this may disregard potentially clinically relevant findings). *ICF* model was used to categorize outcome measures (the potential for artificial segregation and overlap of constructs exists). Only specific categories of outcomes within *ICF* categories were used, causing them to extract the variables of interest from the context of individual studies.

(Continued)

Table D3. Evidence on Occupational Therapy-Related Interventions for People With Parkinson's Disease (Cont.)

Author/Year	Study Objectives	Level/Design/Participants	Intervention and Outcome Measures	Results	Study Limitations
			Participation: QoL Quigong, music therapy, resistance training, aerobic exercise, range of motion/stretching, treadmill training, and postural control tasks were performed for 6–13 wk, 1–7×/wk, for a total intervention time of 9.2–42 hr. *Outcome Measures* EuroQol (EQ–5D), PDQ–39, Parkinson's Disease QoL Scale (PDQUALIF), SF–36, and SIP.		
http://dx.doi.org/10.1097/NPT.0b013e3181990fcc					
Dibble, Hale, et al. (2009)	To compare the effects of a chronic, high-intensity eccentric intervention with an evidence-based exercise program on measures of clinical bradykinesia and QoL in persons with mild to moderate PD	Level II Two groups, nonrandomized, quasiexperimental study $N = 20$ persons with PD (age range = 45–85 yr, HY Stages 1–3).	*Intervention* Interventions of 45–60 min, 3 days/wk, for 12 wk. *Eccentric exercise group:* Received high-force eccentric training. *Active control group:* Received evidence-based rehabilitation program consisting of resistance strength training. *Outcome Measures* Quadriceps muscle force, clinical bradykinesia measures (gait speed, TUG), and PDQ–39.	Significant Time × Group interaction effects for gait speed, TUG, and the composite PDQ–39 score ($p < .05$) were found. Muscle force, bradykinesia, and QoL were improved to a greater degree in those who performed high-intensity eccentric resistance training compared with the active control group.	Sample size was small. The study did not include randomization of allocation to the 2 groups. The study did not include follow-up measures.
http://dx.doi.org/10.1016/j.parkreldis.2009.04.009					

(Continued)

Table D3. Evidence on Occupational Therapy–Related Interventions for People With Parkinson's Disease (*Cont.*)

Author/Year	Study Objectives	Level/Design/ Participants	Intervention and Outcome Measures	Results	Study Limitations
Dixon et al. (2007) http://dx.doi.org/10.1002/14651858.CD002813.pub2	To compare the efficacy and effectiveness of OT with placebo or no interventions in patients with PD	Level I Systematic review of 2 studies (both RCTs) Patients with PD of all ages on any drug therapy for any duration of treatment (*M* age = 63–76 yr).	*Intervention* OT, a placebo control intervention, or no intervention. *Treatment group:* Received OT and/or PT and group treatment. *Control group:* Received no treatment or PT and was treated individually. *Outcome Measures* Adverse effects, caregiver outcomes, economic analysis, and both short-term and long-term (6–12 mo) effects of intervention. • *Motor impairments:* UPDRS and PDQ-39 • *ADLs:* UPDRS • *Handicap and QoL measures:* PDQ-39 and SF-36 • *Depression:* Hospital Anxiety and Depression Scale (HADS).	Both trials claimed a positive effect of OT in PD; however, the improvements were small, and it is doubtful whether they are clinically or statistically significant. It is unsafe to draw any conclusions regarding the efficacy of OT in persons with PD.	The study had methodological flaws, small sample sizes, and the possibility of publication bias. The study had inclusion criteria that excluded most potential studies.
Elkis-Abuhoff, Goldblatt, Gaydos, & Corrato (2008) http://dx.doi.org/10.1080/07421656.2008.10129596	To determine whether patients with PD would experience a decrease in the somatic and emotional symptoms of the disease by engaging in the manipulation of clay	Level III Pretest–posttest *n* = 22 persons with PD (*M* age = 71.4 yr; HY stage not reported); *n* = 19 patients without PD.	*Intervention* Manipulation of colored modeling clay into "a shape other than a ball." *Outcome Measures* Brief Symptom Inventory (BSI) for psychological distress about symptoms.	A pre- to postintervention decrease in symptom severity was found across all 9 domains of the BSI for all participants, regardless of PD diagnosis, although the decrease in symptoms was greater for those with PD. The PD group showed greater change in outcome as a result of the clay manipulation.	Intervention was of short duration. Sample size was small. The study did not include follow-up assessments. Non-PD group had lower BSI at pretest than PD group, suggesting a greater potential to benefit from intervention.

(*Continued*)

Table D3. Evidence on Occupational Therapy–Related Interventions for People With Parkinson's Disease (Cont.)

Author/Year	Study Objectives	Level/Design/ Participants	Intervention and Outcome Measures	Results	Study Limitations
Gage & Storey (2004) http://dx.doi.org/10.1191/0269215504cr764oa	To systematically review available evidence on the effectiveness of nonpharmacological interventions for people with PD and identify future research needs	Level I Systematic review of 44 studies reported in 51 papers Participants community-living adults with PD (M age range = 61–74 yr).	*Intervention* There were 44 different interventions: PT, OT, speech therapy, language therapy, psychological counseling and support, and multidisciplinary intervention and education provided in the home or in clinical settings such as outpatient centers. *Outcome Measures* Mobility, functional status, speech, swallowing, and psychological well-being.	A variety of nonpharmacological interventions can improve mobility, functional status, speech, swallowing, and psychological well-being for people with PD. These findings confirm small to moderate effect sizes for measures of mobility and independence reported by other discipline-based reviews.	Most studies had small sample size and had other methodological weaknesses. The study did not include follow-up beyond the completion of treatment.
Gobbi et al. (2009) http://dx.doi.org/10.1016/S1353-8020(09)70780-1	To verify the effectiveness of 2 exercise programs on balance and mobility in people with idiopathic PD	Level III Pretest–posttest 2 interventions, no control group. Group 1 (*n* = 21, intensive exercise program); Group 2 (*n* = 13, adaptive program); HY Stages 1–3.	*Intervention* Intensive exercise program for aerobic capacity, flexibility, strength, motor coordination, and balance was conducted over 6 mo, in 72 sessions, 3×/wk, 60 min per session. Participants of the adaptive exercise program received flexibility, strength, motor coordination, and balance training (6 m, 24 sessions, 1×/wk, 60/session). *Outcome Measures* UPDRS, modified TUG, and BBS.	Both groups were affected by the exercise intervention. There were no significant differences between groups in either mobility or balance results. Both the intensive and adaptive exercise programs improved balance and mobility in patients with PD.	Sample size was small. The study did not include a control group. The study did not include follow-up assessments.

(Continued)

Table D3. Evidence on Occupational Therapy–Related Interventions for People With Parkinson's Disease (Cont.)

Author/Year	Study Objectives	Level/Design/ Participants	Intervention and Outcome Measures	Results	Study Limitations
Goodwin, Richards, Taylor, Taylor, & Campbell (2008) http://dx.doi.org/10.1002/mds.21922	To systematically review RCTs reporting on the effectiveness of exercise interventions on outcomes for people with PD	Level I Systematic review of 14 studies $N = 495$ (range = 11–142; 67% men). All except 2 studies had participants in HY Stages 2–3.	*Intervention* Exercise/physical activity; frequency of intervention between 6–36 hr spread over 4–12 wk. All were outpatient, except 1 home-based setting and 1 leisure setting. All except 4 studies reported that service delivery included PTs. A corrective therapist, student nurse with a black belt in karate, and a trained exercise leader also provided services. Six studies used group intervention, and 8 used individual intervention. *Outcome Measures* HRQoL: Physical, psychological, and social functioning; UPDRS; Northwestern University Disability Scale (NUDS); Self-assessment Parkinson's Disease Disability Scale (SPDDS); Brown's Disablity Scale (BDS); PDQ–39; SIP–68; EQ–5D; BBS; SOT; functional reach; Geriatric depression scale; and BDI.	Evidence supports exercise as being beneficial with regards to physical functioning, HRQoL, strength, balance, and gait speed for people with PD. There is currently insufficient evidence to support or refute the value of exercise in reducing falls, depression, or its safety with people with PD.	Methodological details reported in the articles were often varied and poor. Included studies were offered only in English language. Most studies had small sample sizes.
Hackney & Earhart (2009a)	To compare the effects of 3 distinct, socially interactive physical activities and no intervention on HRQoL in people with PD	Level I RCT $N = 61$ participants with PD (HY Stages 1–3). Tango group, $n = 14$; waltz/foxtrot group, $n = 17$; tai chi group, $n = 13$; no intervention group, $n = 17$.	*Intervention* Intervention groups: 20 1-hr sessions of Argentine tango, combined waltz and foxtrot, or tai chi, over 13 wk. Control group: No intervention. *Outcome Measures* PDQ–39.	The tango group reported significant improvements on the PDQ–39 Mobility, Social Support, and Summary Index scales at posttest. No significant changes in PDQ–39 scores were noted in the waltz/foxtrot, tai chi, or no-intervention groups.	No follow-up measures were used. Attrition was high (75 participants were enrolled in the study and randomized). The tai chi group had higher dyskinesia scores at baseline compared with the other 3 groups.

(Continued)

Table D3. Evidence on Occupational Therapy–Related Interventions for People With Parkinson's Disease (Cont.)

Author/Year	Study Objectives	Level/Design/ Participants	Intervention and Outcome Measures	Results	Study Limitations
Hackney & Earhart (2009b)	To prospectively compare the effects of 3 distinct, socially interactive, physical activities with no intervention on HRQoL in those with PD	Level I RCT $N = 75$ persons with PD (HY Stages 1–3) assigned to 4 conditions.	*Intervention* 20 1-hr sessions (2×/wk) over 5 wk for each of 2 groups. *Leisure movement group:* Argentine tango (tango), combined waltz and foxtrot lessons (waltz/foxtrot; 30 min waltz, 30 min foxtrot), or tai chi. *Control group:* No intervention. *Outcome Measures* UPDRS III, PDQ–39, and a PDQ–39 summary index.	Tango significantly improved mobility, social support, and the PDQ–39 summary index at posttest. No significant changes in HRQoL were noted in the waltz/foxtrot, tai chi, or no-intervention conditions. Tango may be helpful for improving HRQoL in PD because it addresses balance and gait deficits in the context of a social interaction that requires working closely with a partner.	The study did not include follow-up measures. Attrition rate was high. Some differences found at baseline for dyskinesia between tai chi and remaining groups.
http://dx.doi.org/10.1016/j.parkreldis.2009.03.003					
Hackney & Earhart (2009c)	To determine the acceptability and feasibility of a high-dosage social dance program for those with mild to moderate PD To determine the effects of short-duration, intensive tango lessons on functional mobility in people with PD	Level III Within-subject, prospective, repeated-measures design $N = 14$ persons with idiopathic PD (M HY Stage = 2.4).	*Intervention* Short-duration, intensive Argentine tango dancing with a partner who did not have PD (10 1.5-hr dance lessons over 2 wk); lessons provided by an experienced instructor. *Outcome Measures* BBS, UPDRS, TUG, 6-min walking test (6MWT), gait velocity, step length, stance, swing percentage, stance percentage, forward walking, backward walking.	The program proved to be feasible and acceptable. Significant improvements were seen on the UPDRS and BBS, whereas nonsignificant improvements were seen on the TUG and 6MWT. Significant decrease in percentage of forward gait cycle spent in stance. Nonsignificant improvements were seen in other aspects of forward and backward gait.	Sample size was small. A nonrandomized controlled design was used. The study did not include follow-up measures.
http://dx.doi.org/10.1016/j.ctim.2008.10.005					

(Continued)

Table D3. Evidence on Occupational Therapy–Related Interventions for People With Parkinson's Disease (*Cont.*)

Author/Year	Study Objectives	Level/Design/Participants	Intervention and Outcome Measures	Results	Study Limitations
Jöbges et al. (2004) http://dx.doi.org/10.1136/jnnp.2003.016550	To develop a method of repetitive training of compensatory steps to enhance protective postural responses by using training strategies based on recent neurophysiological research	Level III Pretest–posttest $N = 14$ persons with PD (HY Stages 2.5–4).	*Intervention* Training in an ambulant setting for 14 days, 2 sessions 20 min/day. Repetitive postural training by physiotherapist. *Outcome Measures* PDQ–39, length and initiation of compensatory steps, step length, cadence and double support, SOT, and Limits of Stability Test (LOS).	After training, the length of compensatory steps increased and the step initiation shortened. In a gait analysis, the cadence and the step length increased, gait velocity improved, and the period of double support shortened. The mobility subscore of PDQ–39 also improved. All changes were significant ($p < .05$). These effects were stable for 2 mo without additional training.	Sample size was small. Heterogeneous sample used. Time resolution of the gait analysis was 20 Hz.
Keus et al. (2007) http://dx.doi.org/10.1002/mds.21244	To facilitate the uniformity and efficacy of PT intervention in PD by analyzing current evidence and making practice recommendations	Level I Systematic review of articles published from 1997 through 2003 in MEDLINE, CINHAL, EMBASE, and Cochrane. Part of the Dutch ParkNet project to train expert therapists in PD rehabilitation	*Intervention* Included analysis of 6 systematic reviews and 23 RCTs that involved OT intervention. *Outcome Measures* Gait, transfer quality, balance, joint mobility, and muscle power.	Treatment recommendations include • Cueing strategies to improve gait, • Cognitive movement strategies to improve transfers, • Exercises to improve balance, and • Training of joint mobility and muscle power to improve physical capacity.	Evidence is suggestive of effectiveness but inconclusive on the basis of the studies' small sample size, methodological flaws of primary studies, and possible publication bias. This study is not a meta-analysis and may have Type II (low power) errors.

(*Continued*)

Table D3. Evidence on Occupational Therapy–Related Interventions for People With Parkinson's Disease (Cont.)

Author/Year	Study Objectives	Level/Design/Participants	Intervention and Outcome Measures	Results	Study Limitations
Kwakkel, de Goede, & van Wegen (2007) http://dx.doi.org/10.1016/S1353-8020(08)70053-1	To determine the impact of PT for PD	Level I Systematic review Includes 6 systematic reviews and 23 RCTs involving 1,063 patients.	*Intervention* Task-specific training to improve postural control and balance; gait and gait-related activities with and without cueing; physical condition improvement by individual, group strength, or endurance training; and training in transfers and ADLs. *Outcome Measures* Gait, balance, reach, rotation, and UPDRS.	Results of the trials suggest that effects of PT are task- and context-specific, indicating that tasks that are trained tend not to generalize to related activities not directly trained in the rehabilitation program itself. The decline in treatment effects after intervention completion has been observed. There is moderate to strong evidence for exercise improving physical function and moderate evidence that PT improves transfer ability.	Insufficient statistical power (Type II error). Poor methodological quality because of inadequate randomization and blinding procedures. Insufficient contrast in dosage and treatment between experimental and control groups. Lack of appropriate measurement instruments able to identify clinically meaningful changes according to *ICF*.
Lee, Lam, & Ernst (2008) http://dx.doi.org/10.1016/j.parkreldis.2008.02.003	To assess the effectiveness of tai chi as a treatment option for PD	Level I Systematic review of 7 studies	*Intervention* Tai chi programs for people with PD. *Outcome Measures* Motor function, falling, locomotor ability, UPDRS, PDQ–39, and TUG.	The evidence is insufficient to suggest tai chi as an effective intervention for PD.	Potential incompleteness of evidence reviewed. Poor methodological qualities of studies. No mention of which type of tai chi was used as intervention.
Mehrholz et al. (2010) http://dx.doi.org/10.1002/14651858.CD007830.pub2	To evaluate the effectiveness of treadmill training to improve gait in persons with PD	Level I Meta-analysis of 8 trials Review of databases through March 2009, including Cochrane Movement Disorders Group, Specialised Register, Cochrane Central Register of Controlled Trials, MEDLINE, and EMBASE.	*Intervention* RCTs were included that compared treadmill training to no treadmill training. *Outcome Measures* Walking speed, stride length, walking distance, and cadence.	The results indicate that treadmill training improves gait speed, stride length, and walking distance. There was no difference for cadence at the completion of the studies.	Variations between trials in patient characteristics, duration and amount of training, and types of treatment.

(Continued)

Table D3. Evidence on Occupational Therapy–Related Interventions for People With Parkinson's Disease (*Cont.*)

Author/Year	Study Objectives	Level/Design/ Participants	Intervention and Outcome Measures	Results	Study Limitations
Morris, Iansek, & Kirkwood (2009) http://dx.doi.org/10.1002/mds.22295	To compare the effects of movement strategy training and exercise therapy in hospitalized patients with PD	Level I RCT $N = 28$ participants with PD (M age = 67 yr, HY Stages 2–3). Movement strategy group, $n = 14$; exercise group, $n = 14$.	*Intervention* 2-wk inpatient therapy; follow-up 3 mo postdischarge. *Movement strategy group*: Cognitive strategies to enhance functional mobility and ADL performance. *Exercise group*: Exercises to improve strength, joint range of motion, muscle length, endurance, and aerobic capacity. *Outcome Measures* UPDRS Motor and ADL scales, balance, walking speed, endurance, and PDQ–39.	Although in general the movement strategy group experienced larger improvements from pre- to postintervention compared with the exercise group, the only significant difference between groups was a larger improvement in balance in the movement strategy group. In general, both groups improved from pre- to postintervention, but these improvements were not preserved at the 3-mo follow-up (except for improved PDQ–39 scores in the exercise group).	The stated differences between the movement strategy and exercise groups were based on Level III rather than Level I evidence. Sample size was small.
Müller & Muhlack (2010) http://dx.doi.org/10.1136/jnnp.2009.174987	To assess reactivity and motion behavior after cued dopaminergic stimulation (pharmacological) and an interval of rest or of exercise in PD patients	Level I RCT, randomized repeated measures $N = 22$ with idiopathic PD (M age = 61, M HY Stage = 1.9).	*Intervention* Following 12-hr removal of drug therapy, participants were randomly assigned to rest or to endurance exercise (cycle ergometer). The 2nd day participants switched to the other condition. *Outcome Measures* Simple reaction time, tapping, and peg insertion.	Reactivity and execution of both simple and complex tasks were better following exercise condition. Findings suggest that endurance exercise augments the synthesis and release of dopamine during subsequent task performance.	The study did not test the effects of exercise or rest on participants without dopamine substitution; therefore, the explanation of the effect of exercise on dopamine as an explanation for increased task performance is speculative.

(*Continued*)

Table D3. Evidence on Occupational Therapy–Related Interventions for People With Parkinson's Disease (*Cont.*)

Author/Year	Study Objectives	Level/Design/Participants	Intervention and Outcome Measures	Results	Study Limitations
Nocera, Horvart, & Ray (2009)	To evaluate the effectiveness of a home-based exercise intervention on postural control, together with the use of sensory information, to maintain balance in individuals with PD	Level II 2 groups of nonrandomized controlled trials $N = 10$ persons with PD living in the community (M age = 73.4 yr, HY Stages 2–3). Age-matched controls (AMC) = 10.	*Intervention* 10-wk home-based exercise program supervised by a PT (abdominal crunch, wall squat, lunge, standing calf raise, knee flexion and extension, and step-up), along with sensory information. *Outcome Measures* *Postural control:* Computerized dynamic posturography, SOT.	Individuals with PD showed increased scores from pretest to posttest on the SOT. Although individuals with PD had lower balance scores at pretest than AMC, at posttest there were no statistical differences in balance between individuals with PD and AMC, indicating that the PD group had progressed to same level of balance as AMC. A home exercise program may be an effective method of improving postural control in individuals with PD.	Comparison to non-PD control group does not provide as strong a test of the effect of exercise on PD as would a PD control group.
http://dx.doi.org/10.1016/j.parkreldis.2009.07.002					
Qutubuddin et al. (2007)	To evaluate the effectiveness of Computerized Dynamic Posturography (CDP) and standard PT for persons with mild to moderate PD	Level I RCT $N = 21$ persons with mild to moderate PD (HY stage not reported). $n = 12$ CDP, $n = 9$ PT.	*Intervention* CDP: Balance and mobility training in 30-min sessions 2×/wk for 4 wk using Longforce plate of the Smart Balance Master. Standard PT: Balance and gait training for same frequency and duration. *Outcome Measures* BBS and subscales of the CDP system.	There were no significant differences between groups on outcome measures. Both groups improved on the CDP Limits of Stability subscale.	Sample size was small. High attrition rate. Practice effects on the posttest for those in CDP group.

(*Continued*)

Table D3. Evidence on Occupational Therapy-Related Interventions for People With Parkinson's Disease (Cont.)

Author/Year	Study Objectives	Level/Design/ Participants	Intervention and Outcome Measures	Results	Study Limitations
Rao (2010)	To appraise the literature from the past decade on the effectiveness of OT intervention in patients with PD	Level I Systematic review of 8 studies $N = 17–153$ (total = 503).	*Intervention* Training of functional activities with or without the use of external visual or auditory cues (functional training with external visual or auditory cues ranged over 3–6 wk). OT as part of multidisciplinary intervention (OT task-related training ranged over 4–8 wk). *Outcome Measures* ADL measures, QoL measures, UPDRS, and Functional Reach (FR) Test.	OT is well-tolerated by PD patients and leads to gains in motor function and QoL, at least for the duration of therapy; however, lack of RCTs with large number of participants, lack of consistency in outcome measures, and differences in structure and length of intervention indicate that there is insufficient evidence to refute or support effectiveness of OT in PD.	Lack of RCTs with large sample size. Lack of consistency in outcome measures. Differences in structure and length of intervention.

http://dx.doi.org/10.1002/mds.22784

(Continued)

Table D3. Evidence on Occupational Therapy–Related Interventions for People With Parkinson's Disease (Cont.)

Author/Year	Study Objectives	Level/Design/ Participants	Intervention and Outcome Measures	Results	Study Limitations
Rochester et al. (2010)	To evaluate the effectiveness of a home PT program based on rhythmical cueing using participant's preferred type of cue vs. no attention control on gait parameters, suggestive of motor learning in PD (RESCUE trial)	Level I Single-blind, crossover, randomized *N* = 153 participants with PD (age range = 41–80 yr, HY Stages 2–4). Early intervention group, *n* = 76; late intervention group, *n* = 77.	*Intervention* A 3-wk home cueing program using the participant's preferred method of cueing (audio, with beep to earpiece; video, with flash to glasses; or somatosensory, with vibration to wristband) during functional mobility tasks. *Early group:* Cueing program for 3 wk followed by 3 wk without training (control period). *Late group:* Same intervention and control period, in reverse order. *Both groups:* After initial 6 wk, 6-wk follow-up without training. *Outcome Measures* Accelerometers measured walking speed, step length, step frequency during 4 cueing conditions: no cue at baseline vs. 3 randomized cueing conditions (auditory, visual, and somatosensory) during single and dual tasks in the lab. Follow-up measures conducted at home.	There was a significant increase in walking speed and step length during each cueing condition, including no cue, during performance of single- and dual-task gait, with effects retained after the home training had ended. Any type of cue training in the home (whether auditory, visual, or somatosensory) generalized to improved gait during the gait assessment in the lab. The findings support that home training using cues improves motor learning.	The home intervention was compared with a no-attention wait-list control.

http://dx.doi.org/10.1016/j.brainres.2010.01.001

(Continued)

Table D3. Evidence on Occupational Therapy–Related Interventions for People With Parkinson's Disease (Cont.)

Author/Year	Study Objectives	Level/Design/ Participants	Intervention and Outcome Measures	Results	Study Limitations
Rossi-Izquierdo et al. (2009) http://dx.doi.org/10.1080/09638280902846384	To assess the effectiveness of a vestibular rehabilitation program to improve overall stability in persons with PD	Level III Pretest–posttest $N = 10$ persons with PD at high risk of falls (HY Stages 3–4).	*Intervention* Vestibular rehabilitation program using CDP for exercises in 9 sessions over 1 mo, with 1-yr follow-up. *Outcome Measures* TUG, CDP, Dizziness Handicap Inventory (DHI), and SOT.	There were significant improvements on limits of stability and rhythmic weight shift tests as measured by CDP, DHI, and TUG. There was also a significant improvement on SOT. Improvements continued at 1-yr follow-up.	Sample size was small. Lack of control group. Lack of randomization.
Sage & Almeida (2010) http://dx.doi.org/10.1002/mds.22886	To evaluate the effect of increased attention to sensory feedback during exercise for persons with PD	Level I RCT $N = 26$ persons with idiopathic PD (M age $= 66.5$ yr; HY stage not reported). $n = 13$ persons received PD SAFEx, $n = 13$ received non-SAFE.	*Intervention* During PD SAFEx, participants, with eyes closed in dim lighting, focused their attention on the sensory feedback of specific portions of nonaerobic gait and chair exercises. The non-SAFE program mirrored PD SAFEx, but instructions did not focus attention on sensory feedback, and lights were on. Both were provided 3×/wk over 12 wk, with 6-wk follow-up. *Outcome Measures* UPDRS–III Motor Section and functional measures: grooved pegboard (GP), TUG, and velocity and step length of self-paced gait.	Only SAFEx improved in motor symptoms (UPDRS) and maintained that improvement at 6 wk. Motor symptoms significantly worsened during the 6-wk period for non-SAFE. Both groups significantly improved in functional performance (TUG, GP, velocity, and step length) and maintained after 6 wk.	Sample size was small.

(Continued)

Table D3. Evidence on Occupational Therapy–Related Interventions for People With Parkinson's Disease (Cont.)

Author/Year	Study Objectives	Level/Design/Participants	Intervention and Outcome Measures	Results	Study Limitations
Smania et al. (2010)	To evaluate the effect of balance training on postural instability (PI) for persons with PD	Level I RCT $N = 55$ persons with PI and PD living in the community (age range = 50–79 yr; HY Stages 3–4). Balance training, $n = 28$; general physical exercise, $n = 27$.	*Intervention* *Balance training group:* Exercises to emphasize feedforward and feedback postural training. *General physical exercise group:* Exercises not specifically to emphasize the improvement of postural reactions. *Outcome Measures* BBS, Activities-Specific Balance Confidence (ABC), postural transfer test, self-destabilization of the center of foot pressure test, number of falls, UPDRS, Geriatric Depression Scale (GDS), and HY.	At the end of treatment, those in the balance training group showed significant improvement on all measures except for the UPDRS and HY Scale. At 1-mo follow-up, significant improvements were maintained, except for the GDS. No significant changes were observed in the control group.	Limited follow-up. No assessment of QoL and fear of falling.
http://dx.doi.org/10.1177/1545968310376057					
Stankovic (2004)	To evaluate the effect of PT on balance of people with PD	Level III Pretest–posttest $N = 60$ persons over age 50; $n = 40$ persons with PD (HY Stage 3) over age 50; $n = 20$ healthy controls of same age.	*Intervention* A 30-day PT program for the participants with PD included strategy of movements of daily activities, fall prevention, education, physical and sports activity, and maintaining an upright posture. *Outcome Measures* Functional reaching, tandem stance, one-leg stance, step test, and external perturbation. Results were compared descriptively (no inferential statistics) with the control group's nonintervention performance.	From pretest to posttest, participants with PD who had no history of falls had significant improvement for tandem stance. For those with a history of falls, there were significant improvements in both tandem and single-leg stance. With the addition of perturbation to the balance tests, those with and without fall history improved on step and external perturbation tests. Those with a history of falls also improved on functional reach.	The study included limited follow-up. No control group conditions included in analysis. Validity and reliability of outcome measures not reported.
http://dx.doi.org/10.1097/00004356-200403000-00007					

(Continued)

Table D3. Evidence on Occupational Therapy–Related Interventions for People With Parkinson's Disease (*Cont.*)

Author/Year	Study Objectives	Level/Design/ Participants	Intervention and Outcome Measures	Results	Study Limitations
Stewart & Crosbie (2009)	To critically appraise available evidence from studying the effects of increased aerobic capacity in persons with PD and make recommendations for best clinical practice based on findings	Level I Systematic review of 7 studies *N* = 2–26 (age range 47–78 yr; HY Stages 0–4).	*Intervention* Treadmill and cycle ergometer training. *Length of intervention:* 7 wk–6 mo. *Level I and II studies:* Cycling, walking, and walking activities; large-muscle movements to music for 20–50 min, 2–3×/wk for 7–16 wk; intensity ranged from 50%–85% of max heart rate. *Level III and IV studies:* Walking, cycling, treadmill training for 24–50 min, 3×/wk for 12 wk; intensity between 40%–70% of max heart rate or rate of perceived exertion >14. *Level V studies:* Cycle and upper-limb ergometers for 15–30 min, 3×/wk for 12 wk. *Outcome Measures* Classified according to the *ICF*.	Aerobic exercise positively affects people with PD in terms of functional ability. Cycling and walking seem to be most the effective interventions for aerobic fitness. The study suggests that independence in ADLs and QoL is also affected by aerobic exercise, yet little evidence is offered.	Sample size was small. None of Level I and II studies performed power calculations; therefore, generalizability is unknown. American Academy for Cerebral Palsy and Developmental Medicine (AACPDM) guidelines recommend that 2 people review the literature independently to reduce possible bias, but this was not possible. All measured outcomes at body structure/function level, and all except 1 measured them at participation level. None assessed contextual factors, which is necessary to obtain the full picture of the disease and its impact and how exercise can influence this. None conducted long-term follow-up of gains (>1 yr).

http://dx.doi.org/10.1002/mds.22293

(*Continued*)

Table D3. Evidence on Occupational Therapy–Related Interventions for People With Parkinson's Disease (Cont.)

Author/Year	Study Objectives	Level/Design/ Participants	Intervention and Outcome Measures	Results	Study Limitations
Tanaka et al. (2009)	To analyze the effects of a multimodal exercise program on executive function in older people with PD	Level II 2 groups, nonrandomized controlled trial $N = 20$ persons with PD without dementia (M age = 65.4 yr, HY Stages 1–3). Training group, $n = 10$ (5 men, 5 women); control group, $n = 10$ (6 women, 4 men).	*Intervention* *Training group:* Multimodal physical exercise and activity program (aerobic, strength training, recreational activities, complex sequencing of movements) for 6 mo, done in 6 increasingly challenging phases, each lasting a month. Each phase consisted of 12 group sessions, for 60 min, 3×/wk, under the supervision of 3 physical education professionals at a time. *Control group:* Regular daily routine with no exercise program. *Outcome Measures* Wisconsin Card Sorting Test (WCST)—abstraction, mental flexibility, attention; Wechsler Adult Intelligence Scale III (WAIS–III)—concentrated attention.	Training group showed significantly greater improvement than control group on the abstraction and mental flexibility subtests of the WCST. No difference shown for the attention subtest. The findings support the benefit of multimodal exercise and activity on executive functioning in PD.	Sample size was small. No randomization. No follow-up test for maintenance of results.

http://dx.doi.org/10.1016/j.bandc.2008.09.008

(Continued)

Table D3. Evidence on Occupational Therapy–Related Interventions for People With Parkinson's Disease (Cont.)

Author/Year	Study Objectives	Level/Design/Participants	Intervention and Outcome Measures	Results	Study Limitations
Tassorelli et al. (2009) http://dx.doi.org/10.1016/j.parkreldis.2009.03.006	To evaluate the effect of rehabilitation on functional impairments following bilateral deep brain stimulation (DBS) on persons with PD	Level III Pretest–posttest $N = 34$ persons hospitalized with functional impairments who underwent DBS (M age = 58 yr, HY Stages 1–5). Divided into 3 subgroups based on time from surgery: $n = 13$ acute (1 mo), $n = 8$ postacute (1 mo–1 yr), $n = 13$ stabilized (1 yr+).	*Intervention* The individualized rehabilitation program included exercises for recovery and maintenance of range of motion, active exercises, exercises for coordination and proprioception, dual-task performance, and gait training with sensory cues. Sessions were conducted daily for 4–8 wk. *Outcome Measures* UPDRS, FIM™, modified Barthel Index (MBI), walking, and standing balance.	There were significant improvements on the FIM, MBI, and the independent walking ability and motor examination section of UPDRS for the total group. There was a significant improvement on functional independence as seen in the FIM and MBI for persons in the acute group. These improvements were not observed in postacute and stabilized group.	Sample size was small. Lack of control group.
van Eijkeren et al. (2008) http://dx.doi.org/10.1002/mds.22293	To evaluate both the immediate and long-term effects of a Nordic walking exercise program	Level III Pretest–posttest $N = 19$ persons with idiopathic PD (M age = 67 yr, M disease duration = 5 yr, M HY Stage 1.6). Divided into 2 training groups, both of which received the same intervention.	*Intervention* 6-wk Nordic walking exercise program in a city park with walking poles, delivered by 2 PTs qualified as Nordic walking instructors. 2×/wk, 1-hr sessions consisted of warming up, practicing Nordic walking competence, improving intensity and distance, and cooling down. Social partners also offered a training course of 5 sessions. *Outcome Measures* Timed 10-min walking test (10MWT), TUG, 6MWT, PDQ–39; assessments at baseline (T1), immediately after completion of training (T2), and after 5 mo for a subgroup of patients.	All 4 outcome measures showed clear and significant improvement at T2. In the subgroup of 9 patients who were retested 5 mo later, all treatment effects had persisted.	Neither patients nor raters were blinded. On the basis of no control group, effect of placebo/attention cannot be ruled out. Results cannot be extrapolated to more severe PD.

(Continued)

Table D3. Evidence on Occupational Therapy–Related Interventions for People With Parkinson's Disease (Cont.)

Author/Year	Study Objectives	Level/Design/Participants	Intervention and Outcome Measures	Results	Study Limitations
Yousefi, Tadibi, Khoei, & Montazeri (2009)	To examine the effects of an exercise therapy program on ADLs and perceived health status in persons with PD	Level I RCT $N = 24$ persons with PD (M age $= 59.8$ yr, HY Stages 2–3). Experimental, $n = 12$; control, $n = 12$.	*Intervention* *Experimental group:* 1-hr exercise therapy sessions 4×/wk, including range of movement, strengthening, functional transitions (sit, stand) and relaxation exercises. *Control group:* No exercise. Both groups received pharmacological therapy. *Outcome Measures* Short Parkinson Evaluation Scale/Scale for Outcomes in Parkinson's Disease (SPES/SCOPA)–ADL Parkinson's Disease Quality of Life (PDQL)–perceived health status.	The experimental group showed significantly greater improvement than the control group in PD symptoms, systemic symptoms, social functioning, and overall scores on PDQL and SPES/SCOPA–ADL. There were no differences between groups for emotional functioning.	Sample size was small. Study sample included only men. Intervention received over short period. The study did not include follow-up after completion of intervention.

http://dx.doi.org/10.1186/1745-6215-10-67

Environmental Cues, Stimuli, and Objects to Improve Task and Occupational Performance

| Bächlin et al. (2010) | To develop and evaluate a system that provides cueing automatically only in the context of freezing of gait | Level III

Single-group before-and-after

$N = 10$ patients with idiopathic PD with a history of freezing of gait, able to walk unassisted in the off period of medication cycle (M age $= 66.5$ yr, M HY Stage $= 2.7$). | *Intervention*

Wearable FOG detection system. 2 sessions, each with 3 walking tasks: straight baseline walking, random walking, and walking related to ADL. First session used FOG detection and deactivated rhythmic auditory stimulation (RAS); second session used activated RAS under observation of 2 PTs.

Outcome Measures

Visual Analog Scale (VAS) to evaluate system's operation and Clinical Global Impression Change Scale (CGICS). | 96.2% of the identified FOG episodes (237) were detected online by the wearable device. Of those who experienced FOG during the study, 5/8 patients thought they had fewer freezing events with the device. Five patients had the impression their freezing episodes have been shorter with the device. Some suggestions were made by the PTs and the patients to accommodate for the variable experiences and to optimize specificity and sensitivity. | Laboratory set-up instead of natural set-up.

Short duration of protocol.

Sample size was small. |

http://dx.doi.org/10.3414/ME09-02-0003

(Continued)

Table D3. Evidence on Occupational Therapy–Related Interventions for People With Parkinson's Disease (Cont.)

Author/Year	Study Objectives	Level/Design/ Participants	Intervention and Outcome Measures	Results	Study Limitations
Bryant, Rintala, Lai, Raines, & Protas (2009) http://dx.doi.org/10.1080/17483100903038576	To compare walking characteristics of individuals who have PD when using a new walking aid, the WalkAbout, with usual walking	Level III Single-group before-and-after $N = 15$ persons with PD (M age = 75.3 yr, HY Stages 2–4).	*Intervention* The WalkAbout walking aid is a wide-based wheeled rolling walker that completely encircles the walker. *Outcome Measures* GAITRite—Speed, cadence, step length. 5-min walk test using portable metabolic analyzer—Gait endurance and oxygen consumption. Questionnaire—Self-report feedback about the WalkAbout.	Persons with PD who were older with slower gait speeds, poorer gait endurance, and more severe disease (responders) benefited more from using the WalkAbout than those who were younger, with faster gait speeds, better gait endurance, and less severe disease (nonresponders).	Functional use of the device in various settings not assessed. Testing done only in a single session. No randomization of sequence of testing (HY Stage 4 is severe).
Elston, Honan, Powell, Gormley, & Stein (2010) http://dx.doi.org/10.1177/0269215509360646	To evaluate the effect of acoustic cueing using metronomes on HRQoL in people with moderate to severe PD	Level I Pragmatic, single-blind, randomized crossover trial $N = 42$ participants with PD (age range = 18–85 yr, HY Stages 2–4). Early intervention group, $n = 21$; late intervention group, $n = 21$.	*Intervention* Walking with a metronome set to a comfortable frequency over 4 wk, with limited support (5–10 min of training and on-demand telephone assistance). *Early group:* Used metronome for 4 wk followed by 6 wk without metronome. *Late group:* Received metronome at 10 wk. *Outcome Measures* PDQ–39, SF–36 Version 2, and falls diary.	Positive effects were found in 6 domains of the SF–36 and 8 domains of the PDQ–39. None of these changes were statistically significant, and the only effect deemed clinically important was improvement in the role limitation (emotional) domain of the SF–36. No statistically significant differences were found in fall rates over the study period. Ten participants wanted to continue using their metronome at the end of the study.	The crossover design could have resulted in the early-group participants becoming disappointed when asked to give up their metronomes and possibly reduced their HRQoL scores at follow-up. Sample size was small, resulting in low power.

(Continued)

Table D3. Evidence on Occupational Therapy-Related Interventions for People With Parkinson's Disease (Cont.)

Author/Year	Study Objectives	Level/Design/ Participants	Intervention and Outcome Measures	Results	Study Limitations
Lim et al. (2005) http://dx.doi.org/10.1191/0269215505cr906oa	To review studies evaluating the effects of external rhythmic cueing on gait in patients with PD	Level I Systematic review of 24 studies (2 RCTs) Included articles published from 1996 to January 2005 in MEDLINE, PiCarta, PEDro, Cochran, DocOnline, CINAHL, and SUMSEARCH.	*Intervention* Studies of gait and cueing (auditory, visual, tactile, and combination). *Outcome Measures* Walking speed stride length, cadence, number of freezing episodes.	There was strong evidence for auditory cues helping to improve walking speed, but insufficient evidence for visual and somatosensory cueing.	Description of cueing was not clear in some studies. Studies not conducted in home/community environments. Majority of studies used a preexperimental design.
Ma, Hwang, & Lin (2009) http://dx.doi.org/10.1177/0269215508098896	To examine the effect of 2 different auditory stimuli on functional arm movement in people with PD	Level I RCT; counterbalanced repeated-measures design with randomization of condition order $N = 20$ participants with PD (M age = 66.5 yr, HY Stages 1–3).	*Intervention* Upper-extremity functional task (reaching for a spoon to scoop beans and transfer them to a bowl) while marching music or a weather forecast played; 3 conditions in each auditory stimulus: listen to auditory stimulus, ignore auditory stimulus, and no auditory stimulus present. *Outcome Measures* Kinematic variables of arm movement, including movement time, peak velocity, deceleration time, and number of movement units.	No differences were found in reaching kinematics between conditions for the marching music. However, movement was slower, less forceful, and less efficient when participants listened to the weather forecast than when they ignored it. Thus, attending to the weather forecast was detrimental to reaching kinematics.	Sample size was small. Practice and test trials occurred in only 1 session.

(Continued)

Table D3. Evidence on Occupational Therapy–Related Interventions for People With Parkinson's Disease (Cont.)

Author/Year	Study Objectives	Level/Design/ Participants	Intervention and Outcome Measures	Results	Study Limitations
Ma, Trombly, Tickle-Degnen, & Wagenaar (2004)	To determine whether a single auditory cue affected movement kinematics of >1 step in a sequential upper-limb task in people with PD	Level I RCT; counterbalanced repeated-measures design with randomization to condition order $N = 32$ (age range = 40–75 yr). PD group, $n = 16$ men (HY Stages 2–3). Control group, $n = 16$ age-matched men and women.	*Intervention* 3-step upper-extremity task (pick up a pen, bring the pen to the paper, and write down a short telephone message) performed under 2 conditions: • *Signal-present condition:* A bell ring signaled movement initiation. • *Signal-absent condition:* Participants initiated movement when ready. *Outcome Measures* Kinematic measurements for the first 2 task steps (e.g., movement time, peak velocity, movement variability).	When picking up the pen (Step 1) and bringing it to the paper (Step 2), participants with PD produced faster and more forceful movement in the signal-present than in the signal-absent condition, as reflected in shorter movement time and higher peak velocity. The signal-present condition evoked a more energy-efficient and stable movement in Step 1 but a less-smooth movement in Step 2. The single auditory cue did not affect movement kinematics of the controls.	Sample size was small. The PD group included only men. Practice and test trials were done in only 1 session.

http://dx.doi.org/10.1097/01.PHM.0000130032.97113.E0

| Mak & Hui-Chan (2008) | To examine whether a task-specific training program using auditory and visual cues would be more effective than conventional exercise or no intervention in improving sit-to-stand (STS) in people with PD | Level I

RCT

$N = 52$ participants with PD (M age = 65 yr, M HY Stage = 2.7).

Audiovisual cued task-specific training group (AV), $n = 19$; conventional exercise group (Ex), $n = 19$; control group, $n = 14$. | *Intervention*
4-wk training program.

AV group: Cued STS training using part to whole training principle (20 min, 3×/wk).

Ex group: 45 min of conventional mobility and strengthening exercises for trunk, hips, knees, and ankles, followed by STS practice (45 min, 2×/wk).

Control group: No intervention.

Outcome Measures
Peak horizontal and vertical velocity of the body center of movement during STS, time taken to complete STS and peak torques, and time-to-peak torques from STS onset. | After 2 wk of training, the AV group significantly increased in peak horizontal velocity of STS compared with the Ex group. After 4 wk of training, the AV group increased both peak horizontal and vertical velocities and reduced the time taken to complete STS. The Ex group also showed improvement; however, the effects were not as large as those of the AV group. | Sample size was small.

Results lack generalizability to PD patients in advanced stages and with cognitive deficits. |

http://dx.doi.org/10.1002/mds.21509

(Continued)

Table D3. Evidence on Occupational Therapy–Related Interventions for People With Parkinson's Disease (Cont.)

Author/Year	Study Objectives	Level/Design/ Participants	Intervention and Outcome Measures	Results	Study Limitations
Nieuwboer et al. (2007)	To evaluate the effectiveness of a home PT program based on rhythmical cueing on gait and gait-related activity in people with PD (RESCUE trial)	Level I Single-blind, randomized, crossover trial $N = 153$ participants with PD (age range = 41–80 yr, HY Stages 2–4). Early intervention group, $n = 76$; late intervention group, $n = 77$.	*Intervention* A 3-wk home cueing program using the participant's preferred method of cueing (audio, with beep to earpiece; video, with flash to glasses; or somatosensory, with vibration to wristband) during functional mobility tasks. *Early group:* Cueing program for 3 wk followed by 3 wk without training (control period). *Late group:* Same intervention and control period, in reverse order. *Both groups:* After initial 6 wk, 6-wk follow-up without training. *Outcome Measures* *Posture and gait:* Composite of UPDRS gait and balance items *Gait and balance measures:* Freezing of Gait Questionnaire, TUG *Activity:* NEADL, Falls Efficacy Scale, falls diary *Participation:* PDQ–39, Carer Strain Index.	The intervention was associated with small but significant improvements in PG, gait speed, step length, and balance and a reduction of freezing in freezers only. Improvement was found in falls efficacy, but no other effects were observed in the activity and participation domains. The effects of the intervention were stable 3 wk postintervention but had been reduced by 6-wk follow-up.	Treatment duration was limited. The home intervention group was compared with a no-attention wait-list control group.

http://dx.doi.org/10.1136/jnnp.200X.097923

(Continued)

Table D3. Evidence on Occupational Therapy–Related Interventions for People With Parkinson's Disease (Cont.)

Author/Year	Study Objectives	Level/Design/ Participants	Intervention and Outcome Measures	Results	Study Limitations
Rochester, Burn, Woods, Godwin, & Nieuwboer (2009)	To evaluate the effectiveness of auditory cues to improve gait in person with PD and cognitive impairment (PD–CI)	Level II Repeated-measures design comparing 2 conditions, nonrandomized $N = 9$ persons with PD and MMSE score of 15–26 (M age = 75 yr, HY Stages 2.5–4).	*Intervention* One session in a clinical setting where participants walked with and without auditory cues using two strategies: cue with temporal instruction to "step in time to the beat" and spatiotemporal instruction to "take a big step in time to the beat." *Outcome Measures* Gait assessed using GAITRite, walking speed, stride amplitude, step frequency, and variability of step, and double-limb support time.	Cueing that focused attention on temporal and spatial parameters of gait significantly improved single- and dual-task walking speed and stride amplitude in people with PD and mild cognitive impairment. The most effective cue focused attention on step length while participants were externally prompted to maintain step frequency.	Sample size was small. Participants had modest levels of cognitive impairment, and it is unknown if those with more cognitive impairment would respond similarly.
http://dx.doi.org/10.1002/mds.22400					
Rochester et al. (2005)	To evaluate the effect of audio vs. video vs. no rhythmic cues on gait during simple-task vs. dual-task functional activity in the home by people with PD	Level II Repeated-measures partially randomized; complexity of task not randomized; audio and video conditions randomized; no cue condition not randomized; video cues randomized $n = 20$ persons with idiopathic PD (HY Stages 1.5–4). $n = 10$ persons without PD matched on age, sex, education.	*Intervention* During a single session, participants performed a simple functional task in home that included walking and dual-motor task (picking up a tray with cups and carrying it to another room and sitting down). Tasks were performed with no cues, audio only (tone was delivered to ear phone), or video only (flash was delivered to eye glasses). *Outcome Measures* Walking speeds, mean step length, and step frequency.	There was a significant increase in step length for persons with PD during dual-task performance with auditory cues compared with no cues. The positive effect of audio cues was significantly greater for the dual task than for the simple walking task, suggesting that the cues reduce the effect of cognitive interference caused by dual task on gait performance. Video cues did not have as large an effect on step length (nonsignificant), but there was no significant difference between audio vs. video cues. There were no effects of cueing on walking speed and step frequency under the 2 task conditions.	Sample size was small. Variation in home environments and walking distance.
http://dx.doi.org/10.1016/j.apmr.2004.10.040					

(*Continued*)

Table D3. Evidence on Occupational Therapy–Related Interventions for People With Parkinson's Disease (Cont.)

Author/Year	Study Objectives	Level/Design/Participants	Intervention and Outcome Measures	Results	Study Limitations
Takahashi, Tickle-Degnan, Coster, & Latham (2010)	To determine whether qualities of interview context are associated with the motivational behavior of a client with PD during an interview	Level II Nonrandomized 2 interview conditions, repeated measures N = 106 persons with PD (M age = 67 yr, HY stages 2–3).	*Intervention* Positive topic interview question vs. negative topic interview question. *Outcome Measures* Expressive behavior, including active facial expressivity as rated in videotapes of interview responses.	There was significantly greater active facial expressivity in the face of participants when they were responding to a positive topic question than to a negative topic question.	Not clear whether the findings would generalize to other positive or negative contexts. The majority of participants were White Americans; therefore, it is unknown if facial responses would occur across various cultures and ethnicities.

http://dx.doi.org/10.5014/ajot.2010.09078

Integration of Self-Management and Cognitive–Behavioral Strategies Into Daily Life to Improve Occupational Performance and QoL

| A'Campo, Spliethoff-Kamminga, Macht, & Roos (2010) | The formative evaluation of a standardized psychosocial education program for patients with PD and their caregivers | Level III

Single group, pretest–posttest

PD caregivers, n = 137; persons with PD, n = 151.

M age = 64 yr; HY Sstages 1–5. Participants from 7 European countries. | *Intervention*
Patient Education Program Parkinson (PEPP). Groups of 4–7 members met for 8 weekly sessions of 90 min. Patients and caregivers had separate groups. Trainers were mostly psychologists. Method based on cognitive–behavioral therapy and self-management education.

Outcome Measures
• *Belastungsfragebogen Parkinson Kurzversion* (BELA-P-K): Psychosocial problems, need for help.
• Mood Visual Analogue Scale (Mood VAS): Patients and caregiver rating of mood.
• EuroQol Five-Dimension Visual Analogue Scale (EQ–5D VAS): Caregiver's present health state.
• PDQ-39
• Self-Rating Depression Scale (SDS). | The program was successfully applied in different settings and cultural contexts. BELA-P/A–k diminished significantly for caregivers. Mood VAS showed significant improvement in mood after each session for patients and caregivers. EQ–5D VAS, PDQ-39, and caregiver and patient SDS showed no significant improvement after participation in the PEPP. | No control group was included.

There were missing values in the data.

Although BELA-P/A-k was translated into the languages of the 7 countries for administering, it was only validated in Dutch.

No follow-up measurements were used. |

http://dx.doi.org/10.1007/s11136-009-9559-y

(Continued)

D Übersicht zur Evidenz 153

Table D3. Evidence on Occupational Therapy–Related Interventions for People With Parkinson's Disease (Cont.)

Author/Year	Study Objectives	Level/Design/ Participants	Intervention and Outcome Measures	Results	Study Limitations
Carne et al. (2005) http://dx.doi.org/10.1682/JRRD.2005.03.0054	To examine the impact of multidisciplinary clinical management of the PD Research, Education, and Clinical Center program on PD progression	Level III Retrospective medical chart review $N = 49$ community-living persons with PD (M age $= 71.2$ yr, HY stage not reported). Divided into 3 groups on the basis of timing of most recent follow-up: 12 mo, 24 mo, 36 mo ± 4 mo.	*Intervention* Multidisciplinary intervention by neurologist, nursing, physiatrist, psychologist, rehabilitation therapists (OT, PT, speech–language pathologist), support group, home exercise program, health and wellness education. *Outcome Measures* Part III Motor Examination subscale of UPDRS.	Overall, the entire sample showed a mean improvement in UPDRS score. In the 1-yr follow-up group, 78.6% improved and 21.4% worsened. In the 2-yr follow-up group, 66.7% improved and 33.3% worsened. In the 3-yr follow-up group, 83.3% improved and only 16.7% worsened.	Control over all potentially confounding variables was difficult. Post hoc chart analysis prevented the establishment of a strict schedule for follow-up appointments.
Gharari & Packer (2012)	To evaluate effectiveness of a face-to-face and an online fatigue self-management program and to compare these with 2 control groups (information only and no intervention) in adults with neurological conditions reporting extreme fatigue Data analysis includes Gharari, Packer, & Passmore (2010) data.	Level II Nonequivalent pretest– posttest control group with partial randomization and 3-mo follow-up $N = 95$ with neurological disorders ($n = 23$ with PD, HY stage not reported). Participants who could not travel to face-to-face intervention were randomized to 3 conditions: $n = 34$, online fatigue self-management; $n = 28$, information-only and $n = 33$, no intervention control. Participants who could travel to face-to-face intervention received face-to-face self-management (no randomization).	*Intervention* Online self-management group: An orientation week was followed by 6 wk of self-management (importance of rest, communication, body mechanics, rearranging activity stations, setting priorities and standards, and balancing a schedule) facilitated actively by OTs. Participants were involved in interactive online activities and discussions using self-management principles. Information-only group: Attention control condition. Same written material as online self-management, but no interactive online activities and no discussions following self-management principles. Facilitator had passive, technical role. Control group: Routine care.	In comparison with the control group, participants in the face-to-face version had decreased fatigue levels, while those in the online version were better able to self-manage depression and stress and to improve their self-efficacy. Generally, these effects persisted at 3-mo follow-up.	Low power statistics for a powerful design—inflating Type II error.

(Continued)

Table D3. Evidence on Occupational Therapy–Related Interventions for People With Parkinson's Disease (Cont.)

Author/Year	Study Objectives	Level/Design/ Participants	Intervention and Outcome Measures	Results	Study Limitations
Ghahari & Packer (2012) (Cont.) http://dx.doi.org/10.3109/09638288.2011.613518			*Outcome Measures* Fatigue Impact Questionnaire, Personal Wellbeing index, Activity Card Sort, secondary measures of Depression Anxiety & Stress Scale, Duke Social Support Index, and Generalized Self-Efficacy Scale.		
Guo, Jiang, Yatsuya, Yoshida, & Sakamoto (2009)	To evaluate the effects of a group education program with personal rehabilitation for people with PD	Level I RCT $N = 44$ participants with PD (M age = 63.6 yr, M HY Stage = 2.2). Intervention group, $n = 23$; control group, $n = 21$	*Intervention* Intervention group: 8-wk multidisciplinary intervention (including neurology, OT, PT, dietitian, psychologist, and nurse) consisting of 3 group education lectures (45 min each), and 24 sessions (30 min each) of an empowerment and self-management rehabilitation program. Control group: No intervention. *Outcome Measures* PDQ-39, UPDRS Motor and ADL, Schwab and England ADL scale (SEADL), Zung Self-Rating Depression Scale (SDS), and global patient's mood status (PMS).	Compared with the control group, the intervention group showed significant improvement in PDQ-39, UPDRS Motor and ADL, and PMS. No significant differences were found between groups for SEADL or SDS.	No active control intervention was used.

(Continued)

Table D3. Evidence on Occupational Therapy–Related Interventions for People With Parkinson's Disease (Cont.)

Author/Year	Study Objectives	Level/Design/Participants	Intervention and Outcome Measures	Results	Study Limitations
Johnston & Chu (2010)	To determine whether attendance at an outpatient multidisciplinary community rehabilitation program for people with PD produces quantitative short-term or long-term improvements	Level I Systematic review Persons with diagnosed PD on a stable medication regimen (M age range = 68–73.1 yr).	*Intervention* Multidisciplinary rehabilitation provided in outpatient setting for not more than 3 mo. *Outcome Measures* HRQoL, functional measures, and physical measures.	There is no high-level evidence to support or reject that multidisciplinary programs produce short-term improvements in people with PD. There is insufficient high-level evidence to support or reject that there are long-term improvements following multidisciplinary rehabilitation.	Studies were inconsistent in outcomes and measurement scales used. Studies showed inconsistency in reporting and timing of measurements in relation to medication cycles. Not all studies were of high quality—2 studies were very old (1981, 1982).
Tickle-Degnen, Ellis, Saint-Hilaire, Thomas, & Wagenaar (2010) http://dx.doi.org/10.3233/NRE-2010-0575	To determine whether increasing hours of self-management rehabilitation had increasing benefits for HRQoL in people with PD, whether effects persisted at 2- and 6-mo follow-up, and whether targeted domains of HRQoL were more responsive to therapy than nontargeted domains	Level I RCT N = 116 participants with PD (M age = 66.3 yr, HY Stages 2–3). 0-hr rehabilitation group (medications only), n = 40; 18-hr rehabilitation group, n = 37; 27-hr rehabilitation group, n = 39.	*Intervention* Rehabilitation over 6 wk, with follow-up at 2 and 6 mo. *18-hr rehabilitation group:* 18 hr of in-clinic group rehabilitation (conducted by PT, OT, and speech therapist emphasizing self-management of PD) and 9 hr of attention control social sessions. *27-hr rehabilitation group:* 18 hr of in-clinic group rehabilitation and 9 hr of individual home and community sessions designed to foster transfer of clinic training to locations of daily living. *0-hr rehabilitation group (control):* No rehabilitation. *Outcome Measures* PDQ–39.	At 6 wk, both 18 and 27 hr of rehabilitation resulted in significantly greater gains in HRQoL than 0 hr of rehabilitation. More hours of rehabilitation resulted in progressively greater gains in HRQoL, although the difference between 18 and 27 hr was not significant. Rehabilitation effects were largest for the Communication and Mobility subscales of the PDQ–39. Gains were retained at 2- and 6-mo follow-up. More concerns with mobility and ADLs at baseline predicted greater benefit from rehabilitation.	Results do not differentiate the active contributions of various rehabilitation disciplines or methods (e.g., group clinic vs. individualized home-based intervention) to the outcomes.

(Continued)

Table D3. Evidence on Occupational Therapy-Related Interventions for People With Parkinson's Disease (Cont.)

Author/Year	Study Objectives	Level/Design/ Participants	Intervention and Outcome Measures	Results	Study Limitations
White, Wagenaar, Ellis, & Tickle-Degnen (2009)	To evaluate changes in walking activity and endurance after an interdisciplinary self-management rehabilitation program for people with PD	Level I RCT N = 108 people with PD (subset of participants from Tickle-Degnen et al., 2010). 0-hr rehabilitation group, n = 36; 18-hr rehabilitation group, n = 35; 27-hr rehabilitation group, n = 37.	*Intervention* Rehabilitation over 6 wk, with follow-up at 2 and 6 mo. *18-hr rehabilitation group:* 18 hr of in-clinic group rehabilitation (conducted by PT, OT, and speech therapist emphasizing self-management of PD) and 9 hr of attention control social sessions. *27-hr rehabilitation group:* 18 hr of in-clinic group rehabilitation and 9 hr of individual home and community sessions designed to foster transfer of clinic training to locations of daily living. *0-hr rehabilitation group (control):* No rehabilitation. *Outcome Measures* Walking activity estimated with an activity monitor (AM) and 2-min walk test (2MWT).	No differences in improvements in AM and 2MWT were found across the different doses of rehabilitation. Higher doses of rehabilitation resulted in significant improvements in 2MWT for participants with low baseline walking endurance and in AM for those with high baseline walking activity.	Many AM records were unusable because of malfunction of the AM sensors. Use of AM to measure typical daily activity has not been well-studied or validated in PD.

http://dx.doi.org/10.1016/j.apmr.2008.06.034

Note. ADL/ADLs = activity/activities of daily living; HRQoL = health-related quality of life; HY = Hoehn and Yahr Scale; ICF = International Classification of Functioning, Disability and Health; M = mean; min = minute/minutes; mo = month/months; MS = multiple sclerosis; OT = occupational therapy/therapist; PD = Parkinson's disease; PT = physical therapy/therapist; QoL = quality of life; RCT = randomized controlled trial; WHO = World Health Organization; yr = year/years.

This revised table is a product of AOTA's Evidence-Based Practice Project and was previously published in the *American Journal of Occupational Therapy.* Copyright © 2014 by the American Occupational Therapy Association. It may be freely reproduced for personal use in clinical or educational settings as long as the source is cited. All other uses require written permission from the American Occupational Therapy Association. To apply, visit http://www.copyright.com.

Table D4. Evidence for the Effectiveness of Occupational Therapy Interventions for People With Amyotrophic Lateral Sclerosis

Author/Year	Study Objectives	Level/Design/Participants	Intervention and Outcome Measures	Results	Study Limitations
Aksu, Karaduman, Yakut, & Tan (2002)	To determine the effects of 2 exercise programs over 1 yr for people with ALS	Level II Nonrandomized controlled trial $N = 26$ patients with ALS ≤5 yr duration; supervised exercise group, $n = 13$; home exercise program, $n = 13$.	*Intervention* *Supervised exercise program:* 3 days/wk for 2 mo, followed by home program. *Home program:* Provided to those not living in the city where held (Ankara, Turkey) or who could not attend supervised program. *Outcome Measures* • Range of motion • Muscle strength and shortness • Grip strength • Functional activities—Modified Norris Limb Scale.	The supervised exercise program resulted in significant but short-lived improvements in joint limitation, muscle strength, and muscle shortness. Over time, the difference between the 2 groups in these areas was not significant. Functional capacity was better sustained in the supervised exercise program than in the home program. The home exercise program was effective in maintaining joint mobility and preventing muscle shortness and contractures but had no effect on sustaining muscle strength and functional capacity.	Small sample size. Lack of randomization.
Albert, Murphy, Del Bene, & Rowland (1999)	To prospectively evaluate palliative care in people with ALS	Level II Prospective cohort study $N = 121$ participants with ALS (M age = 59.7 yr).	*Intervention* Participants with ALS followed in a multidisciplinary clinic. Baseline was within 1 yr of diagnosis. During 4-mo follow-up appointments, patients were asked about palliative care methods such as tracheostomy; use of OT, PT, and speech therapy; use of skilled nursing facility; use of hospice; and having a signed health care proxy and a health care directive. *Outcome Measures* Death during follow-up period.	Those who died within the follow-up period were more likely than those who were still alive to have used hospice, to have used home care and a wheelchair, and to have had a health care proxy as well as a DNR order in the chart. They were less likely to have participated in an ALS support group. No differences were found for having a living will and being seen by an OT practitioner.	Limited information on role of occupational therapy. Small sample size. Variation in the length of time before diagnosis.

http://dx.doi.org/10.1016/S0022-510X(99)00227-0

(Continued)

Table D4. Evidence for the Effectiveness of Occupational Therapy Interventions for People With Amyotrophic Lateral Sclerosis (*Cont.*)

Author/Year	Study Objectives	Level/Design/Participants	Intervention and Outcome Measures	Results	Study Limitations
Bohannon (1983)	To determine the effects of a resistive exercise protocol on specific muscle groups in people with ALS	Level IV Single-subject design $N = 1$ woman age 56 yr.	*Intervention* Proprioceptive neuromuscular facilitation patterns; slow reversals resistance techniques; sessions 5×/week for 10 wk by therapist and at home. *Outcome Measures* • Muscle strength measured with Chatillon push–pull gauge. • Data compared with those for 10 unimpaired participants in a matched control group.	Improvement in static muscle strength in 14 muscle groups was reported without significant change in the functional skills. An intensive home exercise program, monitored by a therapist, may be effective in reducing muscle wasting.	Small sample size. Lack of control group. Learning effect and familiarity with the testing protocol may have influenced outcomes.
Dal Bello-Haas et al. (2007) http://dx.doi.org/10.1212/01.wnl.0000264418.92308.a4	To evaluate the effects of resistance exercise on function, fatigue, and QoL of people with ALS	Level I RCT $N = 27$ participants with diagnosis of clinically definite, probable, or laboratory-supported ALS, forced vital capacity (FVC) ≥90%, and an ALS Functional Rating Scale (ALSFRS) score ≥30. $n = 13$ exercise program, $n = 14$ usual care.	*Intervention* *Resistance exercise program:* Home exercise program consisting of daily stretching and resistance exercises 3×/wk. *Control:* usual care; included only stretching. *Outcome Measures* • ALSFRS • Fatigue Severity Scale (FSS) • SF–36 • FVC, maximum voluntary isometric contraction (MVIC) • Completed at baseline and monthly for 6 mo.	Eight resistance exercise and 10 usual-care participants completed the study. At 6 mo, those in the resistance exercise group had significantly higher ALSFRS and SF–36 Physical Function subscale scores. There were no adverse events, and FVC and MVIC indicated no negative effects.	Small sample size. High dropout rate as a result of disease progression.

(*Continued*)

D Übersicht zur Evidenz   159

Table D4. Evidence for the Effectiveness of Occupational Therapy Interventions for People With Amyotrophic Lateral Sclerosis (*Cont.*)

Author/Year	Study Objectives	Level/Design/Participants	Intervention and Outcome Measures	Results	Study Limitations
Drory, Goltsman, Reznik, Mosek, & Korczyn (2001) http://dx.doi.org/10.1016/S0022-510X(01)00610-4	To evaluate the effectiveness of moderate daily exercise on functional performance of people with ALS	Level I RCT $N = 25$; exercise program, $n = 14$; control, $n = 11$.	*Intervention* Individualized exercise program to improve muscle endurance; designed to last 15 min and done 2×/day at home. Controls instructed to not perform physical activity in addition to daily life requirements. *Outcome Measures* Outcomes at 3, 6, 9, and 12 mo. • Manual Muscle Test (MMT) • Modified Ashworth Scale (MAS) • ALSFRS, Fatigue, Pain • SF–36.	Statistical analysis was available only at 3 and 6 mo because of the high dropout rate. Although both groups declined over time for all outcomes, those in the intervention group had significantly more functional activity and lower spasticity at 3 mo than those in the control group.	Small sample size at start of study. High dropout rate as a result of disease progression.
Foley, Timonen, & Hardiman (2012) http://dx.doi.org/10.3109/17482968.2011.607500	To systematically review the evidence related to ALS service users' perspectives on health care and social services	Level I Systematic review Review of databases and journals from 1988 through March 2011.	*Intervention* No intervention. *Outcome Measures* Overall views of, experiences with, and expectations for health care services, use of assistive devices and telemedicine, communication of the diagnosis, and end-of-life decision making.	Limited evidence was provided that telemedicine may be associated with high levels of satisfaction. Even though participants were satisfied with telemedicine, they also reported that face-to-face contact was more highly valued for discussion of psychological and emotional concerns. This systematic review also reported on the results of Trail, Nelson, Van, Appel, and Lai (2001) and Ward et al. (2010).	Use of self-report rather than experimental conditions for assistive devices and telemedicine.

(Continued)

Table D4. Evidence for the Effectiveness of Occupational Therapy Interventions for People With Amyotrophic Lateral Sclerosis (Cont.)

Gruis, Wren, & Huggins (2011)	To survey people with ALS regarding use of and satisfaction with assistive devices	Level III Cross-sectional survey N = 63 adults with ALS attending a single multidisciplinary clinic.	*Intervention* No intervention. *Outcome Measures* Telephone survey assessing frequency of use, perceived usefulness, and satisfaction with 33 assistive devices.	For assistive technologies used "often or always" by 20% of respondents, arm rails by the toilet, elevated toilet seat, shower seat, shower bars, and slip-on shoes were ranked very highly for both usefulness and satisfaction. Ankle brace for ambulation, transfer board, speaker phone, and electronic seating controls were also ranked highly. The buttonhook, dressing stick, and long-handled reaching tool were rated low for both usefulness and satisfaction. A few participants reported using motorized scooters, communication boards, and sound- or voice-activated environmental controls, and satisfaction with how well the devices worked was very high. Although motorized wheelchairs were used by >25% of participants, satisfaction with them was moderate.	Use of a self-report survey design rather than experimental conditions.
http://dx.doi.org/10.1002/mus.21951					

(Continued)

Table D4. Evidence for the Effectiveness of Occupational Therapy Interventions for People With Amyotrophic Lateral Sclerosis *(Cont.)*

Author/Year	Study Objectives	Level/Design/Participants	Intervention and Outcome Measures	Results	Study Limitations
Handa et al. (1995) http://dx.doi.org/10.1620/tjem.175.123	To describe the effects of therapeutic electrical stimulation (TES) on affected muscle groups in people with ALS	Level IV Single-subject design $N = 1$ man age 47 yr.	*Intervention* TES to stimulate alternate flexion and extension movement in upper and lower extremity for total of 3 mo with increasing frequency and duration each week. *Outcome Measures* • Muscle strength (MMT) • Measurement of functional use and density of muscles (CT scan).	After 3 mo, improvement was shown in bilateral hand functions, and hip bridging was achieved. More improvement was observed in right-knee extension than in left-knee extension. The discrepancy in muscle strength between the right and left sides, which existed before the intervention, was eliminated. The CT scan reports indicated improved muscle density and circumference. TES appears to have the potential to reduce some of the wasting associated with ALS.	Potential therapist bias. Small sample size.
Johnson (1988) http://dx.doi.org/10.5014/ajot.42.2.115	To describe the case of an adult with ALS participating in an aquatic therapy program	Level V Case study $N = 1$ man age 62 yr with ALS; during participation in program (3 yr), ALS was stable without evidence of rapid progression.	*Intervention* Aquatic therapy program 1×/wk for 45 min with assistance and an adapted flotation device; exercises for strength and flexibility, overall conditioning, recreation, and socialization. *Outcome Measures* • OT observations • Spouse reports.	The participant swam laps for 45 m. As observed by the OT, no fatigue was reported at the end, the spouse indicated an increase in energy after aquatic therapy sessions, and the participant was able to contribute more transfer assistance after aquatic therapy sessions.	Small sample size. Use of OT and spouse reports as outcome measures.

(Continued)

D Übersicht zur Evidenz 161

Table D4. Evidence for the Effectiveness of Occupational Therapy Interventions for People With Amyotrophic Lateral Sclerosis (Cont.)

Author/Year	Study Objectives	Level/Design/Participants	Intervention and Outcome Measures	Results	Study Limitations
Lancioni et al. (2012) http://dx.doi.org/10.3109/17518423.2011.633572	To assess a technology-assisted program for increasing leisure participation and communication in people with ALS	Level IV Single-subject design $N = 1$ man age 51 yr with ALS (duration = approximately 3.5 yr) living in a medical care center in Italy; before intervention, participant used boards with letters to communicate using eye blink.	*Intervention* The intervention included a laptop computer equipped with Clicker 5 software and an optic microswitch and interface device. Participant could choose between 2 leisure options (songs and videos) and could write messages through a virtual keyboard and microswitch. Intervention sessions lasted 20 min 3×–8×/day. *Outcome Measures* • Number of words • Number of messages • Video or song activations.	Use of the computer program increased the frequency of words written to about 15 per 20-minute session during the 2nd intervention phase, with a mean of 2 messages per session. The participant also listened to songs and watched videos. All tasks were performed independently.	Small sample size.
Trail, Nelson, Van, Appel, & Lai (2001) http://dx.doi.org/10.1053/apmr.2001.18062	To determine the types and features of wheelchairs that are most beneficial to people with ALS	Level III Cross-sectional survey $N = 43$ people with ALS using wheelchairs (M age = 53.9 yr, range = 32–79 yr).	*Intervention* No intervention. *Outcome Measures* A 39-item questionnaire developed at a neurology clinic assessing features of both motorized and manual wheelchairs, ALS status, functional performance, and other assistive devices.	Of 42 participants, 41 reported that wheelchairs allowed them to have greater interaction in community. Supports (for the head, neck, trunk, and extremities) and improved maneuverability were desirable features. Sling backs and sling seats, nonremovable static leg rests, and large frames were undesirable. Motorized wheelchairs offered a greater sense of independence and improved well-being.	Small sample size. Limited number of participants from 1 geographic area.

(Continued)

Table D4. Evidence for the Effectiveness of Occupational Therapy Interventions for People With Amyotrophic Lateral Sclerosis *(Cont.)*

Author/Year	Study Objectives	Level/Design/Participants	Intervention and Outcome Measures	Results	Study Limitations
Traynor, Alexander, Corr, Frost, & Hardiman (2003) http://dx.doi.org/10.1136/jnnp.74.9.1258	To evaluate the effectiveness of multidisciplinary care for patients with ALS	Level II Cohort study Data on all ALS cases diagnosed in Ireland over a 5-yr period from the Irish ALS Registry. *N* = 344 people with ALS; 82 (24%) people in a multidisciplinary ALS clinic, 262 (76%) people in a general neurology clinic.	*Intervention* The team at the multidisciplinary clinic included neurologists; specialist nurses; OT, PT, and speech therapists; pulmonologists; nutritionists; psychologist; and social worker. A voluntary organization also participated. All services were provided at no cost to the patient. Patients were reviewed every 6 wk and contacted by telephone ≥1×/mo. *Outcome Measures* • Survival.	Mean follow-up time was 1.5 yr. Patients in the multidisciplinary clinic were more likely to be younger, to have familial ALS, and to have been prescribed riluzole. The median survival of the participants at the multidisciplinary ALS clinic was significantly longer (7.5 mo) than for patients in the general neurology group. One-yr mortality rate was decreased by 29.7%. Attendance at the multidisciplinary ALS clinic was an independent covariate of survival.	Difficulty separating the role of OT in a multidisciplinary program.
Van den Berg et al. (2005) http://dx.doi.org/10.1212/01.wnl.0000180717.29273.12	To examine the effects of multidisciplinary ALS care on the QoL of patients with ALS and their caregivers	Level III Cross-sectional survey *N* = 208 ALS patients and their caregivers. Exclusion criteria were cognitive deficits and lack of knowledge of the Dutch language. Criteria for multidisciplinary ALS care included a consultant in rehabilitation and team consisting of at least an OT, PT, speech–language pathologist, dietitian, and social worker; use of the Dutch ALS consensus guidelines for ALS care; and ≥6 ALS patients per year. Other care was considered general care.	*Intervention* Face-to-face interview in a structured format with an experienced research nurse blinded for type of care during home visits and at outpatient clinic. *Outcome Measures* • QoL: SF–36 • ALSFRS • Life satisfaction and well-being Visual Analog Scales (VASs).	133 patients received multidisciplinary care, and 75 received general care. Participants in the multidisciplinary programs had a significantly higher percentage of adequate aids and appliances than those in the general care group. No differences were found between groups for visits to professional caregivers. Those in the multidisciplinary group also had better QoL in social functioning and mental health than those in the general group. No differences were found between groups for physical functioning, VASs, or QoL of caregivers.	Difficulty separating the role of OT in a multidisciplinary program.

(Continued)

D Übersicht zur Evidenz   163

Table D4. Evidence for the Effectiveness of Occupational Therapy Interventions for People With Amyotrophic Lateral Sclerosis (Cont.)

Ward et al. (2010)	To determine power wheelchair (PWC) features selected most frequently and satisfaction with those features of people with ALS	Level III Cross-sectional survey $N = 45$ patients with ALS and motor neuron disease who were PWC users (age range = 27–85 yr).	*Intervention* No intervention. *Outcome Measures* Cross-sectional survey (31 questions) examining patient pattern of selection and measuring the use of and satisfaction with PWC.	63% used mid-wheel-drive PWCs, and 38% used front-wheel-drive PWCs. 79% of PWC users were satisfied with overall comfort, and 72% were satisfied with ease of use. 88% would get the same type of chair with the same features again. Features frequently used include tilt, recline, power elevating leg rests, the ability to run power features through the joystick with upgraded electronics, air or gel cushion, height-adjustable armrests (flat, gel, or contoured), soft headrest, and seatbelt.	Small sample size. Use of 1-clinic survey participants. Potential recall bias because study was retrospective.

http://dx.doi.org/10.1016/j.apmr.2009.10.023

Note. ALS = amyotrophic lateral sclerosis; CT = computed tomography; DNR = do not resuscitate; M = mean; mo = month/months; OT = occupational therapist/therapy; PT = physical therapist/therapy; QoL = quality of life; RCT = randomized controlled trial; wk = week/weeks; yr = year/years.

This revised table is a product of AOTA's Evidence-Based Practice Project and an earlier version was published in the *American Journal of Occupational Therapy*. Copyright © 2014 by the American Occupational Therapy Association. May be freely reproduced for personal use in clinical or educational settings as long as the source is cited. All other uses require written permission from the American Occupational Therapy Association. To apply, visit http://www.copyright.com.

Literatur

American Occupational Therapy Association. (2010b). Standards of practice for occupational therapy. *American Journal of Occupational Therapy, 64*, 106-111. http://dx.doi.org/10.5014/ajot.2010.64S106

American Occupational Therapy Association. (2013a). Guidelines for documentation of occupational therapy. *American Journal of Occupational Therapy, 67*, 32-38. http://dx.doi.org/10.5014/ajot.2013.67S32

American Occupational Therapy Association. (2013b). Occupational therapy in the promotion of health and well-being. *American Journal of Occupational Therapy, 67*, 47-59. http://dx.doi.org/10.5014/ajot.2013.67S47

American Occupational Therapy Association. (2014). Occupational therapy practice framework: Domain and process (3rd ed.). *American Journal of Occupational Therapy, 68* (Suppl. 1), 1-48. http://dx.doi.org/10.5014/ajot.2014.682006

Asano, M., Dawes, D. J., Arafah, A., Moriello, C. & Mayo, N. E. (2009). What does a structured review of the effectiveness of exercise interventions for persons with multiple sclerosis tell us about the challenges of designing trials? *Multiple Sclerosis, 15,* 412-421. http://dx.doi.org/10.1177/1352458508101877

Atkins, G., Amor, S., Fletcher, J. M. & Mills, K. H. G. (2012). *Biology of multiple sclerosis.* West Nyack, NY: Cambridge University Press.

Ay'an P'erez, C., Martin S'anchez, V., de Souza Teixeira, F. & De Paz Fern'andez, J. A. (2007). Effects of a resistance training program in multiple sclerosis Spanish patients: A pilot study. *Journal of Sport Rehabilitation, 16,* 143-153.

Bächlin, M., Plotnik, M., Roggen, D., Giladi, N., Hausdorff, J. M. & Tröster, G. (2010). A wearable system to assist walking of Parkinson's disease patients. *Methods of Information in Medicine, 49,* 88-95. http://dx.doi.org/10.3414/ME09-02-0003

Baron, K. & Kielhofner, G. (2006). *A user's manual for the occupational self assessment* (Version 2.2). Chicago: University of Illinois at Chicago.

Batson, G. (2010). Feasibility of an intensive trial of modern dance for adults with Parkinson disease. *Complementary Health Practice Review, 15,* 65-83. http://dx.doi.org/10.1177/1533210110383903

Baum, C. M. & Edwards, D. (2008). *Activity Card Sort* (2nd ed.). Bethesda, MD: AOTA Press.

Baum, C., Morrison, T., Hahn, M. & Edwards, D. (2003). *Executive Function Performance Test: Test protocol booklet* (Program in Occupational Therapy). Washington University School of Medicine, St. Louis, MO

Berg, K. O., Wood-Dauphinee, S. O., Williams, J. I. & Gayton, D. (1989). Measuring balance in the elderly: Preliminary development of an instrument. *Physiotherapy Canada/Physiotherapie Canada, 41,* 304-311. http://dx.doi.org/10.3138/ptc.41.6.304

Bhat, A., Naguwa, S., Cheema, G. & Gershwin, M. E. (2010). The epidemiology of transverse myelitis. *Autoimmunity Reviews, 9,* 395-399. http://dx.doi.org/10.1016/j.autrev.2009.12.007

Bjarnadottir, O. H., Konradsdottir, A. D., Reynisdottir, K. & Olafsson, E. (2007). Multiple sclerosis and brief moderate exercise. A randomised study. *Multiple Sclerosis, 13,* 776-782. http://dx.doi.org/10.1177/1352458506073780

Blikman, L. J., Huisstede, B. M., Kooijmans, H., Stam, H. J., Bussmann, J. B. & van Meeteren, J. (2013). Effectiveness of energy conservation treatment in reducing fatigue in multiple sclerosis: A systematic review and meta-analysis. *Archives of Physical Medicine and Rehabilitation, 94,* 1360-1376. http://dx.doi.org/10.1016/j.apmr.2013.01.025

Bohannon R. W. (1983). Results of resistance exercise on a patient with amyotrophic lateral sclerosis: A case report. *Physical Therapy, 63,* 965-968.

Bombardier, C. H., Cunniffe, M., Wadhwani, R., Gibbons, L. E., Blake, K. D. & Kraft, G. H. (2008). The efficacy of telephone counselling for health promotion in people with multiple sclerosis: A randomized controlled trial. *Archives of Physical Medicine and Rehabilitation, 89,* 1849-1856. http://dx.doi.org/10.1016/j.apmr.2008.03.021

Bovend'Eerdt, T. J., Dawes, H., Sackley, C., Izadi, H. & Wade, D. T. (2010). An integrated motor imagery program to improve functional task performance in neurorehabilitation: A single-blind randomized controlled trial. *Archives of Physical Medicine and Rehabilitation, 91,* 939-946. http://dx.doi.org/10.1016/j.apmr.2010.03.008

Braveman, B., Robson, M., Velozo, C., Kielhofner, G., Fisher, G.,... Kerschbaum, J. (2005). *Worker Role Inter-*

view (WRI), Version 10.0. Chicago: University of Illinois at Chicago.

Brenk, A., Laun, K. & Haase, C. G. (2008). Shortterm cognitive training improves mental efficiency and mood in patients with multiple sclerosis. *European Neurology, 60,* 304–309. http://dx.doi.org/10.1159/000157885

Brittle, N., Brown, M., Mant, J., McManus, R., Riddoch, J. & Sackley, C. (2008). Short-term effects on mobility, activities of daily living, and health-related quality of life of a Conductive Education programme for adults with multiple sclerosis, Parkinson's disease, and stroke. *Clinical Rehabilitation, 22,* 329–337. http://dx.doi.org/10.1177/0269215507082334

Bryant, M. S., Rintala, D. H., Lai, E. C., Raines, M. L. & Protas, E. J. (2009). Evaluation of a new device to prevent falls in persons with Parkinson's disease. *Disability and Rehabilitation: Assistive Technology, 4,* 357–363. http://dx.doi.org/10.1080/17483100903038576

Cakit, B. D., Nacir, B., Genc, H., Sarac, o, M., Karagöz, A.,... Ergün, U. (2010). Cycling progressive resistance training for people with multiple sclerosis: A randomized controlled study. *American Journal of Physical Medicine and Rehabilitation, 89,* 446–457. http://dx.doi.org/10.1097/PHM.0b013e3181d3e71f

Canning, C. G., Ada, L. & Woodhouse, E. (2008). Multiple-task walking training in people with mild to moderate Parkinson's disease: A pilot study. *Clinical Rehabilitation, 22,* 226–233. http://dx.doi.org/10.1177/0269215507082341

Carne, W., Cifu, D. X., Marcinko, P., Baron, M., Pickett, T.,... Mutchler, B. (2005). Efficacy of multidisciplinary treatment program on long-term outcomes of individuals with Parkinson's disease. *Journal of Rehabilitation Research and Development, 42,* 779–786. http://dx.doi.org/10.1682/JRRD.2005.03.0054

Carpinella, I., Cattaneo, D., Abuarqub, S. & Ferrarin, M. (2009). Robot-based rehabilitation of the upper limbs in multiple sclerosis: Feasibility and preliminary results. *Journal of Rehabilitation Medicine, 41,* 966–970. http://dx.doi.org/10.2340/16501977-0401

Cattaneo, D., Jonsdottir, J., Zocchi, M. & Regola, A. (2007). Effects of balance exercises on people with multiple sclerosis: A pilot study. *Clinical Rehabilitation, 21,* 771–781. http://dx.doi.org/10.1177/0269215507077602

Cattaneo, D., Marazzini, F., Crippa, A. & Cardini, R. (2002). Do static or dynamic AFOs improve balance? *Clinical Rehabilitation, 16,* 894–899. http://dx.doi.org/10.1191/0269215502cr547oa

Centers for Medicare and Medicaid Services. (2014). *ICD-9-CM diagnosis and procedure codes: Abbreviated and full code titles.* Retrieved from http://www.cms.gov/Medicare/Coding/ICD-9ProviderDiagnosticCodes/index.html

Chaudhuri, K. R., Clough, C. G. & Sethi, K. D. (2011). *Fast facts: Parkinson's disease* (3rd ed.). Abingdon, England: GBR Health Press.

Chen, C. C. & Bode, R. K. (2010). Psychometric validation of the Manual Ability Measure-36 (MAM-36) in patients with neurologic and musculoskeletal disorders. *Archives of Physical Medicine and Rehabilitation, 91,* 414–420. http://dx.doi.org/10.1016/j.apmr.2009.11.012

Chiaravalloti, N. D., DeLuca, J., Moore, N. B. & Ricker, J. H. (2005). Treating learning impairments improves memory performance in multiple sclerosis: A randomized clinical trial. *Multiple Sclerosis, 11,* 58–68. http://dx.doi.org/10.1191/1352458505ms1118oa

Chiaravalloti, N. D., Demaree, H., Gaudino, E. A. & DeLuca, J. (2003). Can the repetition effect maximize learning in multiple sclerosis? *Clinical Rehabilitation, 17,* 58–68. http://dx.doi.org/10.1191/0269215503cr586oa

Clemson, L. (1997). *Home fall hazards: A guide to identifying fall hazards in the homes of elderly people and an accompaniment to the assessment tool, the Westmead Home Safety Assessment.* West Brunswick, Victoria, Australia: Co-ordinates.

Cohen, J. A. & Rudick, R. A. (2011). *Multiple sclerosis therapeutics* (4th ed.). Cambridge, England: Cambridge University Press, Committee on the Review of the Scientific Literature on Amyotrophic Lateral Sclerosis in Veterans.

Costello, E., Raivel, K. & Wilson, R. (2009). The effects of a twelve-week home walking program on cardiovascular parameters and fatigue perception of individuals with multiple sclerosis: A pilot study. *Cardiopulmonary Physical Therapy Journal, 20,* 5–12.

Craig, J., Young, C. A., Ennis, M., Baker, G. & Boggild, M. (2003). A randomised controlled trial comparing rehabilitation against standard therapy in multiple sclerosis patients receiving intravenous steroid treatment. *Journal of Neurology, Neurosurgery, and Psychiatry, 74,* 1225–1230. http://dx.doi.org/10.1136/jnnp.74.9.1225

Crizzle, A. M. & Newhouse, I. J. (2006). Is physical exercise beneficial for persons with Parkinson's disease? *Clinical Journal of Sport Medicine, 16,* 422–425. http://dx.doi.org/10.1097/01.jsm.0000244612.55550.7d

Cwik, V. A. (2009). What is amyotrophic lateral sclerosis? In H. Mitsumoto (Ed.), *Amyotrophic lateral sclerosis: A guide for patients and families* (pp. 3–19). New York: Demos Medical.

Dal Bello-Haas, V., Florence, J. M., Kloos, A. D., Scheirbecker, J., Lopate, G.,... Mitsumoto, H. (2007). A randomized controlled trial of resistance exercise in individuals with ALS. *Neurology, 68,* 2003–2007. http://dx.doi.org/10.1212/01.wnl.0000264418.92308.a4

DeBolt, L. S. & McCubbin, J. A. (2004). The effects of home-based resistance exercise on balance, power, and mobility in adults with multiple sclerosis. *Archives of Physical Medicine and Rehabilitation, 85,* 290–297. http://dx.doi.org/10.1016/j.apmr.2003.06.003

Dereli, E. E. & Yaliman, A. (2010). Comparison of the effects of a physiotherapist-supervised exercise programme and a self-supervised exercise programme on quality of life in patients with Parkinson's disease. *Clin-*

ical Rehabilitation, 24, 352–362. http://dx.doi.org/10.1177/0269215509358933

de Souza-Teixeira, F., Costilla, S., Ay'an, C., Garcia-L'opez, D., Gonz'alez-Gallego, J. & de Paz, J. A. (2009). Effects of resistance training in multiple sclerosis. International Journal of Sports Medicine, 30, 245–250. http://dx.doi.org/10.1055/s-0028-1105944

Dettmers, C., Sulzmann, M., Ruchay-Plössl, A., Gütler, R. & Vieten, M. (2009). Endurance exercise improves walking distance in MS patients with fatigue. Acta Neurologica Scandinavica, 120, 251–257. http://dx.doi.org/10.1111/j.1600-0404.2008.01152.x

Dibble, L. E., Addison, O. & Papa, E. (2009). The effects of exercise on balance in persons with Parkinson's disease: A systematic review across the disability spectrum. Journal of Neurologic Physical Therapy, 33, 14–26. http://dx.doi.org/10.1097/NPT.0b013e3181990fcc

Dibble, L. E., Hale, T. F., Marcus, R. L., Gerber, J. P. & LaStayo, P. C. (2009). High intensity eccentric resistance training decreases bradykinesia and improves quality of life in persons with Parkinson's disease: A preliminary study. Parkinsonism and Related Disorders, 15, 752–757. http://dx.doi.org/10.1016/j.parkreldis.2009.04.009

Dixon, L., Duncan, D., Johnson, P., Kirkby, L., O'Connell, H.,… Deane, K. H. (2007). Occupational therapy for patients with Parkinson's disease. Cochrane Database of Systematic Reviews, 2007, CD002813. http://dx.doi.org/10.1002/14651858.CD002813.pub2

Drory, V. E., Goltsman, E., Reznik, J. G., Mosek, A. & Korczyn, A. D. (2001). The value of muscle exercise in patients with amyotrophic lateral sclerosis. Journal of the Neurological Sciences, 191, 133–137. http://dx.doi.org/10.1016/S0022-510X(01)00610-4

Dunn, W., McClain, L. H., Brown, C. & Youngstrom, M. J. (1998). The ecology of human performance. In M. E. Neistadt & E. B. Crepeau (Eds.), Williard and Spackman's occupational therapy (9th ed.) (pp. 525–535). Philadephia: Lippincott Williams & Wilkins.

Elkis-Abuhoff, D., Goldblatt, R., Gaydos, M. & Corrato, S. (2008). Effects of clay manipulation on somatic dysfunction and emotional distress in patients with Parkinson's disease. Art Therapy, 25, 122–128. http://dx.doi.org/10.1080/07421656.2008.10129596

Elston, J., Honan, W., Powell, R., Gormley, J. & Stein, K. (2010). Do metronomes improve the quality of life in people with Parkinson's disease? A pragmatic, singleblind, randomized cross-over trial. Clinical Rehabilitation, 24, 523–532. http://dx.doi.org/10.1177/0269215509360646

Ennis, M., Thain, J., Boggild, M., Baker, G. A. & Young, C. A. (2006). A randomized controlled trial of a health promotion education programme for people with multiple sclerosis. Clinical Rehabilitation, 20, 783–792. http://dx.doi.org/10.1177/0269215506070805

Esnouf, J. E., Taylor, P. N., Mann, G. E. & Barrett, C. L. (2010). Impact on activities of daily living using a functional electrical stimulation device to improve dropped foot in people with multiple sclerosis, measured by the Canadian Occupational Performance Measure. Multiple Sclerosis, 16, 1141–1147. http://dx.doi.org/10.1177/1352458510366013

Finkelstein, J., Lapshin, O., Castro, H., Cha, E. & Provance, P. G. (2008). Home-based physical telerehabilitation in patients with multiple sclerosis: A pilot study. Journal of Rehabilitation Research and Development, 45, 1361–1373. http://dx.doi.org/10.1682/JRRD.2008.01.0001

Finlayson, M. (2005). Pilot study of an energy conservation education program delivered by telephone conference call to people with multiple sclerosis. NeuroRehabilitation, 20, 267–277.

Finlayson, M. & Holberg, C. (2007). Evaluation of a teleconference-delivered energy conservation education program for people with multiple sclerosis. Canadian Journal of Occupational Therapy, 74, 337–347. http://dx.doi.org/10.2182/cjot.06.0018

Finlayson, M., Preissner, K., Cho, C. & Plow, M. (2011). Randomized trial of a teleconferencedelivered fatigue management program for people with multiple sclerosis. Multiple Sclerosis, 17, 1130–1140. http://dx.doi.org/10.1177/1352458511404272

Fisher, A. G. & Griswold, L. A. (2014). Performance skills: Implementing performance analyses to evaluate quality of occupational performance. In B. A. Boyt Schell, G. Gillen & M. Scaffa (Eds.), Willard and Spackman's occupational therapy (12th ed.) (pp. 249–264). Philadelphia: Lippincott Williams & Wilkins.

Fisher, A. G. & Jones, K. B. (2012). Assessment of Motor and Process Skills (7th ed.). Fort Collins, CO: Three Star Press.

Flavia, M., Stampatori, C., Zanotti, D., Parrinello, G. & Capra, R. (2010). Efficacy and specificity of intensive cognitive rehabilitation of attention and executive functions in multiple sclerosis. Journal of the Neurological Sciences, 288, 101–105. http://dx.doi.org/10.3109/10.1016/j.jns.2009.09.024

Foley, G., Timonen, V. & Hardiman, O. (2012). Patients' perceptions of services and preferences for care in amyotrophic lateral sclerosis: A review. Amyotrophic Lateral Sclerosis, 13, 11–24. http://dx.doi.org/10.3109/17482968.2011.607500

Forman, A. C. & Lincoln, N. B. (2010). Evaluation of an adjustment group for people with multiple sclerosis: A pilot randomized controlled trial. Clinical Rehabilitation, 24, 211–221. http://dx.doi.org/10.1177/0269215509343492

Forsyth, K., Salamy, M., Simon, S. & Kielhofner, G. (1998). The Assessment of Communication and Interaction Skill (ACIS), Version 4.0. Chicago: University of Illinois at Chicago.

Forwell, S. J., Copperman, L. F. & Hugos, L. (2008). Neurodegenerative diseases. In M. V. Radomski & C. A. T. Latham (Eds.), Occupational therapy for physical dysfunction (6th ed.) (pp. 1079–1105). Philadelphia: Lippincott Williams & Wilkins.

Fragoso, Y. D., Santana, D. L. B. & Pinto, R. C. (2008). The positive effects of a physical activity program for multiple sclerosis patients with fatigue. *NeuroRehabilitation, 23*, 153–157.

Freeman, J. & Allison, R. (2004). Group exercise classes in people with multiple sclerosis: A pilot study. *Physiotherapy Research International, 9*, 104–107. http://dx.doi.org/10.1002/pri.307

Gage, H. & Storey, L. (2004). Rehabilitation for Parkinson's disease: A systematic review of available evidence. *Clinical Rehabilitation, 18*, 463–482. http://dx.doi.org/10.1191/0269215504cr764oa

Gardarsd'ottir, S. & Kaplan, S. (2002). Validity of the Arnad'ottir OT-ADL Neurobehavioral Evaluation (A-ONE): Performance in activities of daily living and neurobehavioral impairments of persons with left and right hemisphere damage. *American Journal of Occupational Therapy, 56*, 499–508. http://dx.doi.org/10.5014/ajot.56.5.499

Geddes, E. L., Costello, E., Raivel, K. & Wilson, R. (2009). The effects of a twelve-week home walking program on cardiovascular parameters and fatigue perception of individuals with multiple sclerosis: A pilot study. *Cardiopulmonary Physical Therapy Journal, 20*, 5–12.

Ghahari, S. & Packer, T. (2012). Effectiveness of online and face-to-face fatigue self-management programmes for adults with neurological conditions. *Disability and Rehabilitation, 34*, 564–573. http://dx.doi.org/10.3109/09638288.2011.613518

Ghahari, S., Packer, T. & Passmore, A. E. (2010). Effectiveness of an online fatigue self-management programme for people with chronic neurological conditions: A randomized controlled trial. *Clinical Rehabilitation, 24*, 727–744. http://dx.doi.org/10.1177/0269215509360648

Gobbi, L. T., Oliveira-Ferreira, M. D., Caetano, M. J., Lirani-Silva, E., Barbieri, F. A.,... Gobbi, S. (2009). Exercise programs improve mobility and balance in people with Parkinson's disease. *Parkinsonism and Related Disorders, 15* (3), 49–52. http://dx.doi.org/10.1016/S1353-8020(09)70780-1

Goodwin, V. A., Richards, S. H., Taylor, R. S., Taylor, A. H. & Campbell, J. L. (2008). The effectiveness of exercise interventions for people with Parkinson's disease: A systematic review and meta-analysis. *Movement Disorders, 23*, 631–640. http://dx.doi.org/10.1002/mds.21922

Goverover, Y., Chiaravalloti, N. & DeLuca, J. (2008). Self-generation to improve learning and memory of functional activities in persons with multiple sclerosis: Meal preparation and managing finances. *Archives of Physical Medicine and Rehabilitation, 89*, 1514–1521. http://dx.doi.org/10.1016/j.apmr.2007.11.059

Goverover, Y., Hillary, F. G., Chiaravalloti, N., Arango-Lasprilla, J. C. & DeLuca, J. (2009). A functional application of the spacing effect to improve learning and memory in persons with multiple sclerosis. *Journal of Clinical and Experimental Neuropsychology, 31*, 513–522. http://dx.doi.org/10.1080/13803390802287042

Grasso, M. G., Troisi, E., Rizzi, F., Morelli, D. & Paolucci, S. (2005). Prognostic factors in multidisciplinary rehabilitation treatment in multiple sclerosis: An outcome study. *Multiple Sclerosis, 11*, 719–724. http://dx.doi.org/10.1191/1352458505ms1226oa

Gronwall, D. M. (1977). Paced auditory serialaddition task: A measure of recovery from concussion. *Perceptual and Motor Skills, 44*, 367–373. http://dx.doi.org/10.2466/pms.1977.44.2.367

Gruis, K. L., Wren, P. A. & Huggins, J. E. (2011). Amyotrophic lateral sclerosis patients' selfreported satisfaction with assistive technology. *Muscle and Nerve, 43*, 643–647. http://dx.doi.org/10.1002/mus.21951

Guo, L., Jiang, Y., Yatsuya, H., Yoshida, Y. & Sakamoto, J. (2009). Group education with personal rehabilitation for idiopathic Parkinson's disease. *Canadian Journal of Neurological Sciences, 36*, 51–59.

Hackney, M. E. & Earhart, G. M. (2009a). Effects of dance on movement control in Parkinson's disease: A comparison of Argentine tango and American ballroom. *Journal of Rehabilitation Medicine, 41*, 475–481.

Hackney, M. E. & Earhart, G. M. (2009b). Healthrelated quality of life and alternative forms of exercise in Parkinson disease. *Parkinsonism and Related Disorders, 15*, 644–648. http://dx.doi.org/10.1016/j.parkreldis.2009.03.003

Hackney, M. E. & Earhart, G. M. (2009c). Short duration, intensive tango dancing for Parkinson disease: An uncontrolled pilot study. *Complementary Therapies in Medicine, 17*, 203–207. http://dx.doi.org/10.1016/j.ctim.2008.10.005

Handa, I., Matsushita, N., Ihashi, K., Yagi, R., Mochizuki, R.,... Itoyama, Y. (1995). A clinical trial of therapeutic electrical stimulation for amyotrophic lateral sclerosis. *Tohoku Journal of Experimental Medicine, 175*, 123–134. http://dx.doi.org/10.1620/tjem.175.123

Hanson, L. J. & Cafruny, W. A. (2002). Current concepts in multiple sclerosis: Part I. *South Dakota Journal of Medicine, 55*, 433–436.

Holberg, C. & Finlayson, M. (2007). Factors influencing the use of energy conservation strategies by persons with multiple sclerosis. *American Journal of Occupational Therapy, 61*, 96–107. http://dx.doi.org/10.5014/ajot.61.1.96

Hughes, R. B., Robinson-Whelen, S., Taylor, H. B. & Hall, J. W. (2006). Stress self-management: An intervention for women with physical disabilities. *Women's Health Issues, 16*, 389–399. http://dx.doi.org/10.1016/j.whi.2006.08.003

Hugos, C. L., Copperman, L. F., Fuller, B. E., Yadav, V., Lovera, J. & Bourdette, D. N. (2010). Clinical trial of a formal group fatigue program in multiple sclerosis. *Multiple Sclerosis, 16*, 724–732. http://dx.doi.org/10.1177/1352458510364536

Huijgen, B. C., Vollenbroek-Hutten, M. M., Zampolini, M., Opisso, E., Bernabeu, M.,... Hermens, H. J. (2008). Feasibility of a home-based telerehabilitation system compared to usual care: Arm/hand function in patients with stroke, traumatic brain injury and multiple sclerosis. *Journal of Telemedicine and Telecare, 14,* 249–256. http://dx.doi.org/10.1258/jtt.2008.080104

Jöbges, M., Heuschkel, G., Pretzel, C., Illhardt, C., Renner, C. & Hummelsheim, H. (2004). Repetitive training of compensatory steps: A therapeutic approach for postural instability in Parkinson's disease. *Journal of Neurology, Neurosurgery, and Psychiatry, 75,* 1682–1687. http://dx.doi.org/10.1136/jnnp.2003.016550

Johnson, C. R. (1988). Aquatic therapy for an ALS patient. *American Journal of Occupational Therapy, 42,* 115–120. http://dx.doi.org/10.5014/ajot.42.2.115

Johnston, M. & Chu, E. (2010). Does attendance at a multidisciplinary outpatient rehabilitation program for people with Parkinson's disease produce quantitative short term or long term improvements? A systematic review. *NeuroRehabilitation, 26,* 375–383. http://dx.doi.org/10.3233/NRE-2010-0575

Kellor, M., Frost, J., Silberberg, N., Iversen, I. & Cummings, R. (1971). Hand strength and dexterity. *American Journal of Occupational Therapy, 25,* 77–83.

Kenealy, S. J., Pericak-Vance, M. A. & Haines, J. L. (2003). The genetic epidemiology of multiple sclerosis. *Journal of Neuroimmunology, 143,* 7–12. http://dx.doi.org/10.1016/j.jneuroim.2003.08.005

Keus, S. H., Bloem, B. R., Hendriks, E. J., Bredero-Cohen, A. B. & Munneke, M. (2007). Evidencebased analysis of physical therapy in Parkinson's disease with recommendations for practice and research. *Movement Disorders, 22,* 451–460. http://dx.doi.org/10.1002/mds.21244

Khan, F., Ng, L. & Turner-Stokes, L. (2009). Effectiveness of vocational rehabilitation intervention on the return to work and employment of persons with multiple sclerosis. *Cochrane Database of Systematic Reviews, 2009,* CD007256. http://dx.doi.org/10.1002/14651858.CD007256.pub2

Khan, F., Pallant, J. F., Brand, C. & Kilpatrick, T. J. (2008). Effectiveness of rehabilitation intervention in persons with multiple sclerosis: A randomised controlled trial. *Journal of Neurology, Neurosurgery, and Psychiatry, 79,* 1230–1235. http://dx.doi.org/10.1136/jnnp.2007.133777

Khan, F., Turner-Stokes, L., Ng, L. & Kilpatrick, T. (2008). Multidisciplinary rehabilitation for adults with multiple sclerosis. *Journal of Neurology, Neurosurgery, and Psychiatry, 79,* 114. http://dx.doi.org/10.1136/jnnp.2007.127563

Kielhofner, G., Mallinson, T., Crawford, C., Nowak, M., Rigby, M.,… Walens, D. (2004). *The Occupational Performance History Interview-II, Version 2.1.* Chicago: University of Illinois at Chicago.

Kos, D., Duportail, M., D'hooghe, M. B., Nagel, G. & Kerckhofs, E. (2007). Multidisciplinary fatigue management programme in multiple sclerosis: A randomized clinical trial. *Clinical Neurology, 13,* 996–1003. http://dx.doi.org/10.1177/1352458507078392

Krupp, L. B., LaRocca, N. G., Muir-Nash, J. & Steinberg, A. D. (1989). The Fatigue Severity Scale. Application to patients with multiple sclerosis and systemic lupus erythematosus. *Archives of Neurology, 46,* 1121–1123. http://dx.doi.org/10.1001/archneur.1989.00520460115022

Kwakkel, G., de Goede, C. J. & van Wegen, E. E. (2007). Impact of physical therapy for Parkinson's disease: A critical review of the literature. *Parkinsonism and Related Disorders, 13* (3), 478–487. http://dx.doi.org/10.1016/S1353-8020(08)70053-1

Lancioni, G. E., Singh, N. N., O'Reilly, M. F., Ferlisi, G., Blotta, I.,… Oliva, D. (2012). A technology-aided program to support leisure engagement and communication by a man with amyotrophic lateral sclerosis. *Developmental Neurorehabilitation, 15,* 149–153. http://dx.doi.org/10.3109/17518423.2011.633572

Lang, A. E. & Lozano, A. M. (1998). Parkinson's disease. First of two parts. *New England Journal of Medicine, 339,* 1044–1053.

Law, M., Baptiste, S., McColl, M. A., Carswell, A., Polatajko, H. & Pollock, N. (2005). *Canadian Occupational Performance Measure* (4th ed.). Ottawa, Ontario: CAOT Publications ACE.

Lee, D., Newell, R., Ziegler, L. & Topping, A. (2008). Treatment of fatigue in multiple sclerosis: A systematic review of the literature. *International Journal of Nursing Practice, 14,* 81–93. http://dx.doi.org/10.1111/j.1440-172X.2008.00670.x

Lee, M. S., Lam, P. & Ernst, E. (2008). Effectiveness of tai chi for Parkinson's disease: A critical review. *Parkinsonism and Related Disorders, 14,* 589–594. http://dx.doi.org/10.1016/j.parkreldis.2008.02.003

Lieberman, D. & Scheer, J. (2002). AOTA's Evidence-Based Literature Review Project: An overview. *American Journal of Occupational Therapy, 56,* 344–349. http://dx.doi.org/10.5014/ajot.56.3.344

Liepold, A. & Mathiowetz, V. (2005). Reliability and validity of the self-efficacy for performing energy conservation strategies assessment for persons with multiple sclerosis. *Occupational Therapy International, 12,* 234–249. http://dx.doi.org/10.1002/oti.5

Lim, I., van Wegen, E., de Goede, C., Deutekom, M., Nieuwboer, A.,… Kwakkel, G. (2005). Effects of external rhythmical cueing on gait in PATIENTS with Parkinson's disease: A systematic review. *Clinical Rehabilitation, 19,* 695–713. http://dx.doi.org/10.1191/0269215505cr906oa

Ma, H. I., Hwang, W. J. & Lin, K. C. (2009). The effects of two different auditory stimuli on functional arm movement in persons with Parkinson's disease: A dual-task paradigm. *Clinical Rehabilitation, 23,* 229–237. http://dx.doi.org/10.1177/0269215508098896

Ma, H. I., Trombly, C. A., Tickle-Degnen, L. & Wagenaar, R. C. (2004). Effect of one single auditory cue on movement kinematics in patients with Parkinson's disease. *American Journal of Physical Medicine and Rehabilitation,*

83, 530–536. http://dx.doi.org/10.1097/01.PHM.0000130032.97113.E0

Mahoney, F. I. & Barthel, D. W. (1965). Functional evaluation: The Barthel Index. *Maryland State Medical Journal, 14,* 61–65.

Maitra, K., Hall, C., Kalish, T., Anderson, M., Dugan, E.,... Zeitlin, D. (2010). Five-year retrospective study of inpatient occupational therapy outcomes for patients with multiple sclerosis. *American Journal of Occupational Therapy, 64,* 689–694. http://dx.doi.org/10.5014/ajot.2010.090204

Mak, M. K. & Hui-Chan, C. W. (2008). Cued task-specific training is better than exercise in improving sit-to-stand in patients with Parkinson's disease: A randomized controlled trial. *Movement Disorders, 23,* 501–509. http://dx.doi.org/10.1002/mds.21509

Malcomson, K. S., Dunwoody, L. & Lowe-Strong, A. S. (2007). Psychosocial interventions in people with multiple sclerosis: A review. *Journal of Neurology, 254,* 1–13. http://dx.doi.org/10.1007/s00415-006-0349-y

Mark, V. W., Taub, E., Bashir, K., Uswatte, G., Delgado, A.,... Cutter, G. R. (2008). Constraint-induced movement therapy can improve hemiparetic progressive multiple sclerosis. Preliminary findings. *Multiple Sclerosis, 14,* 992–994. http://dx.doi.org/10.1177/1352458508090223

Mathiowetz, V. G., Finlayson, M. L., Matuska, K. M., Chen, H. Y. & Luo, P. (2005). Randomized controlled trial of an energy conservation course for persons with multiple sclerosis. *Multiple Sclerosis, 11,* 592–601. http://dx.doi.org/10.1191/1352458505ms1198oa

Mathiowetz, V. G., Matuska, K. M., Finlayson, M. L., Luo, P. & Chen, H. Y. (2007). One-year follow-up to a randomized controlled trial of an energy conservation course for persons with multiple sclerosis. *International Journal of Rehabilitation Research, 30,* 305–313. http://dx.doi.org/10.1097/MRR.0b013e3282f14434

Mathiowetz, V., Weber, K., Kashman, N. & Volland, G. (1985). Adult norms for the Nine Hole Peg Test of finger dexterity. *OTJR: Occupation, Participation and Health, 5,* 24–38.

McAuley, E., Motl, R. W., Morris, K. S., Hu, L., Doerksen, S. E.,... Konopack, J. F. (2007). Enhancing physical activity adherence and well-being in multiple sclerosis: A randomised controlled trial. *Multiple Sclerosis, 13,* 652–659. http://dx.doi.org/10.1177/1352458506072188

McCullagh, R., Fitzgerald, A. P., Murphy, R. P. & Cooke, G. (2008). Long-term benefits of exercising on quality of life and fatigue in multiple sclerosis patients with mild disability: A pilot study. *Clinical Rehabilitation, 22,* 206–214. http://dx.doi.org/10.1177/0269215507082283

Mehrholz, J., Friis, R., Kugler, J., Twork, S., Storch, A. & Pohl, M. (2010). Treadmill training for patients with Parkinson's disease. *Cochrane Database of Systematic Reviews, 2010,* CD007830. http://dx.doi.org/10.1002/14651858.CD007830.pub2

Mills, R. J., Yap, L. & Young, C. A. (2007). Treatment for ataxia in multiple sclerosis. *Cochrane Database of Systematic Reviews, 2007,* CD005029. http://dx.doi.org/10.1002/14651858.CD005029.pub2

Mohr, D. C., Hart, S. L. & Goldberg, A. (2003). Effects of treatment for depression on fatigue in multiple sclerosis. *Psychosomatic Medicine, 65,* 542–547. http://dx.doi.org/10.1097/01.PSY.0000074757.11682.96

Morris, M. E., Iansek, R. & Kirkwood, B. (2009). A randomized controlled trial of movement strategies compared with exercise for people with Parkinson's disease. *Movement Disorders, 24,* 64–71. http://dx.doi.org/10.1002/mds.22295

Morrison, M. T., Giles, G. M., Ryan, J. D., Baum, C. M., Dromerick, A. W.,... Edwards, D. F. (2013). Multiple Errands Test-Revised (MET-R): A performance-based measure of executive function in people with mild cerebrovascular accident. *American Journal of Occupational Therapy, 67,* 460–468. http://dx.doi.org/10.5014/ajot.2013.007880

Moyers, P. & Dale, L. (2007). *The guide to occupational therapy practice* (2nd ed.). Bethesda, MD: AOTA Press.

Müller, T. & Muhlack, S. (2010). Effect of exercise on reactivity and motor behaviour in patients with Parkinson's disease. *Journal of Neurology, Neurosurgery, and Psychiatry, 81,* 747–753. http://dx.doi.org/10.1136/jnnp.2009.174987

Multiple Sclerosis Council for Clinical Practice Guidelines. (1998). *Fatigue and multiple sclerosis: Evidence-based management for fatigue in multiple sclerosis.* Washington, DC: Multiple Sclerosis Council for Clinical Practice Guidelines.

National Institute of Neurological Disorders and Stroke. (2013a). *Amyotrophic lateral sclerosis fact sheet.* Retrieved from http://www.ninds.nih.gov/disorders/amyotrophiclateralsclerosis/detail_ALS.htm

National Institute of Neurological Disorders and Stroke. (2013b). *Transverse myelitis fact sheet.* Retrieved from http://www.ninds.nih.gov/disorders/transversemyelitis/detail_transversemyelitis.htm

National Multiple Sclerosis Society. (2012). *Fatigue: What you should know: A guide for people with multiple sclerosis. Consumer guide to clinical practice guidelines.* Retrieved from http://www.nationalmssociety.org/download.aspx?id=54

National Multiple Sclerosis Society. (2013a). *Cognitive dysfunction.* Retrieved from http://www.nationalmssociety.org/about-multiple-sclerosis/what-we-know-about-ms/symptoms/cognitivedysfunction/index.aspx

National Multiple Sclerosis Society. (2013b). *Symptoms.* Retrieved from http://www.nationalmssociety.org/about-multiple-sclerosis/what-we-knowabout-ms/symptoms/index.aspx

National Multiple Sclerosis Society. (2013c). *What is multiple sclerosis?* Retrieved from http://www.nationalmssociety.org/about-multiple-sclerosis/what-we-know-about-ms/what-is-ms/index.aspx

National Multiple Sclerosis Society. (2013d). *Who gets MS?* Retrieved from http://www.nationalmssociety.org/about-multiple-sclerosis/what-weknow-about-ms/who-gets-ms/index.aspx

National Research Council. (2006). *Amyotrophic lateral sclerosis in veterans: Review of the scientific literature.* Washington, DC: National Academies Press.

Nieuwboer, A., Kwakkel, G., Rochester, L., Jones, D., van Wegen, E.,... Lim, I. (2007). Cueing training in the home improves gait-related mobility in Parkinson's disease: The RESCUE trial. *Journal of Neurology, Neurosurgery, and Psychiatry, 78,* 134–140. http://dx.doi.org/10.1136/jnnp.200X.097923

Nocera, J., Horvat, M. & Ray, C. T. (2009). Effects of home-based exercise on postural control and sensory organization in individuals with Parkinson disease. *Parkinsonism and Related Disorders, 15,* 742–745. http://dx.doi.org/10.1016/j.parkreldis.2009.07.002

Oakley, F., Kielhofner, G. & Barris, R. (1985). An occupational therapy approach to assessing psychiatric patients' adaptive functioning. *American Journal of Occupational Therapy, 39,* 147–154. http://dx.doi.org/10.5014/ajot.39.3.147

Oger, J. & Al-Araji, A. (2006). *World Federation of Neurology Seminars in Clinical Neurology: Vol. 5. Multiple sclerosis for the practicing neurologist.* New York: Demos Medical.

Oken, B. S., Kishiyama, S., Zajdel, D., Bourdette, D., Carlsen, J.,... Mass, M. (2004). Randomized controlled trial of yoga and exercise in multiple sclerosis. *Neurology, 62,* 2058–2064. http://dx.doi.org/10.1212/01.WNL.0000129534.88602.5C

Okun, M. S., Fernandez, H. H., Grosset, D. G. & Grosset, K. A. (2009). *Parkinson's disease: Clinican's desk reference.* London: Manson.

Oliver, R., Blathwayt, J., Brackley, C. & Tamaki, T. (1993). Development of the Safety Assessment of Function and the Environment for Rehabilitation (SAFER) tool. *Canadian Journal of Occupational Therapy, 60,* 78–82. http://dx.doi.org/10.1177/000841749306000204

Packer, T., Brink, N. & Sauriol, A. (1995). *Managing fatigue: A six-week course for energy conservation.* Tucson, AZ: Therapy Skill Builders.

Parkinson, S., Forsyth, K. & Kielhofner, G. (2006). *The Model of Human Occupation Screening Tool (MOHOST), Version 2.0.* Chicago: University of Illinois at Chicago.

Patti, F., Ciancio, M. R., Cacopardo, M., Reggio, E., Fiorilla, T.,... Thompson, A. J. (2003). Effects of a short outpatient rehabilitation treatment on disability of multiple sclerosis patients—A randomised controlled trial. *Journal of Neurology, 250,* 861–866. http://dx.doi.org/10.1007/s00415-003-1097-x

Patti, F., Ciancio, M. R., Reggio, E., Lopes, R., Palermo, F.,... Reggio, A. (2002). The impact of outpatient rehabilitation on quality of life in multiple sclerosis. *Journal of Neurology, 249,* 1027–1033. http://dx.doi.org/10.1007/s00415-002-0778-1

Pendleton, H. M. & Schultz-Krohn, W. (Eds.).(2013). *Pedretti's occupational therapy: Practice skills for physical dysfunction.* St. Louis, MO: Mosby/Elsevier.

Plow, M. A., Mathiowetz, V. & Lowe, D. A. (2009). Comparing individualized rehabilitation to a group wellness intervention for persons with multiple sclerosis. *American Journal of Health Promotion, 24,* 23–26. http://dx.doi.org/10.4278/ajhp.071211128

Qutubuddin, A. A., Cifu, D. X., Armistead-Jehle, P., Carne, W., McGuirk, T. E. & Baron, M. S. (2007). A comparison of computerized dynamic posturography therapy to standard balance physical therapy in individuals with Parkinson's disease: A pilot study. *NeuroRehabilitation, 22,* 261–265.

Radomski, M. V. & Latham, C. A. T. (Eds.).(2008). *Occupational therapy for physical dysfunction* (6th ed.). Baltimore: Lippincott Williams & Wilkins.

Rajput, M. L., Rajput, A. H. & Rajput, A. (2007). Epidemiology. In S. A. Factor & W. J. Weiner (Eds.), *Parkinson's disease: Diagnosis and medical management* (2nd ed.). New York: Demos Medical.

Rao, A. K. (2010). Enabling functional independence in Parkinson's disease: Update on occupational therapy intervention. *Movement Disorders, 25* (1), 146–151. http://dx.doi.org/10.1002/mds.22784

Ratchford, J. N., Shore, W., Hammond, E. R., Rose, J. G., Rifkin, R.,... Kerr, D. A. (2010). A pilot study of functional electrical stimulation cycling in progressive multiple sclerosis. *Neuro Rehabilitation, 27,* 121–128. http://dx.doi.org/10.3233/NRE-2010-0588

Rietberg, M. B., Brooks, D., Uitdehaag, B. M. & Kwakkel, G. (2004). Exercise therapy for multiple sclerosis. *Cochrane Database of Systematic Reviews, 2004,* CD003980. http://dx.doi.org/10.1002/14651858.CD003980.pub2

Rigby, S. A., Thornton, E. W. & Young, C. A. (2008). A randomized group intervention trial to enhance mood and self-efficacy in people with multiple sclerosis. *British Journal of Health Psychology, 13,* 619–631. http://dx.doi.org/10.1348/135910707X241505

Rochester, L., Baker, K., Hetherington, V., Jones, D., Willems, A. M.,... Nieuwboer, A. (2010). Evidence for motor learning in Parkinson's disease: Acquisition, automaticity, and retention of cued gait performance after training with external rhythmical cues. *Brain Research, 1319,* 103–111. http://dx.doi.org/10.1016/j.brainres.2010.01.001

Rochester, L., Burn, D. J., Woods, G., Godwin, J. & Nieuwboer, A. (2009). Does auditory rhythmical cueing improve gait in people with Parkinson's disease and cognitive impairment? A feasibility study. *Movement Disorders, 24,* 839–845. http://dx.doi.org/10.1002/mds.22400

Rochester, L., Hetherington, V., Jones, D., Nieuwboer, A., Willems, A. M., & Van Wegen, E. (2005). The effect of external rhythmic cues (auditory and visual) on walking during a functional task in homes of people with Parkinson's disease. *Archives of Physical Medicine and Rehabilitation, 86, 999–1006. http://dx.doi.org/10.1016/j.apmr.2004.10.040

Roehrs, T. G. & Karst, G. M. (2004). Effects of an aquatics exercise program on quality of life measures for individuals with progressive multiple sclerosis. *Journal of Neurologic Physical Therapy, 28,* 63–71. http://dx.doi.org/10.1097/01.NPT.0000281186.94382.90

Rogers, J. C. & Holm, M. B. (1994). *Performance Assessment of Self-Care Skills, Version 3.1.* Chicago: PASS.

Romberg, A., Virtanen, A., Ruutiainen, J., Aunola, S., Karppi, S.-L., … Seppänen, A. (2004). Effects of a 6-month exercise program on patients with multiple sclerosis: A randomized study. *Neurology, 63,* 2034–2038. http://dx.doi.org/10.1212/01.WNL.0000145761.38400.65

Rosenthal, R. & Rosnow, R. L. (2008). *Essentials of behavioral research: Methods and data analysis* (3rd ed.). New York: McGraw-Hill.

Rossi-Izquierdo, M., Soto-Varela, A., Santos-Pe'rez, S., Sesar-Ignacio, A., Labella-Caballero, T., … Labella-Caballero, T. (2009). Vestibular rehabilitation with computerised dynamic posturography in patients with Parkinson's disease: Improving balance impairment. *Disability and Rehabilitation, 31,* 1907–1916. http://dx.doi.org/10.1080/09638280902846384

Rowland, L. P. & Shneider, N. A. (2001). Amyotrophic lateral sclerosis. *New England Journal of Medicine, 344,* 1688–1700. http://dx.doi.org/10.1056/NEJM200105313442207

Sackett, D. L., Rosenberg, W. M., Muir Gray, J. A., Haynes, R. B. & Richardson, W. S. (1996). Evidence-based medicine: What it is and what it isn't. *British Medical Journal, 312,* 71–72. http://dx.doi.org/10.1136/bmj.312.7023.71

Sage, M. D. & Almeida, Q. J. (2010). A positive influence of vision on motor symptoms during sensory attention focused exercise for Parkinson's disease. *Movement Disorders, 25,* 64–69. http://dx.doi.org/10.1002/mds.22886

Sauter, C., Zebenholzer, K., Hisakawa, J., Zeitlhofer, J. & Vass, K. (2008). A longitudinal study on effects of a six-week course for energy conservation for multiple sclerosis patients. *Multiple Sclerosis, 14,* 500–505. http://dx.doi.org/10.1177/1352458507084649

Schaber, P. (2010). *Occupational therapy practice guidelines for adults with Alzheimer's disease and related disorders* (2nd ed.). Bethesda, MD: American Occupational Therapy Association.

Schultz-Krohn, W. & Pendleton, H. M. (2013). Application of the *Occupational Therapy Practice Framework* to physical dysfunction. In H. M. Pendleton & W. Schultz-Krohn (Eds.), *Pedtretti's occupational therapy: Practice skills for physical dysfunction* (7th ed.) (pp. 28–54). St. Louis, MO: Mosby/Elsevier.

Schulz, K. H., Gold, S. M., Witte, J., Bartsch, K., Lang, U. E., … Heesen, C. (2004). Impact of aerobic training on immuneendocrine parameters, neurotrophic factors, quality of life, and coordinative function in multiple sclerosis. *Journal of the Neurological Sciences, 225,* 11–18. http://dx.doi.org/10.1016/j.jns.2004.06.009

Shatil, E., Metzer, A., Horvitz, O. & Miller, A. (2010). Home-based personalized cognitive training in MS patients: A study of adherence and cognitive performance. *NeuroRehabilitation, 26,* 143–153. http://dx.doi.org/10.3233/NRE-2010-0546

Smania, N., Corato, E., Tinazzi, M., Stanzani, C., Fiaschi, A., … Gandolfi, M. (2010). Effect of balance training on postural instability in patients with idiopathic Parkinson's disease. *Neurorehabilitation and Neural Repair, 24,* 826–834. http://dx.doi.org/10.1177/1545968310376057

Snook, E. M. & Motl, R. W. (2009). Effect of exercise training on walking mobility in multiple sclerosis: A meta-analysis. *Neurorehabilitation and Neural Repair, 23,* 108–116. http://dx.doi.org/10.1177/1545968308320641

Solari, A., Motta, A., Mendozzi, L., Pucci, E., Forni, M., … Pozzilli, C. (2004). Computer-aided retraining of memory and attention in people with multiple sclerosis: A randomized, double-blind controlled trial. *Journal of the Neurological Sciences, 222,* 99–104. http://dx.doi.org/10.1016/j.jns.2004.04.027

Solway, S., Beaton, D. E., McConnell, S., Bombardier, C., Hudak, P. & Amadio, P. (1997). *Disabilities of the Arm, Shoulder, and Hand Questionnaire.* Toronto: Institute for Work and Health.

Sosnoff, J., Motl, R. W., Snook, E. M. & Wynn, D. (2009). Effect of a 4-week period of unloaded leg cycling exercise on spasticity in multiple sclerosis. *NeuroRehabilitation, 24,* 327–331. http://dx.doi.org/10.3233/NRE-2009-0486

Souza, A., Kelleher, A., Cooper, R., Cooper, R. A., Iezzoni, L. I. & Collins, D. M. (2010). Multiple sclerosis and mobility-related assistive technology: Systematic review of literature. *Journal of Rehabilitation Research and Development, 47,* 213–223. http://dx.doi.org/10.1682/JRRD.2009.07.0096

Stankovic, I. (2004). The effect of physical therapy on balance of patients with Parkinson's disease. *International Journal of Rehabilitation Research, 27,* 53–57. http://dx.doi.org/10.1097/00004356-200403000-00007

Stark, S. L., Somerville, E. K. & Morris, J. C. (2010). In-Home Occupational Performance Evaluation (I-HOPE). *American Journal of Occupational Therapy, 64,* 580–589. http://dx.doi.org/10.5014/ajot.2010.08065

Steultjens, E. M., Dekker, J., Bouter, L. M., Leemrijse, C. J. & van den Ende, C. H. (2005). Evidence of the efficacy of occupational therapy in different conditions: An overview of systematic reviews. *Clinical Rehabilitation, 19,* 247–254. http://dx.doi.org/10.11191/0269215505cr870oa

Stewart, A. & Crosbie, J. (2009). Aerobic fitness in people with Parkinson's disease: A review of the evidence. *Physiotherapy Practice and Research, 30,* 21–26. http://dx.doi.org/10.3233/PPR-2009-30206

Storr, L. K., Sørensen, P. S. & Ravnborg, M. (2006). The efficacy of multidisciplinary rehabilitation in stable multiple sclerosis patients. *Multiple Sclerosis, 12*, 235–242. http://dx.doi.org/10.1191/135248506ms1250oa

Surakka, J., Romberg, A., Ruutiainen, J., Aunola, S., Virtanen, A., Karppi, S. L. & Mäentaka, K. (2004). Effects of aerobic and strength exercise on motor fatigue in men and women with multiple sclerosis: A randomized controlled trial. *Clinical Rehabilitation, 18*, 737–746. http://dx.doi.org/10.1191/0269215504cr780oa

Takahashi, K., Tickle-Degnen, L., Coster, W. J. & Latham, N. K. (2010). Expressive behavior in Parkinson's disease as a function of interview context. *American Journal of Occupational Therapy, 64*, 484–495. http://dx.doi.org/10.5014/ajot.2010.09078

Tanaka, K., Quadros, A. C., Jr., Santos, R. F., Stella, F., Gobbi, L. T. & Gobbi, S. (2009). Benefits of physical exercise on executive functions in older people with Parkinson's disease. *Brain and Cognition, 69*, 435–441. http://dx.doi.org/10.1016/j.bandc.2008.09.008

Tassorelli, C., Buscone, S., Sandrini, G., Pacchetti, C., Furnari, A.,... Martignoni, E. (2009). The role of rehabilitation in deep brain stimulation of the subthalamic nucleus for Parkinson's disease: A pilot study. *Parkinsonism and Related Disorders, 15*, 675–681. http://dx.doi.org/10.1016/j.parkreldis.2009.03.006

Thomas, P. W., Thomas, S., Hillier, C., Galvin, K. & Baker, R. (2006). Psychological interventions for multiple sclerosis. *Cochrane Database of Systematic Reviews, 2006*, CD004431. http://dx.doi.org/10.1002/14651858.CD004431.pub2

Thomson, L. K. (1993). *KELS: The Kohlman Evaluation of Living Skills* (3rd ed.). Bethesda, MD: AOTA Press.

Tickle-Degnen, L., Ellis, T., Saint-Hilaire, M. H., Thomas, C. A. & Wagenaar, R. C. (2010). Selfmanagement rehabilitation and health-related quality of life in Parkinson's disease: A randomized controlled trial. *Movement Disorders, 25*, 194–204. http://dx.doi.org/10.1002/mds.22940

Trail, M., Nelson, N., Van, J. N., Appel, S. H. & Lai, E. C. (2001). Wheelchair use by patients with amyotrophic lateral sclerosis: A survey of user characteristics and selection preferences. *Archives of Physical Medicine and Rehabilitation, 82*, 98–102. http://dx.doi.org/10.1053/apmr.2001.18062

Traynor, B. J., Alexander, M., Corr, B., Frost, E. & Hardiman, O. (2003). Effect of a multidisciplinary amyotrophic lateral sclerosis (ALS) clinic on ALS survival: A population based study, 1996–2000. *Journal of Neurology, Neurosurgery, and Psychiatry, 74*, 1258–1261. http://dx.doi.org/10.1136/jnnp.74.9.1258

Trombly, C. A. (1995). Occupation: Purposefulness and meaningfulness as therapeutic mechanisms (Eleanor Clarke Slagle Lecture). *American Journal of Occupational Therapy, 49*, 960–972. http://dx.doi.org/10.5014/ajot.49.10.960

Uniform Data System for Medical Rehabilitation. (1997). *Guide for the Uniform Data Set for Medical Rehabilitation (including the FIMTM instrument), Version 5.1*. Buffalo: State University of New York at Buffalo.

Van den Berg, J. P., Kalmijn, S., Lindeman, E., Veldink, J. H., de Visser, M.,... Van den Berg, L. H. (2005). Multidisciplinary ALS care improves quality of life in patients with ALS. *Neurology, 65*, 1264–1267. http://dx.doi.org/10.1212/01.wnl.0000180717.29273.12

van Eijkeren, F. J. M., Reijmers, R. S. J., Kleinveld, M. J., Minten, A., Bruggen, J. & Bloem, B. R. (2008). Nordic walking improves mobility in Parkinson's disease. *Movement Disorders, 23*, 2239–2243. http://dx.doi.org/10.1002/mds.22293

Velikonja, O., Curicˇ, K., Ozura, A. & Jazbec, S. S. (2010). Influence of sports climbing and yoga on spasticity, cognitive function, mood and fatigue in patients with multiple sclerosis. *Clinical Neurology and Neurosurgery, 112*, 597–601. http://dx.doi.org/10.1016/j.clineuro.2010.03.006

Vikman, T., Fielding, P., Lindmark, B. & Fredrikson, S. (2008). Effects of inpatient rehabilitation in multiple sclerosis patients with moderate disability. *European Journal of Physiotherapy, 10*, 58–65. http://dx.doi.org/10.1080/14038190701288785

Ward, A. L., Sanjak, M., Duffy, K., Bravver, E., Williams, N.,... Brooks, B. R. (2010). Power wheelchair prescription, utilization, satisfaction, and cost for patients with amyotrophic lateral sclerosis: Preliminary data for evidence-based guidelines. *Archives of Physical Medicine and Rehabilitation, 91*, 268–272. http://dx.doi.org/10.1016/j.apmr.2009.10.023

Ward, C. D., Turpin, G., Dewey, M. E., Fleming, S., Hurwitz, B.,... Lymbery, M. (2004). Education for people with progressive neurological conditions can have negative effects: Evidence from a randomized controlled trial. *Clinical Rehabilitation, 18*, 717–725. http://dx.doi.org/10.1191/0269215504cr792oa

White, D. K., Wagenaar, R. C., Ellis, T. D. & Tickle-Degnen, L. (2009). Changes in walking activity and endurance following rehabilitation for people with Parkinson disease. *Archives of Physical Medicine and Rehabilitation, 90*, 43–50. http://dx.doi.org/10.1016/j.apmr.2008.06.034

White, L. J., McCoy, S. C., Castellano, V., Gutierrez, G., Stevens, J. E.,... Vandenborne, K. (2004). Resistance training improves strength and functional capacity in persons with multiple sclerosis. *Multiple Sclerosis, 10*, 668–674. http://dx.doi.org/10.1191/1352458504ms1088oa

Widener, G. L., Allen, D. D. & Gibson-Horn, C. (2009). Randomized clinical trial of balancebased torso weighting for improving upright mobility in people with multiple sclerosis. *Neurorehabilitation and Neural Repair, 23*, 784–791. http://dx.doi.org/10.1177/1545968309336146

World Health Organization. (1986). The Ottawa Charter for Health Promotion. *Health Promotion, 1*,iii–v.World Health Organization. (2001). *International classification of functioning, disability and health*. Geneva: Author.

Yousefi, B., Tadibi, V., Khoei, A. F. & Montazeri, A. (2009). Exercise therapy, quality of life, and activities of daily living in patients with Parkinson disease: A small scale quasi-randomised trial. *Trials, 10,* 67. http://dx.doi.org/10.1186/1745-6215-10-67

Yu, C. & Mathiowetz, V. (2014a). Systematic review of occupational therapy-related interventions for people with multiple sclerosis: Part 1. Activity and participation level. *American Journal of Occupational Therapy, 68,* 27–32. http://dx.doi.org/10.5014/ajot.2014.008672

Yu, C. H. & Mathiowetz, V. (2014b). Systematic review of occupational therapy-related interventions for people with multiple sclerosis: Part 2. Impairment. *American Journal of Occupational Therapy, 68,* 33–38. http://dx.doi.org/10.5014/ajot.2014.008680

Zhang, Y., Dawson, V. L. & Dawson, T. M. (2000). Oxidative stress and genetics in the pathogenesis of Parkinson's disease. *Neurobiology of Disease, 7,* 240–250. http://dx.doi.org/10.1006/nbdi.2000.0319

Sachwortverzeichnis

A

Abschluss 37
Abschlussevaluierungen 37
Activity Card Sort 26
ADLs 15, 24, 25, 28, 29, 30, 42, 47, 51
Aerobic 50
AgeLine 64
Aktivitätenanforderungen
– Assessmentinstrumente 26
Aktivitäten, komplexe und multimodale 51
Aktivitätenrhythmus 34
Aktivitätsanalyse 24
Aktivitätsanforderungen 16, 24
– Anpassung 36
Aktivitätsmuster 33
ALS 20, 30, 48, 65
Alter 34
Alzheimer-Krankheit 54
Amyotrophic Lateral Sclerosis Functional Rating Scale 48
Ankleidehilfen 49, 51
Anlassidentifikation 26
AOTA 13, 63
AOTA-EBP-Projekte 63
AOTA-Evidenzstandard 63
Arbeit 15, 25
Arbeitsplatzanpassung 42
Arbeitstätigkeit 42
Arthritis 34
Assessmentinstrumente 25
Assessment of Motor and Process 53
Assessment of Motor and Process Skills 29, 37
Assessments 25
– Anpassen 35
–, formelle 26
–, standardisierte 25
– Überlegungen 35
Atemmuskulatur, schwache 21
Atemstillstand 21

Aufmerksamkeit 44, 50
Ausbildung 53
Ausdauertraining 44, 50
Autoimmunerkrankungen 21
Axone 19

B

BADLs 15
Basalganglien 20, 47
Beeinträchtigung, wechselnde 34
Berg-Balance-Scale 53
Best Practice 39
Betätigung 14, 15, 25
Betätigungsanforderungen 26
Betätigungsbedürfnisse 16
Betätigungsbereiche
– Evaluation 32
Betätigungsbereiche identifizieren 26
Betätigungsgeschichte 26
Betätigungsperformanz 16, 46
– Analyse 24, 32
– Evaluation 17
Betätigungsprofil 15
– Evaluation 17, 24, 26
– Fallstudie ALS/Akutbehandlung 30
– Fallstudie IPS/Hausbesuch 29
– Fallstudie MS/Fatigue-Management 27
– Fallstudie MS/Rehabilitationseinrichtung 28
– Fallstudie TM/Rehabilitationseinrichtung, stationäre 31
Betätigungsrollen 26
Bewegungen, verlangsamte 20
Bewegungsübungen, passive 44
Bildsprache 43
Bildung 15, 25, 34
Blasenfehlfunktionen 20, 21
Booster 54
Bottom-Up-Evaluierung 32
Bradykinese 20, 23

C

Campbell Collaboration 64
Canadian Occupational Performance Measure 26
CINAHL 64
Cochrane Database of Systematic Reviews 64
CogniFit Kliental CoachTM 43
Computerprogramme 49, 51
Constraint-Induced Movement Therapy 45
Cues, rhythmische externe 47, 51

D

Darmfehlfunktionen 20, 21
Defizite, sensorische 21
Dehnung 41, 42, 51
Dekubitus 42
Depression 20, 21, 44, 50
Diabetes 34
Dienstleister, gemeindenahe 23
Dopaminmangel 20
Dual-Task-Performanz 46

E

EBP-Projekte 63
Edukation 23
Einführung 13
Einzel-Fallstudien, experimentelle 39
Elektrorollstühle 48, 51
Entlassungsplanung 37
Ergebnisevaluation 37
Ergometer 44
Ergotherapeuten 13, 14
– Qualifikationen 57
Ergotherapie 14
Ergotherapie-Assistenten 13, 14
– Qualifikationen 57
Erhalt 36
Erholung 25
Ernährung 36
Erwartungen 33

Evaluation 15, 17, 24
Evidenz
– Level 39, 63
– Übersicht 67
– Zusammenfassung 39, 49

F
Face-to-Face-Gruppen 40, 50, 53
Fatigue 20, 44
Fatigue-Management 40, 50
– Banking 40
– Budgeting 40
– Face-to-Face-Gruppen 40
– Fatigue
–, Kontrolle übernehmen 40
– gruppenbasiertes bei MS 27
– Programme 50
– Schulung 40
– Telefonkonferenz 40
– Umgang mit/Erhalt von Energie 40
Fatigue Severity Scale 27
Fertigkeiten 16
Fertigkeiten, motorische 15
Fertigkeiten, prozessbezogene 15
FIMT™ 31, 41
Follow-Up 37
Follow-up-Telefonate 42
Forschung 53, 54
Forschungsstudien 39
Framework 14, 15
Freizeit 15, 25
Freizeit-Bewegungs-Aktivitäten 46
Fuss-Orthesen 42

G
Gangprobleme 20
Gang, schleppender 20
Gangtraining 45
Gedächtnisleistungen, verminderte 21
Gedächtnistraining 43, 50
Gegenstandsbereich, ergotherapeutischer 14, 15
– Aspekte 15
Gehgeschwindigkeit 44
Gehirn 19, 20
Gehirnansprechbarkeit 47
Gelenkmobilisation 41, 45
Gemeinschaftsangebote 37
Gender 34
Gesundheit 14, 23
Gesundheitserhaltung 36
Gesundheitsförderung 41

Gesundheitsförderungsprogramme 41, 50
Gesundheitsverantwortung 41
Gewohnheiten 15, 25, 33
Gleichgewichtsprobleme 20
Gleichgewichtstraining 42, 45
Greifwerkzeuge 49, 51
Gruppendiskussionen 44

H
Haltung, gebeugte 20
Haltungsinstabilität 20
Hausaufgaben 44
Heimtrainingsprogramm 51
Hilfsmittel 48, 51
Hilfsmitteln-Training 42
Hydrotherapie 42, 51
Hyperreflexivität 20
Hypomimie 20

I
IADL 15, 24, 25, 28, 29, 31
Interaktionsfertigkeiten, soziale 15
Interessen 26
International Classification of Functioning, Disability and Health 14
Interventionen 15, 17, 23, 35, 54
– Überprüfung/Monitoring 17
– Umsetzung 17
Interventionen/ALS 48
– Empfehlungen 51
– Fallstudie Akutbehandlung 30
– Hilfsmittel und Rollstühle 48
– Palliativpflege 49
– Programme, multidisziplinäre 49
– Stimulation, elektrische 49
– Übung 48
Interventionen/IPS 45
– Aktivität, körperliche u. Übung 45
– Betätigungsperformanz 46
– Empfehlungen 51
– Fallstudie Hausbesuch 29
– Objekte und Stimuli 47
– Performanzfertigkeiten 45
– Reize, umweltbedingte 47
– Selbstmanagement 47
– Verhaltensstrategien, kognitive 47
Interventionen/MS 39
– Aktivität und Partizipation 40
– Empfehlungen 50
– Erschöpfung
–, *siehe* Fatigue-Management 40
– Fallstudie 27

– Fallstudie Rehabilitationseinrichtung 28
– Fertigkeiten, prozessbezogene 43
– Fertigkeiten, soziale 43
– Fertigkeitstraining, motorisches 45
– Gesundheitsförderung 41
– Mobilität, funktionelle 42
– Performanzfertigkeiten 43
– Programme für Settings 42
– Programme für zu Hause 42
– Rehabilitation, ambulante 41
– Rehabilitation, berufliche 42
– Rehabilitation, stationäre 41
– Übungen, motorische u. prozessbezogene 44
Interventionen/TM 31
– Fallstudie Rehabilitationseinrichtung, stationäre 31
Interventionsimplementierung 36
Interventionsplan 17, 36
Interventionsüberprüfung 36
IPS 20, 29, 45, 51, 65
Iyengar Yoga 44

K
Kauprobleme 20
Klientenakten 24
Klientenfaktoren 15, 16, 24
– Assessmentinstrumente 26
– Evaluation 33
Klientenidentifikation 26
Klientenprioritäten 26
Klientenziele 26
Knopflochhilfen 49, 51
Kognitionstrainingsprogramme 43
Kohorten Studie 39
Kommunikation, digitale 49
Kommunikationsboards 49
Kommunikationsfähigkeit 42
Kontextanpassung 36
Kontext und Umwelt 15, 16
– Assessmentinstrumente 25
– Evaluation 33
–, klientenbezogen 34
–, kulturell 15, 33
–, personenbezogen 15
–, physisch 15, 34
–, sozial 15, 34
–, virtuell 15, 35
–, zeitlich 15, 34
Körperfunktionen 15, 26, 33
Körperstrukturen 15, 26, 33
Kostenträger 24
Kräftigungsübungen 42

Krämpfe 20
Krankheiten, neurodegenerative
– siehe NDK 19

L
Lack of Bias 66
Lateralsklerose, amyotrophe
– siehe ALS 20
Lebenserfahrungen 26
Lebensphasen 34
Lebensstilmodifikation 51
Lebensstils, gesunder 36
Lebenszeit 34
Leitlinie Aktives Altern zuhause 54
Leitlinie der Ergotherapie Alzheimer-Krankheit 54
Leitlinie Fahr- und Gemeindemobilität 54
Leitlinien der Ergotherapie 54
Leitlinie Wohnraumanpassung 54
Lou-Gehrig-Syndrom 20

M
Maskengesicht 20
Medikamentenroutinen 36
Medline 64
Mobilität 28, 29, 42, 50
Mobilitätstraining 46
Model of Human Occupation Screening Tool 37
Motoneuronen 20
MS 19, 27, 28, 39, 50, 65
Multiple Sklerose
– siehe MS 19
Muskelatrophie 20
Muskelkraft 45
Muskelkrämpfe 20
Muskelschwäche 20
Muskelstarre 20
Myelitis, transverse
– siehe TM 21

N
Nachsorge 37
Narbengewebe 19
NDK 19, 23
–, chronisch fortschreitende 20
–, entzündliche 21
–, entzündliche fortschreitende 19
–, schnell fortschreitende 20
– Überblick 19
Nervenfasern, entzündete 21
Nerven, kraniale 19
Nervensystem 19
Netzwerk, soziales 34

Neuronen 19, 20
Nine-Hole Peg Test 53

O
Objekte 51
Occupational Self Assessment 26
Occupational Therapy Practice Framework: Domain und Process 13, 14
OPHI-II 26, 53
OTseek 64
Outcome 15, 17

P
Packer`s Managing Fatigue program 40
PADLs 15
Palliativpflege 49
Parkinsonsyndrom, idiopathisches
– siehe IPS 20
Partizipation 14, 23, 40, 50
Performanz 14
Performanzerhalt 36
Performanzfertigkeiten 15, 24, 43, 45
– Assessmentinstrumente 25
– Evaluation 33
Performanzmuster 15, 16, 24
– Assessmentinstrumente 25
– Evaluation 33
–, frühere 26
Persönlichkeitseinsatz, eigener 36
Pilates 44
Plaques 19
PNS 19
Prävention: 36
Praxis 53
Praxis, evidenzbasierte 63
Praxisleitlinien 13
Programme, multidisziplinäre 51
Prozess, ergotherapeutischer 14, 15, 16
– bei NDK 23
– Dienstleistung Überblick 17
Psychoedukation 44
PsycINFO 64

R
RCTs 39
Re-Evaluation 36
Regulation, emotionale 44, 50
RehabComTM 43
Rehabilitation, ambulante 50
Rehabilitation, berufliche 50
Rehabilitation, multidisziplinäre 50
Rehabilitation, robotikbasierte 45

Rehabilitationsprogramme 41
Rehabilitation, stationäre 50
Reize, umweltbedingte 47
Reviews, systematische 39, 63
– Datenbanken/Websites 64
– Methodik 64
– Suchstrategie 65
Rigor 20
Rituale 15, 25, 33
Rollen 15, 25, 32, 33
Rollstühle 48
Rollstühle, handbetriebene 48, 51
Routinen 15, 25, 33
Rückenmark 19
Rückenmarksfasern, entzündete 21
Rückenmarksinfarkte 21
Ruhe und Schlaf 15

S
Safety Assessment of Function and the Environment for Rehabilitation 53
Schlafen 25
Schluckprobleme 20
Schlussfolgerung 53
– Bildung 53
– Forschung 54
– Praxis 53
Schmerzen 20
Schwäche, beidseitige 21
Schwindel 20
Screening 24
Sehprobleme 20
Selbstbild 35
Selbsthilfegruppen 37
Selbstmanagement 47
Selbstmanagement-Schulungen 41
Selbstpflegetraining 46
Selbstwirksamkeit 40, 44, 50
Selected CPT TM Codes 59
Self-Efficacy for Energy Conservation Questionnaire 27
Settings 23
–, gemeindenahe 23
–, medizinische 23
SF-36 physical functional scale 48
Single-Task-Interventionen 51
sling back 49, 51
sling seats 49, 51
Spastizität 20
Spiel 15
Spiritualität 15, 26, 33
Sprechprobleme 20
Stabilitätstraining 45
Status, sozioökonomischer 34
Sterbebegleitung 49

Stimuli 47, 51
Stressabbau 50
Stressmanagement 41, 42
Stretching 44, 48
Studien ohne Kontrollgruppen 39
Studierende 53
Sturzgefahr 42
Sturzprophylaxe 47
Substantia nigra 20
Supervision 47

T
Tai-Chi 46
Tanzen 46, 51
Tastatur, virtuelle 49
Taubheit 20
Technologien, digitale moderne 35
Teilhabe, soziale 15, 25
Telekonferenz 42, 50
Telemedizin 49, 51
Telerehabilitationsprogramm 42
TM 21, 31, 66
Tonmanipulationsaufgaben 46
Top-Down-Evaluierung 32
Training, aerobes 44, 45

Training, computergestütztes kognitives 43, 50
Training, motorisches 45, 50
Trainingsprogramm, überwachtes 51
Transfer-Training 46
Tremor 20

U
Überweisung 24
Überzeugungen 15, 26, 33
Übungen, repetitive körperliche 51
Umweltanpassung 36
Umwelteinflüsse, ablenkende 51
Umweltkontrollboards 49
Uniform Terminology for Occupational Therapy 14
use of the therapeutic self 36

V
Veränderungen, emotionale 20
Veränderungen, kognitive 20, 21
Veränderungen, mentale 20
Veränderungen, sexuelle 20
Verhaltensstandards 33

Verhaltensstrategien, kognitive 47
Verhaltenstheorie 44
Versicherungsgesellschaften 24
Virusinfektionen 21
Visualisierung 43
Vorlieben 34

W
Walking 47
Wassergymnastik 44
Wellness 51
Werte 15, 26, 33
Widerstandstraining 44, 45, 48, 50, 51
Wiederherstellung 36
Willkürkontrolle 20
Willkürmotorik 20
Wohlbefinden 23, 41

Y
Yoga 44

Z
Zittern 20
ZNS 19
Zuckungen 20

Glossar[9]

Adaptation (adaptation): Ergotherapeuten ermöglichen Teilhabe, indem sie Aufgaben, Methoden zur Aufgabenbewältigung und die Umwelt verändern, um das Beteiligen an Betätigung zu fördern (James, 2008).

Aktivitäten (activities): Aktionen, entworfen und ausgewählt zur Unterstützung der Entwicklung von Performanzfertigkeiten und Performanzmustern, um das Beteiligen an Betätigung zu fördern.

Aktivitäten des täglichen Lebens (ADLs) (activities of daily living): Aktivitäten, die darauf gerichtet sind, den eigenen Körper zu versorgen (nach Rogers & Holm, 1994). ADLs werden auch als *Basis-Aktivitäten des täglichen Lebens (BADLs)* und *persönliche Aktivitäten des täglichen Lebens (PADLs)* bezeichnet. Diese Aktivitäten sind „grundlegend für das Leben in einer sozialen Welt; sie ermöglichen elementares Überleben und Wohlbefinden" (Christiansen & Hammecker, 2001, S. 156).

Aktivitätsanalyse (activity analysis). Analyse der „typischen Anforderungen einer Aktivität, der für die Performanz benötigten Fertigkeiten und der verschiedenen kulturellen Bedeutungen, die ihnen beigemessen werden" (Crepeau, 2003, S. 192).

Aktivitätsanforderungen (activity demands). Aspekte einer Aktivität oder Betätigung, die für die Ausführung benötigt werden, einschließlich Relevanz und Wichtigkeit für den Klienten, der verwendeten Gegenstände und deren Eigenschaften, der räumlichen Anforderungen, sozialen Anforderungen, von Sequenzieren und Timing, benötigter Aktionen und Performanzfertigkeiten und benötigter zugrundeliegender Körperfunktionen und -strukturen.

Arbeit (work): „Körperliche Arbeit oder Anstrengung; Gegenstände machen, konstruieren, herstellen, bilden, gestalten, formen; Dienstleistungen oder Lebens- oder Leitungsprozesse planen, strukturieren oder evaluieren; engagierte Betätigungen, die mit oder ohne Vergütung ausgeführt werden" (Christiansen & Townsend, 2010, S. 423).

Assessments (assessments): „Spezielle Werkzeuge oder Instrumente, die im Evaluationsprozess eingesetzt werden" (American Occupational Therapy Association [AOTA], 2010, S. 107).

Aufgabe (task): Was Menschen tun oder getan haben (z.B. Autofahren, einen Kuchen backen, sich anziehen, das Bett machen; A. Fisher[10]).

Betätigung (occupation): Alltägliche Aktivitäten, an denen sich Menschen beteiligen. Betätigung geschieht im Kontext und wird vom Zusammenspiel zwischen den Klientenfaktoren, Performanzfertigkeiten und Betätigungsmustern beeinflusst. Betätigungen geschehen im Lauf der Zeit; sie haben einen Zweck, Bedeutung und empfundenen Nutzen für den Klienten, und sie können von anderen beobachtet werden (z.B. Mahlzeitzubereitung) oder nur der Person selbst bekannt sein (z.B. Lernen durch Lesen eines Lehrbuchs). Betätigungen können die abschließende Ausführung mehrerer Aktivitäten beinhalten und zu verschiedenen Ergebnissen führen. Das *Framework* nennt eine Anzahl von Betätigungen, eingeteilt in Aktivitäten des täglichen Lebens, instrumentelle Aktivitäten des täglichen Lebens, Ruhe, Schlaf, Bildung, Arbeit, Spiel, Freizeit und soziale Teilhabe.

---

[9] Dieses Glossar ist erstellt und erarbeitet von Barbara Dehnhardt, auf der Grundlage ihrer Übersetzung des OTPF (2014).

[10] Persönliche Mitteilung an die Übersetzerin Barbara Dehnhardt am 16.12.2013.

Betätigungsanalyse (occupational analysis): *Siehe Aktivitätsanalyse.*

Betätigungsanforderungen (occupational demands): *Siehe Aktivitätsanforderungen.*

Betätigungsidentität (occupational identity): „Zusammenfassung des Gefühls davon, wer man von der eigenen Betätigungsvorgeschichte her als sich betätigendes Wesen ist und wer man werden möchte" (Boyt Schell et al., 2014a, S. 1238).

Betätigungsgerechtigkeit (occupational justice): „Eine Gerechtigkeit, die Betätigungsrecht für alle Personen in der Gesellschaft anerkennt, unabhängig von Alter, Fähigkeit, Geschlecht, sozialer Klasse oder sonstigen Unterschieden" (Nilsson & Townsend, 2010, S. 58). Zugang zu und Teilhabe an der vollen Bandbreite von bedeutungsvollen und bereichernden Betätigungen für andere, einschließlich Gelegenheit zu sozialer Inklusion und von Ressourcen zur Befriedigung von persönlichen, Gesundheits- und gesellschaftlichen Bedürfnissen (nach Townsend & Wilcock, 2004).

Betätigungsperformanz (occupational performance): Der Akt des Tuns und Ausführens einer ausgewählten Aktion (Performanzfertigkeit), Aktivität oder Betätigung (Fisher, 2009; Fisher & Griswold, 2014, Kielhofner, 2008), der aus der dynamischen Transaktion zwischen Klient, Kontext und Aktivität resultiert. Betätigungsfertigkeiten und -muster zu verbessern oder dazu zu befähigen, führt dazu, sich an Betätigungen oder Aktivitäten zu beteiligen (nach Law et al., 1996, S. 16).

Betätigungsprofil (occupational profile): Zusammenfassung der Betätigungsvorgeschichte, der Erfahrungen, Alltagsmuster, Interessen, Werte und Bedürfnisse eines Klienten.

Beteiligung an Betätigung (engagement in occuption): Ausführung von Betätigungen als Ergebnis von Auswahl, Motivation, und Bedeutung innerhalb von unterstützendem Kontext und unterstützender Umwelt.

Bildung (education)
- *Als Betätigung*: Aktivitäten für Lernen und Teilhaben in der Bildungsumwelt (siehe Tabelle 1).
- *Als Intervention*: Aktivitäten, die Kenntnisse und Informationen zu Betätigung, Gesundheit, Wohlbefinden und Teilhabe umfassen und deren Aneignung durch den Klienten in hilfreichem Verhalten, Gewohnheiten und Alltagsroutinen resultieren, die zur Zeit der Intervention möglicherweise gebraucht werden.

Dienstleistungsmodell (service delivery model): Set von Methoden zum Bereitstellen von Dienstleistungen für oder im Namen von Klienten.

Ergotherapie (occupational therapy): Der therapeutische Einsatz von alltäglichen Aktivitäten (Betätigungen) mit Einzelpersonen oder Gruppen zum Zwecke der Förderung oder Ermöglichung von Teilhabe an Rollen, Gewohnheiten und Routinen zuhause, in der Schule, am Arbeitsplatz, in der Gemeinde oder in anderem Setting. Ergotherapeuten wenden ihre Kenntnisse über die wechselseitigen Beziehungen zwischen der Person, ihrer Beteiligung an wertvollen Betätigungen und dem Kontext an, um betätigungsbasierte Interventionspläne zu erstellen. Diese bahnen Veränderungen oder Entwicklung der Klientenfaktoren (Körperfunktionen, Körperstrukturen, Werte, Überzeugungen und Spiritualität) und Fertigkeiten (motorische, prozessbezogene und soziale Interaktion) an, die für erfolgreiche Teilhabe erforderlich sind. Ergotherapeuten geht es um Partizipation als Endergebnis, sie ermöglichen deshalb Beteiligung durch Adaptation und Modifikation der Umwelt oder von Gegenständen bzw. Objekten innerhalb der Umwelt wenn notwendig. Ergotherapeutische Dienstleistungen werden zu Gesundheitsaufbau und -erhalt (habilitation), Rehabilitation und Förderung von Gesundheit und Wohlbefinden für Klienten mit behinderungsbedingten und nicht-behinderungsbedingtem Bedarf angeboten. Zu diesen Dienstleistungen gehören die Aneignung und der Erhalt der Betätigungsidentität für Menschen, die Krankheit, Verletzung, Störung, Schädigung, Behinderung, Aktivitätseinschränkung oder Eingrenzung der Teilhabe erfahren haben oder die davon bedroht sind (nach AOTA, 2011).

Evaluation (Evaluation): „Prozess des Sammelns und Interpretierens von Daten, die für die Intervention notwendig sind. Dazu gehört das Planen und Dokumentieren des Evaluationsprozesses und der Outcomes" (AOTA, 2011, S. 107).

Freizeit (leisure): „Nicht verpflichtende Aktivität, die intrinsisch motiviert ist und an der man sich in frei verfügbarer Zeit beteiligt, also in der Zeit, die keinen obligatorischen Betätigungen wie Arbeit, Selbstversorgung oder Schlaf dient" (Parham & Fazio, 1997, S. 250).

Fürsprache (advocacy): Bemühungen, Betätigungsgerechtigkeit und Empowerment von Klienten zu fördern, Ressourcen zu suchen und zu finden, damit Klienten ganz an ihren täglichen Betätigungen teilhaben. Anstrengungen des Ergotherapeuten werden als Fürsprache bezeichnet, und diejenigen des Klienten als Vertreten der eigenen Interessen; diese können auch durch den Ergotherapeuten gefördert und unterstützt werden.

Gegenstandsbereich (Domain): Geltungs- und Gegenstandsbereich des Berufes, in dem seine Mitglieder ein gesammeltes Wissen und Erfahrung haben.

Gemeinsame Vorgehensweise (collaborative approach): Ausrichtung, in der die Ergotherapeutin und der Klient im Geiste von Gleichheit und beiderseitiger Teilhabe arbeiten. Gemeinsames Vorgehen beinhaltet, die Klienten zu ermutigen, ihre therapeutischen Anliegen zu beschreiben, ihre eigenen Ziele zu benennen und zu Entscheidungen zu ihrer therapeutischen Intervention beizutragen (Boyt Schell et al., 2014a).

Gesundheit (health): „Zustand kompletten körperlichen, mentalen und sozialen Wohlbefindens und nicht nur die Abwesenheit von Krankheit oder Gebrechen" (WHO, 2006, S. 1).

Gesundheitsaufbau und -erhalt (habilitation): Gesundheitsdienstleistungen, die Menschen helfen, Fertigkeiten, Funktionen oder Performanz zur Partizipation an Betätigungen und alltäglichen Aktivitäten (ganz oder teilweise) aufrecht zu erhalten, zu erwerben, zu verbessern, deren Abbau möglichst klein zu halten oder eine Schädigung zu kompensieren (AOTA policy staff[11]).

Gesundheitsförderung (health promotion)

„Prozess, Menschen zu befähigen, ihre Gesundheit stärker selbst zu steuern und zu verbessern. Um einen Zustand kompletten körperlichen, mentalen und sozialen Wohlbefindens zu erreichen, muss eine Einzelperson oder eine Gruppe fähig sein, das eigene Streben zu erkennen und zu erfassen, Bedürfnisse zu befriedigen und die Umwelt zu verändern oder mit ihr zurecht zu kommen" (WHO, 1986).

Gewohnheiten (habits): „Erworbene Tendenz, in vertrauter Umwelt oder Situation zu reagieren und auf gleichbleibende Weise zu handeln; spezifisches automatisches Verhalten, das wiederholt, relativ automatisch und mit wenig Variation gezeigt wird" (Boyt Schell et al., 2014a, S. 1234). Gewohnheiten können nützlich, dominierend oder verkümmert sein und Performanz in Betätigungsbereichen entweder unterstützen oder behindern (Dunn, 2000).

Gruppe (group): Ansammlung von Einzelpersonen (z. B. Familienmitglieder, Arbeiter, Studenten, Bürger einer Gemeinde).

Gruppenintervention (group intervention): Praktische Kenntnisse und Einsatz von Führungstechniken in unterschiedlichem Setting, um Lernen und Erwerb von Fertigkeiten zur Partizipation durch Klienten über das gesamte Leben anzubahnen, einschließlich grundlegender sozialer Interaktionsfertigkeiten, Instrumenten zur Selbstregulierung, Zielsetzung und positivem Auswählen durch die Dynamik der Gruppe und durch soziale Interaktion. Gruppen können als Methode der Dienstleistung verwendet werden.

Hoffnung (hope): „Empfundene Fähigkeit, Wege zu finden, um erwünschte Ziele zu erreichen und sich selbst zu motivieren, diese Wege zu gehen" (Rand & Cheavens, 2009, S. 323).

Instrumentelle Aktivitäten des täglichen Lebens (IADLs) (instrumental ADLs): Aktivitäten, die das tägliche Leben zuhause und in der Öffentlichkeit unterstützen und die oft komplexere Interaktionen erfordern als ADLs.

Interessen (interests): „Was man gerne und zufriedenstellend macht" (Kielhofner, 2008, S. 42).

Intervention (intervention)
„Gemeinsamer Prozess und praktische Aktionen von Ergotherapeuten und Klienten, um das Beteiligen an Betätigung in Bezug auf die Gesundheit und Partizipation anzubahnen. Eingeschlossen darin sind der Plan, dessen Umsetzung und Überprüfung" (AOTA, 2010, S. 107).

Interventionsansätze (intervention approaches): Spezifische Strategien zur Lenkung des Interven-

---
[11] persönliche Mitteilung an die Übersetzerin Barbara Dehnhardt, 17.12.2013

tionsprozesses auf der Basis der vom Klienten erwünschten Outcomes, Evaluationsdaten und Evidenz.

Klient (client): Person oder Personen (einschließlich derjenigen, die den Klienten versorgen), Gruppe (Ansammlung von Einzelpersonen, z. B. Familien, Arbeitnehmer, Studenten oder Gemeindemitglieder) oder Populationen (Ansammlung von Gruppen oder Einzelpersonen, die in einer ähnlichen Gegend wohnen, z. B. Stadt, Land oder Staat, oder die die gleichen oder ähnliche Anliegen haben).

Klientenzentrierte Versorgung/Praxis (client-centered care/practice): Dienstleistungsansatz, der Respekt für die Klienten und Partnerschaft mit ihnen als aktive Teilnehmer am Therapieprozess umfasst. Dieser Ansatz betont das Wissen und die Erfahrung, Stärken, Auswahlvermögen und allgemeine Autonomie der Klienten (Boyt Schell et al., 2014a, S. 1230).

Klientenfaktoren (client factors): Spezielle Fähigkeiten, Merkmale oder Überzeugungen, die der Person innewohnen und Betätigungsperformanz beeinflussen. Zu Klientenfaktoren gehören Werte, Überzeugungen und Spiritualität, Körperfunktionen und Körperstrukturen.

Klinisches Reasoning (Clinical Reasoning): „Prozess, den Ergotherapeuten zum Planen, Ausrichten, Durchführen und Reflektieren über die Klientenversorgung nutzen" (Boyt Schell et al., 2014a, S. 1231). Der Begriff *professionelles Reasoning* wird gelegentlich genutzt und wird als allgemeinerer Begriff angesehen.

Körperfunktionen (body functions): „Physiologische Funktionen von Körpersystemen (einschließlich psychischer Funktionen)" (World Health Organization [WHO], 2010, S. 107).

Körperstrukturen (body structures): „Anatomische Teile des Körpers wie Organe, Gliedmaßen und ihre Komponenten", die Körperfunktionen unterstützen (WHO, 2001, S. 10).

Ko-Betätigung (co-occupation): Betätigung, die zwei oder mehr Personen umfasst (Boyt Schell et al., 2014a, S. 1232).

Kontext (Kontext): Eine Reihe von miteinander verbundenen Gegebenheiten innerhalb des und um den Klienten herum, die Performanz beeinflussen, auch den kulturellen, personenbezogenen, zeitlichen und virtuellen Kontext.

Kultureller Kontext (cultural context): Von der Gesellschaft, deren Teil der Klient ist, akzeptierte Sitten, Überzeugungen, Aktivitätsmuster, Verhaltensstandards und Erwartungen. Der kulturelle Kontext beeinflusst Identität und Aktivitätsauswahl des Klienten.

Lebensqualität (quality of life): Dynamische Bewertung der Lebenszufriedenheit (Wahrnehmung von Fortschritt in Richtung der herausgefundenen Ziele), des Selbstkonzepts (Überzeugungen und Empfinden über sich selbst), von Gesundheit und Funktionsfähigkeit (z. B. Gesundheitsstatus, Selbstversorgungsfähigkeiten) und von sozioökonomischen Faktoren (z. B. Beruf, Bildung, Einkommen; nach Radomski, 1995).

Motorische Fertigkeiten (motor skills): „Fertigkeiten der Betätigungsperformanz, beobachtet wenn die Person sich selbst und Gegenstände der Aufgabe innerhalb der Aufgabenumwelt bewegt oder mit ihnen interagiert" (z. B. motorische ADL-Fertigkeiten, motorische Schulfertigkeiten; Boyt Schell et al., 2014a, S. 1237).

Organisation (organization): Eine Gesamtheit von Einzelpersonen mit einem gemeinsamen Zweck oder Vorhaben wie eine Gesellschaft, Industrie oder Agentur.

Outcome/Ergebnis (outcome): Endergebnis des ergotherapeutischen Prozesses; was Klienten durch ergotherapeutische Intervention erreichen können.

Partizipation (participation): „Eingebunden-sein in eine Lebenssituation" (WHO, 2001, S. 10).

Performanzanalyse (analysis of occupational performance): Der Schritt der Evaluation, in dem die positiven Aspekte des Klienten und seine Probleme bzw. seine potentiellen Probleme genauer untersucht werden, und zwar mit Hilfe von Assessment-Instrumenten, die beobachten, messen und nach den Faktoren fragen, die Betätigungsperformanz unterstützen oder behindern und mit denen anvisierte Outcomes herausgefunden werden.

Performanzfertigkeiten (performanceskills): Zielgerichtete Aktionen, die als kleine Einheiten der Ausführung von Beteiligung an alltäglichen Betätigungen beobachtbar sind. Sie werden im Laufe der Zeit erlernt und entwickelt und gehören in bestimmte Kontexte oder Umwelten (Fisher & Griswold, 2014).

Performanzmuster (performance patterns): Gewohnheiten, Routineabläufe, Rollen und Rituale bei Betätigungen oder Aktivitäten; diese Muster können Betätigungsperformanz unterstützen oder behindern.

Person (person): Ein Mensch, auch Familienmitglied, Versorger, Lehrer, Angestellter oder wichtige Bezugsperson.

Personenbezogener Kontext (personal context): „Merkmale eines Menschen, die nicht Teil seines Gesundheitszustandes oder -status sind" (WHO, 2001, S. 17). Zum personenbezogenen Kontext gehören Alter, Geschlecht, sozioökonomischer und Bildungsstatus, er kann auch Gruppenmitgliedschaft (z. B. Ehrenamtlicher, Angestellter) oder einer Populationsmitgliedschaft einschließen (z. B. Gesellschaftsmitglied).

Physische Umwelt (physical environment): Natürliche oder hergestellte Umgebung und die Gegenstände darin. Zur natürlichen Umwelt gehören sowohl geografisches Land, Pflanzen und Tiere als auch sensorische Qualitäten der natürlichen Umgebung. Zur hergestellten Umwelt gehören Gebäude, Möbel, Werkzeuge und Geräte.

Population (population): Ansammlung von Gruppen von Einzelpersonen, die an einem ähnlichen Schauplatz leben (z. B. Stadt, Staat, Land) oder die die gleichen oder ähnliche Merkmale oder Anliegen haben.

Prävention (prevention). Bemühungen zur Schulung über oder Förderung von Gesundheit, die das Entstehen oder Auftreten von ungesunden Bedingungen, Risikofaktoren, Krankheiten oder Verletzungen erkennen, reduzieren oder verhüten sollen (AOTA, 2013b).

Prozess (process): Art und Weise, wie Ergotherapeuten ihr Fachwissen für Klienten als Dienstleistung operationalisieren. Zum ergotherapeutischen Prozess gehören Evaluation, Intervention und anvisierten Outcomes; er geschieht auf dem Gebiet des ergotherapeutischen Gegenstandsbereiches und stützt sich auf die Zusammenarbeit zwischen Ergotherapeutin, Ergotherapie-Assistenten und Klient.

Prozessbezogene Fertigkeiten (process skills): „Fertigkeiten der Betätigungsperformanz (z. B. prozessbezogene ADL-Fertigkeiten, Schul-Prozessfertigkeiten), beobachtet, wenn eine Person 1. Werkzeuge der Aufgabe auswählt, mit ihnen interagiert und sie verwendet; 2. einzelne Aktionen und Schritte ausführt; und 3. die Ausführung modifiziert, wenn sich Probleme ergeben" (Boyt Schell et al., 2014a, S. 1239).

Re-Evaluation (re-evaluation): Erneute Bewertung der Performanz und der Ziele eines Klienten, um die Art und das Ausmaß von stattgefundenen Veränderungen festzustellen.

Rehabilitation (rehabilitation): Rehabilitation wird für Klienten bereitgestellt, die Defizite in Schlüsselbereichen von physischen und anderen Funktionen oder Einschränkungen bei Partizipation an alltäglichen Aktivitäten haben. Interventionen werden erstellt, um zum Erreichen und zum Erhalt einer optimalen physischen, sensorischen, intellektuellen, psychischen und sozialen Funktionsebene zu befähigen. Rehabilitation bietet Instrumente und Techniken, die nötig sind, um die erwünschte Ebene von Selbstständigkeit und Selbstbestimmung zu erreichen.

Rituale (rituals): Gruppen von symbolischen Aktionen mit spiritueller, kultureller und sozialer Bedeutung, die zur Identität des Klienten beitragen und seine Werte und Überzeugungen stärken. Rituale haben eine starke affektive Komponente (Fiese, 2007; Fiese et al., 2002, Segal, 2004; siehe Tabelle 4).

Rollen (roles): Sets von Verhalten, die von der Gesellschaft erwartet und von Kultur und Kontext geformt werden; sie können durch den Klienten erweitert und definiert werden.

Routinen (routines). Verhaltensmuster, die beobachtbar und regelmäßig sind, sich wiederholen und den Alltag strukturieren. Sie können befriedigen, fördern oder schädigen. Alltagsabläufe erfordern [nur] kurzen Zeiteinsatz und sind in kulturellen und ökologischen Kontext eingebettet (Fiese, 2007; Segal, 2004).

Soziale Interaktionsfertigkeiten (social interaction skills): „Fertigkeiten der Betätigungsperformanz, beobachtet während des fortlaufenden Stroms von sozialem Austausch" (Boyt Schell et al., 2014a S. 1241).

Soziale Umwelt (social environment). Anwesenheit von, Beziehungen zu und Erwartungen von Personen, Gruppen oder Populationen, mit denen Klienten im Kontakt stehen (z. B. Verfügbarkeit und Erwartungen von wichtigen Menschen wie Ehepartner, Freunde und Betreuer).

Soziale Partizipation/ Teilhabe (social participation) : „Das Verflechten von Betätigungen, um erwünschte Beteiligung an Gemeinde- und Familienaktivitäten sowie an solchen mit Freunden und Bekannten zu unterstützen" (Gillen & Boyt Schell, 2014, 607); eine Untergruppe von Aktivitäten, die soziale Situationen mit anderen beinhalten (Bedell, 2012) und die soziale Wechselbeziehung unterstützen (Magasi & Hammel, 2004). Soziale Teilhabe kann persönlich oder durch Techniken auf die Entfernung wie Telefonanruf, Computerinteraktion oder Videokonferenz stattfinden.

Spiel (play): „Jegliche spontane oder organisierte Aktivität, die Spaß, Unterhaltung, Vergnügen oder Ablenkung bietet" (Parham & Fazio, 1997, S. 525).

Spiritualität (spirituality): „Der Aspekt von Humanität, der sich darauf bezieht, wie Menschen Bedeutung und Zweck suchen und ausdrücken und auf die Art und Weise, wie sie ihre Verbundenheit mit der Gegenwart, mit sich selbst, mit der Natur und mit dem Wesentlichen oder Heiligen erfahren" (Puchalski et al. 2009, S. 887).

Transaktion (transaction): Prozess zwischen zwei oder mehr Personen oder Elementen, die sich fortlaufend und wechselseitig durch die fortdauernde Beziehung beeinflussen (Dickie, Cutchin & Humphry, 2006).

Umwelt (environment): Externe physische und soziale Gegebenheiten um den Klienten herum, in denen sich der Alltag des Klienten abspielt.

Unabhängigkeit/Selbstständigkeit (independence). „Selbstgesteuerter Zustand, gekennzeichnet durch die Fähigkeit eines Menschen, an notwendigen und bevorzugten Betätigungen auf befriedigende Weise teilzuhaben, unabhängig von der Menge oder Art externer erwünschter oder notwendiger Hilfe" (AOTA, 2002a, S. 660).

Vorbereitende Methoden und Aufgaben (preparatory methods and tasks). Methoden und Aufgaben, die den Klienten auf Betätigung vorbereiten, eingesetzt entweder als Teil der Behandlung zur Vorbereitung oder gleichzeitig mit Betätigungen und Aktivitäten oder als häusliche Aktivität zur Unterstützung der täglichen Betätigungsperformanz. Oft sind vorbereitende Methoden Interventionen, die an Klienten vorgenommen werden, ohne dass diese aktiv beteiligt sind; dabei werden Modalitäten, Geräte oder Techniken eingesetzt.

Vertreten eigener Interessen (self-advocacy): Die eigenen Interessen vertreten, einschließlich Entscheidungen über das eigene Leben treffen; lernen, Informationen zu besorgen, um Dinge von persönlichem Interesse oder Wichtigkeit zu verstehen; ein unterstützendes Netzwerk aufbauen; eigene Rechte und Pflichten kennen, anderen bei Bedarf Hilfe anbieten und etwas lernen über Selbstbestimmung.

Virtueller Kontext (virtual context). Umwelt, in der die Kommunikation durch Wellen oder Computer stattfindet, in Abwesenheit von physischem Kontakt. Der virtuelle Kontext schließt simulierte, Echtzeit-, oder zeitnahe Umwelten ein wie Chat-Räume, E-Mail, Videokonferenzen oder Radioübertragungen; Fernüberwachung durch drahtlose Sensoren und computergestützte Datenerhebung.

Wechselbeziehung/Interdependenz (interdependence): „Der Verlass der Menschen untereinander als natürliche Folge des Lebens in Gruppen" (Christiansen & Townsend, 2010, S. 419). „Interdependenz erzeugt ein Gefühl von sozialer Inklusion, gegenseitiger Hilfe und moralischem Einstandspflicht und Verantwortung, Unterschiede anzuerkennen und zu unterstützen" (Christiansen & Townsend, 2010, S. 187).

Wellness (wellness). „Wahrnehmung von und Verantwortlichkeit für psychisches und physisches Wohlbefinden, weil dies zur allgemeinen Zufriedenheit mit der eigenen Lebenssituation beiträgt" (Boyt Schell et al., 2014a, S. 1243).

Werte (values): Erworbene, aus der Kultur abgeleitete Überzeugungen und Selbstverpflichtungen, was gut, richtig und wichtig zu tun ist (Kielhofner, 2008); Prinzipien, Standards oder Qualität, die als lohnend oder wünschenswert von dem Klienten angesehen werden, der sie vertritt (Moyers & Dale, 2007).

Wohlbefinden (well-being): Allgemeiner Begriff für den gesamten menschlichen Lebensbereich mit physischen, mentalen und sozialen Aspekten (WHO, 2006, S. 211).

Zeitlicher Kontext (temporal context). Das Zeiterleben, wie es durch Beteiligung an Betätigungen geformt wird. Die zeitlichen Aspekte von Betätigung, die „zum Muster täglicher Betätigungen beitragen", schließen „Rhythmus ... Tempo ... Synchronisation ... Dauer ... und Sequenz" ein (Larson & Zemke, 2003, S. 82; Zemke, 2004, S. 610). Zum zeitlichen Kontext gehören Lebensstadium, Tages- oder Jahreszeit, Dauer und Rhythmus von Aktivität und die Vorgeschichte.

Ziel (goal): Messbares und bedeutungsvolles, betätigungsbasiertes lang- oder kurzfristiges Ziel, unmittelbar bezogen auf die Fähigkeiten und Bedürfnisse des Klienten, sich an erwünschten Betätigungen zu beteiligen (AOTA, 2013a, S. 35).

Literaturhinweise zum Glossar

American Occupational Therapy Association. (2002a). Broadening the construct of independence [Position Paper]. *American Journal of Occupational Therapy, 56,* 660. http://dx.doi.org/10.5014/ajot.56.6.660

American Occupational Therapy Association. (2010). Standards of practice for occupational therapy. *American Journal of Occupational Therapy, 64*(Suppl.), S106–S111. http://dx.doi.org/10.5014/ajot.2010.64S106

American Occupational Therapy Association. (2011). *Definition of occupational therapy practice for the AOTA Model Practice Act*. Retrieved from http://www.aota.org/-/media/Corporate/Files/ Advocacy/State/Resources /PracticeAct/Model%20 Definition%20of%20OT%20Practice%20 %20Adopted%20 41411.ashx

American Occupational Therapy Association. (2013b). Occupational therapy in the promotion of health and well-being. *American Journal of Occupational Therapy, 67*(Suppl.), S47–S59. http://dx.doi.org/10.5014/ajot.2013.67S47

Bedell, G. M. (2012). Measurement of social participation. In V. Anderson & M. H. Beauchamp (Eds.), *Developmental social neuroscience and childhood brain insult: Theory and practice* (pp. 184–206). New York: Guilford Press.

Boyt Schell, B. A., Gillen, G., & Scaffa, M. (2014a). Glossary. In B. A. Boyt Schell, G. Gillen, & M. Scaffa (Eds.), *Willard and Spackman's occupational therapy* (12th ed., pp. 1229–1243). Philadelphia: Lippincott Williams & Wilkins.

Christiansen, C. H., & Hammecker, C. L. (2001). Self care. In B. R. Bonder & M. B. Wagner (Eds.), *Functional performance in older adults* (pp. 155–175). Philadelphia: F. A. Davis.

Christiansen, C. H., & Townsend, E. A. (2010). *Introduction to occupation: The art and science of living* (2nd ed.). Cranbury, NJ: Pearson Education.

Crepeau, E. (2003). Analyzing occupation and activity: A way of thinking about occupational performance. In E. Crepeau, E. Cohn, & B. A. Boyt Schell (Eds.), *Willard and Spackman's occupational therapy* (10th ed., pp. 189–198). Philadelphia: Lippincott Williams & Wilkins.

Dickie, V., Cutchin, M., & Humphry, R. (2006). Occupation as transactional experience: A critique of individualism in occupational science. *Journal of Occupational Science, 13,* 83–93. http://dx.doi.org/10.1080/14427591.2006.9686573

Dunn, W. (2000). Habit: What's the brain got to do with it? *OTJR: Occupation, Participation and Health, 20*(Suppl. 1), 6S–20S.

Fiese, B. H. (2007). Routines and rituals: Opportunities for participation in family health. *OTJR: Occupation, Participation and Health, 27,* 41S–49S.

Fiese, B. H., Tomcho, T. J., Douglas, M., Josephs, K., Poltrock, S., & Baker, T. (2002). A review of 50 years of research on naturally occurring family routines and rituals: Cause for celebration. *Journal of Family Psychology, 16,* 381–390. http://dx.doi.org/10.1037/0893-3200.16.4.381

Fisher, A. G., & Griswold, L. A. (2014). Performance skills: Implementing performance analyses to evaluate quality of occupational performance. In B. A. Boyt Schell, G. Gillen, & M. Scaffa (Eds.), *Willard and Spackman's occupational therapy* (12th ed., pp. 249–264). Philadelphia: Lippincott Williams & Wilkins.

Gillen, G., & Boyt Schell, B. A. (2014). Introduction to evaluation, intervention, and outcomes for occupations. In B. A. Boyt Schell, G. Gillen, & M. Scaffa (Eds.), *Willard and Spackman's occupational therapy* (12th ed., pp. 606–609). Philadelphia: Lippincott Williams & Wilkins.

James, A. B. (2008). Restoring the role of independent person. In M. V. Radomski & C. A. Trombly Latham (Eds.), *Occupational therapy for physical dysfunction* (pp. 774–816). Philadelphia: Lippincott Williams & Wilkins.

Kielhofner, G. (2008). *The model of human occupation: Theory and application* (4th ed.). Philadelphia: Lippincott Williams & Wilkins.

Larson, E., & Zemke, R. (2003). Shaping the temporal patterns of our lives: The social coordination of occupation. *Journal of Occupational Science, 10,* 80–89. http://dx.doi.org/10.1080/14427591.2003.9686514

Law, M., Cooper, B., Strong, S., Stewart, D., Rigby, P., & Letts, L. (1996). Person-Environment-Occupation Model: A transactive approach to occupational performance. *Canadian Journal of Occupational Therapy, 63,* 9–23. http://dx.doi.org/10.1177/000841749606300103

Magasi, S., & Hammel, J. (2004). Social support and social network mobilization in African American woman who have experienced strokes. *Disability Studies Quarterly, 24*(4). Retrieved from http://dsq-sds.org/article/view/878/1053

Moyers, P. A., & Dale, L. M. (2007). *The guide to occupational therapy practice* (2nd ed.). Bethesda, MD: AOTA Press.

Parham, L. D., & Fazio, L. S. (Eds.). (1997). *Play in occupational therapy for children*. St. Louis, MO: Mosby.

Puchalski, C., Ferrell, B., Virani, R., Otis-Green, S., Baird, P., Bull, J., Sulmasy, D. (2009). Improving the quality of spiritual care as a dimension of palliative care: The report of the Consensus Conference. *Journal of Palliative Medicine, 12,* 885–904. http://dx.doi.org/10.1089/jpm.2009.0142

Radomski, M. V. (1995). There is more to life than putting on your pants. *American Journal of Occupational Therapy, 49,* 487–490. http://dx.doi.org/10.5014/ajot.49.6.487

Segal, R. (2004). Family routines and rituals: A context for occupational therapy interventions. *American Journal of Occupational Therapy, 58,* 499–508. http://dx.doi.org/10.5014/ajot.58.5.499

Townsend, E., & Wilcock, A. A. (2004). Occupational justice and client-centred practice: A dialogue in progress. *Canadian Journal of Occupational Therapy, 71,* 75–87. http://dx.doi.org/10.1177/000841740407100203

World Health Organization. (1986, November 21). *The Ottawa Charter for Health Promotion (First International Conference on Health Promotion, Ottawa)*. Retrieved from http://www.who.int/healthpromotion/conferences/previous/ottawa/en/print.html

World Health Organization. (2001). *International classification of functioning, disability and health*. Geneva: Author.

World Health Organization. (2006). *Constitution of the World Health Organization* (45th ed.). Retrieved from http://www.afro.who.int/index.php?option=com_docman&task=doc_download&gid=19&Itemid=2111WHO2006

Zemke, R. (2004). Time, space, and the kaleidoscopes of occupation (Eleanor Clarke Slagle Lecture). *American Journal of Occupational Therapy, 58,* 608–620. http://dx.doi.org/10.5014/ajot.58.6.608

Personenindex

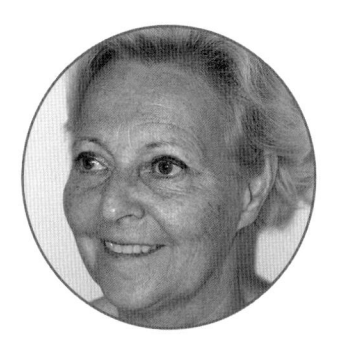

Die internationale Stimme der Ergotherapie – Mieke le Granse ist Herausgeberin der *Leitlinien der Ergotherapie*

Mieke le Granse hat einen Master in Didaktik und den European Master of Science in Occupational Therapy. Nach ihrer beruflichen Tätigkeit als Ergotherapeutin in der Psychiatrie kam sie als Dozentin an die Zuyd Hochschule in Heerlen. Dort war sie von 1999 bis 2017 Koordinatorin der deutschsprachigen Bachelor Studiengänge für deutsche Ergotherapeuten. Im Laufe der Zeit hat sie viel publiziert, national und international. Sie ist Mitherausgeberin und Autorin des niederländischen Buches „Grundlagen der Ergotherapie" und Mitherausgeberin der wissenschaftliche Zeitschrift „ergoscience", des Weiteren ist sie Reviewer bei verschiedenen internationalen Zeitschriften der Ergotherapie. Wegen ihres herausragenden Engagements für die Ergotherapie ist sie Ehrenmitglied des deutschen wie auch des niederländischen Verbands der Ergotherapeutinnen. Für die Niederlande ist sie seit 2010 Delegierte des *World Federation of Occupational Therapists (WFOT)* und damit die internationale Stimme der Ergotherapie.

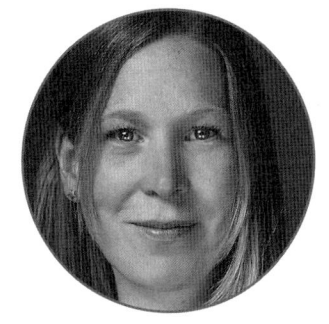

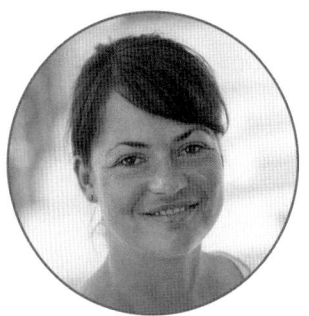

Sabine Brinkmann (links), geb. 1977, ist seit 1999 Ergotherapeutin, seit 2003 B.Sc (HAWK Hildesheim) und M.Sc (Neurorehabilitation, Donau Universität Krems). Ihre beruflichen Schwerpunkte sind Neurologie, medizinisch beruflich orientierte Rehabilitation und Orthopädie. Von 1999-2002 arbeitete sie als Ergotherapeutin in einer ambulanten Praxis für Ergotherapie (Pädiatrie/Neurologie), von 2003-2016 leitete sie die ergotherapeutische Abteilung im Postakut- und Rehabilitationszentrum für Orthopädie und Neurologie in Wilhelmshaven. Seit 2016 ist sie wissenschaftliche Mitarbeiterin in der Lehre an der Hochschule Osnabrück in den Studiengängen: Ergotherapie, Logopädie, Physiotherapie und Ergotherapie, Physiotherapie dual.

Anja Kirchner (rechts), Diplom Ergotherapeutin, arbeitet seit 2007 im Neurologischen Zentrum der Segeberger Kliniken GmbH und dort seit 2011 als wissenschaftliche Mitarbeiterin. Ihr Aufgabengebiet ist: Mitarbeit an einer Multicenter-Studie des Universitätsklinikums Aachen, Einrichtung eines neuen Therapieraumes zur Computer- und Robotik-gestützter Therapie, Mitarbeit an einer Multicenter-Studie des Universitätsklinikums Hamburg-Eppendorf. Sie hat mehrere Fortbildungen absolviert, wie beispielsweise zur ganzheitlichen Behandlung von Klienten mit idiopathischem Parkinson Syndrom, zu Aufmerksamkeits- und Gedächtnisstörungen, Diagnostik und Therapie, zu zerebralen Sehstörungen. Seit Februar 2018 bildet sie sich weiter zur Schmerztherapeutin.